Hepatology: an Update

Editors

ANAND V. KULKARNI
K. RAJENDER REDDY

MEDICAL CLINICS OF NORTH AMERICA

www.medical.theclinics.com

Consulting Editor
JACK ENDE

May 2023 • Volume 107 • Number 3

ELSEVIER

1600 John F. Kennedy Boulevard • Suite 1800 • Philadelphia, Pennsylvania, 19103-2899

http://www.theclinics.com

MEDICAL CLINICS OF NORTH AMERICA Volume 107, Number 3
May 2023 ISSN 0025-7125, ISBN-13: 978-0-443-18322-5

Editor: Taylor Hayes
Developmental Editor: Diana Grace Ang

Medical Clinics of North America (ISSN 0025-7125) is published bimonthly by Elsevier Inc., 360 Park Avenue South, New York, NY 10010-1710. Months of publication are January, March, May, July, September, and November. Business and editorial offices: 1600 John F. Kennedy Boulevard, Suite 1800, Philadelphia, PA 19103-2899. Periodicals postage paid at New York, NY, and additional mailing offices. Subscription prices are USD $332.00 per year (US individuals), $786.00 per year (US institutions), $100.00 per year (US Students), $416.00 per year (Canadian individuals), $1023.00 per year (Canadian institutions), $200.00 per year for (foreign students), $100.00 per year for (Canadian students), $461.00 per year (foreign individuals), and $1023.00 per year (foreign institutions). To receive student/resident rate, orders must be accompanied by name of affiliated institution, date of term, and the signature of program/residency coordinator on institution letterhead. Orders will be billed at individual rate until proof of status is received. Foreign air speed delivery is included in all Clinics' subscription prices. All prices are subject to change without notice. **POSTMASTER:** Send address changes to *Medical Clinics of North America*, Elsevier Health Sciences Division, Subscription Customer Service, 3251 Riverport Lane, Maryland Heights, MO 63043. **Customer Service: Telephone: 1-800-654-2452** (U.S. and Canada); **1-314-447-8871** (outside U.S. and Canada). **Fax: 314-447-8029. E-mail: journalscustomerserviceusa@ elsevier.com** (for print support); **journalsonlinesupport-usa@elsevier.com** (for online support).

Reprints. For copies of 100 or more of articles in this publication, please contact the Commercial Reprints Department, Elsevier Inc., 360 Park Avenue South, New York, NY 10010-1710. Tel.: 212-633-3874; Fax: 212-633-3820; E-mail: reprints@elsevier.com.

Medical Clinics of North America is also published in Spanish by McGraw-Hill Interamericana Editores S. A., P.O. Box 5-237, 06500 Mexico, D.F., Mexico.

Medical Clinics of North America is covered in *MEDLINE/PubMed (Index Medicus), Current Contents, ASCA, Excerpta Medica, Science Citation Index,* and *ISI/BIOMED.*

PROGRAM OBJECTIVE
The goal of the *Medical Clinics of North America* is to keep practicing physicians up to date with current clinical practice by providing timely articles reviewing the state of the art in patient care.

TARGET AUDIENCE
All practicing physicians and other healthcare professionals.

LEARNING OBJECTIVES
Upon completion of this activity, participants will be able to:
1. Review acute and chronic diseases of the hepatic system.
2. Explain varying manifestations of systemic infections or illness on the hepatic system and ranges of severity.
3. Discuss advances and updates in therapy and treatment of hepatitis infections and clinical manifestations.

ACCREDITATION

DISCLOSURE OF CONFLICTS OF INTEREST

Vincent Wai-Sun Wong, MD: Consultant/Advisor: AbbVie, Boehringer Ingelheim, Echosens, Gilead Sciences, Inc., Intercept Pharmaceuticals, Inc., Inventiva, Merck, Novo Nordisk, Pfizer Inc., ProSciento, Sagimet Biosciences, and Target RWE; Speaker: Abbott, AbbVie, Echosens, Gilead Sciences, Inc., Novo Nordisk; Researcher: Gilead Sciences, Inc.; Ownership: Illuminatio Medical Technology Limited

Terry Cheuk-Fung Yip, PhD: Advisor: Gilead Sciences, Inc.

UNAPPROVED/OFF-LABEL USE DISCLOSURE
The EOCME requires CME faculty to disclose to the participants;
1. When products or procedures being discussed are off-label, unlabelled, experimental, and/or investigational (not US Food and Drug Administration [FDA] approved); and
2. Any limitations on the information presented, such as data that are preliminary or that represent ongoing research, interim analyses, and/or unsupported opinions. Faculty may discuss information about pharmaceutical agents that is outside of FDA-approved labelling. This information is intended solely for CME and is not intended to promote off-label use of these medications. If you have any questions, contact the medical affairs department of the manufacturer for the most recent prescribing information.

TO ENROLL
To enroll in the *Medical Clinics of North America* Continuing Medical Education program, call customer service at 1-800-654-2452 or sign up online at http://www.theclinics.com/home/cme. The CME program is available to subscribers for an additional annual fee of USD 324.00.

METHOD OF PARTICIPATION
In order to claim credit, participants must complete the following;
1. Complete enrolment as indicated above.
2. Read the activity.
3. Complete the CME Test and Evaluation. Participants must achieve a score of 70% on the test. All CME Tests and Evaluations must be completed online.

CME INQUIRIES/SPECIAL NEEDS
For all CME inquiries or special needs, please contact elsevierCME@elsevier.com.

MEDICAL CLINICS OF NORTH AMERICA

Contributors

CONSULTING EDITOR

JACK ENDE, MD, MACP
The Schaeffer Professor of Medicine, Perelman School of Medicine, University of Pennsylvania, Philadelphia, Pennsylvania, USA

EDITORS

ANAND V. KULKARNI, MD, DM
Consultant, Department of Hepatology, AIG Hospitals, Hyderabad, India

K. RAJENDER REDDY, MD
Founders Professor of Medicine, Professor of Medicine in Surgery, Division of Gastroenterology and Hepatology, University of Pennsylvania, Philadelphia, Pennsylvania, USA

AUTHORS

AYOOLUWATOMIWA D. ADEKUNLE, MD, MPH
Department of Medicine, University of Kentucky, Lexington, Kentucky, USA

SALEH A. ALQAHTANI, MD
Professor of Medicine, Liver Transplant Centre, King Faisal Specialist Hospital and Research Centre, Riyadh, Saudi Arabia; Associate Professor of Medicine, Division of Gastroenterology and Hepatology, Johns Hopkins University, Baltimore, Maryland, USA

MAHATHI AVADHANAM, MBBS
Department of Emergency Medicine, Queen Elizabeth Hospital, London, United Kingdom

BRYAN D. BADAL, MD, MS
Division of Gastroenterology, Hepatology, and Nutrition, Virginia Commonwealth University, Central Virginia Veterans Healthcare System, Richmond, Virginia, USA

JASMOHAN S. BAJAJ, MD
Division of Gastroenterology, Hepatology, and Nutrition, Virginia Commonwealth University, Central Virginia Veterans Healthcare System, Richmond, Virginia, USA

FERNANDO BESSONE, MD
Professor, Facultad de Ciencias Médicas, Hospital Provincial del Centenario, University of Rosario School of Medicine, Rosario, Argentina

EINAR S. BJÖRNSSON, MD, PhD
Professor, Faculty of Medicine, University of Iceland, Division of Gastroenterology and Hepatology, Department of Internal Medicine, Landspitali University Hospital, Reykjavik, Iceland

PETER D. BLOCK, MD
Gastroenterology Fellow, Section of Digestive Diseases, Yale School of Medicine, New Haven, Connecticut, USA

CHALERMRAT BUNCHORNTAVAKUL, MD
Associate Professor of Medicine, Division of Gastroenterology and Hepatology, Department of Medicine, Rajavithi Hospital, College of Medicine, Rangsit University, Ratchathewi, Bangkok, Thailand

KAI EN CHAN
Division of Gastroenterology and Hepatology, Department of Medicine, National University Hospital, Singapore, Singapore

WAH-KHEONG CHAN, MRCP (UK), MBBS (UM), PhD (Malaya), AM
Gastroenterology and Hepatology Unit, Department of Medicine, University of Malaya, Kuala Lumpur, Malaysia

DOUGLAS CHEE, MBBS (Singapore)
Division of Gastroenterology and Hepatology, Department of Medicine, National University Hospital, Singapore

LUIS ANTONIO DÍAZ, MD
Department of Gastroenterology, Escuela de Medicina, Pontificia Universidad Católica de Chile, Santiago, Chile

GEORGE BOON-BEE GOH, MBBS, MRCP (UK), M Med (Int Med), FAMS (Singapore)
Department of Gastroenterology and Hepatology, Singapore General Hospital, Duke-NUS Medical School, Singapore

HUMBERTO C. GONZALEZ, MD
Division of Gastroenterology and Hepatology, Henry Ford Health, Wayne State University School of Medicine, Detroit, Michigan, USA

STUART C. GORDON, MD
Division of Gastroenterology and Hepatology, Henry Ford Health, Wayne State University School of Medicine, Detroit, Michigan, USA

DANIEL Q. HUANG, MBBS (Singapore), MRCP (UK), MMED (Singapore)
Division of Gastroenterology and Hepatology, Department of Medicine, National University Hospital, Yong Loo Lin School of Medicine, National University of Singapore, National University Centre for Organ Transplantation, National University Health System, Singapore, Singapore

DINESH JOTHIMANI, FRCP
Institute of Liver Disease and Transplantation, Dr Rela Institute and Medical Centre, Chennai, India

PATRICK S. KAMATH, MD
Division of Gastroenterology and Hepatology, Mayo Clinic College of Medicine and Science, Rochester, Minnesota, USA

ANAND V. KULKARNI, MD, DM
Consultant, Department of Hepatology, AIG Hospitals, Hyderabad, India

JOSEPH K. LIM, MD
Professor of Medicine, Section of Digestive Diseases, Yale Liver Center, Yale School of Medicine, New Haven, Connecticut, USA

VICTORIA MAINARDI, MD
Hepatology and Liver Transplant Unit, Hospital Central de Las Fuerzas Armadas, Montevideo, Uruguay

MANUEL MENDIZABAL, MD
Hepatology and Liver Transplant Unit, Hospital Universitario Austral, Pilar, Provincia de Buenos Aires, Argentina

MARK MUTHIAH, MBBS (Singapore), MRCP (UK), MMED (Singapore)
Consultant Gastroenterologist and Hepatologist, Division of Gastroenterology and Hepatology, Department of Medicine, National University Hospital, Yong Loo Lin School of Medicine, National University of Singapore, Singapore, Singapore

CHENG HAN NG
Division of Gastroenterology and Hepatology, Department of Medicine, National University Hospital, Singapore, Singapore

JOSEFINA PAGES, MD
Hepatology and Liver Transplant Unit, Hospital Universitario Austral, Pilar, Provincia de Buenos Aires, Argentina

PRANAV PENNINTI, DO
Division of Gastroenterology and Hepatology, University of Texas Health San Antonio, San Antonio, Texas, USA

SALVATORE PIANO, MD, PhD
Department of Medicine, Unit of Internal Medicine and Hepatology, University of Padova, Padova, Italy

K. RAJENDER REDDY, MD
Founders Professor of Medicine, Professor of Medicine in Surgery, Division of Gastroenterology and Hepatology, University of Pennsylvania, Philadelphia, Pennsylvania, USA

MOHAMED RELA, FRCS
Institute of Liver Disease and Transplantation, Dr Rela Institute and Medical Centre, Chennai, India

ASHWANI K. SINGAL, MD, MS, FACG, FAASLD, AGAF
Professor of Medicine, Director, Hepatology Elective Course, University of South Dakota Sanford School of Medicine, Transplant Hepatologist, Avera Transplant Institute and University Hospital, Avera McKennan University Hospital, Research Scientist, VA Medical Center, Sioux Falls, Sanford, USA

BETHANY NAHRI SO, BA
Division of Gastroenterology and Hepatology, Perelman School of Medicine, University of Pennsylvania, Philadelphia, Pennsylvania, USA

MARK S. SULKOWSKI, MD
Professor, Department of Medicine, Johns Hopkins School of Medicine, Baltimore, Maryland, USA

MARGARET TENG, MBBS (Singapore), MRCP (UK), MMED (Singapore)
Division of Gastroenterology and Hepatology, Department of Medicine, National University Hospital, Yong Loo Lin School of Medicine, National University of Singapore, National University Centre for Organ Transplantation, National University Health System, Singapore, Singapore

MARTA TONON, MD, PhD
Department of Medicine, Unit of Internal Medicine and Hepatology, University of Padova, Padova, Italy

GRACE LAI-HUNG WONG, MD
Department of Medicine and Therapeutics, Medical Data Analytics Centre (MDAC), Institute of Digestive Disease, The Chinese University of Hong Kong, Hong Kong

VINCENT WAI-SUN WONG, MD
Department of Medicine and Therapeutics, Medical Data Analytics Centre (MDAC), Institute of Digestive Disease, The Chinese University of Hong Kong, Hong Kong

TERRY CHEUK-FUNG YIP, PhD
Department of Medicine and Therapeutics, Medical Data Analytics Centre (MDAC), Institute of Digestive Disease, The Chinese University of Hong Kong, Hong Kong

Contents

Chronic liver disease is a major global health threat and is the 11th leading cause of death globally. A liver biopsy is frequently required in assessing the degree of steatosis and fibrosis, information that is important in diagnosis, management, and prognostication. However, liver biopsies have limitations and carry a considerable risk, leading to the development of various modalities of noninvasive testing tools. These tools have been developed in recent years and have improved markedly in diagnostic accuracy. Moving forward, they may change the practice of hepatology.

Hepatitis C virus (HCV) infection contributes significantly to liver cirrhosis and hepatocellular carcinoma (HCC), often requiring liver transplantation. Introducing direct-acting antiviral agents (DAAs) has radically changed HCV treatment. DAAs achieve high rates of sustained virological response (>98%). Even then, resistant-associated substitution and HCC during or after treatment have become prominent clinical concerns. Further, several clinically significant issues remain unresolved after successful HCV eradication by DAAs, including treating patients with chronic kidney disease or decompensated liver cirrhosis. Extensive and large-scale screening and treatment implementation programs are needed to make DAA therapies effective at the population level.

Chronic hepatitis B virus (HBV) infection is a bloodborne infection which affects approximately 1.6 million persons in the U.S. and 292 million persons worldwide and is associated with significant morbidity and mortality due to cirrhosis and hepatocellular carcinoma. HBV disproportionately affects foreign-persons from endemic regions such as sub-Saharan Africa and the Asian-Pacific region. Chronic HBV is diagnosed with positive HBsAg and detectable HBV DNA. Patients with immunoactive disease (elevated HBV DNA and serum ALT) may require antiviral therapy with peg-interferon or oral nucleos(t)ide analogues which suppress viral replication, and are associated with a decreased risk for liver events.

peritonitis, hepatorenal syndrome, recurrent/refractory ascites, and hepatic hydrothorax) further worsen survival. The development of ascites is driven by portal hypertension, systemic inflammation, and splanchnic arterial vasodilation. Etiologic treatment and nonselective beta-blockers can prevent ascites in compensated cirrhosis. The treatment of ascites is currently based on the management of fluid overload (eg, diuretics, sodium restriction, and/or paracenteses). In selected patients, long-term albumin use, norfloxacin prophylaxis, and transjugular intrahepatic portosystemic shunt reduce the risk of further decompensation and improve survival.

Hepatic encephalopathy (HE) is brain dysfunction secondary to liver insufficiency or portosystemic shunting. HE is a major burden on patients and caregivers, impairs quality of life and is associated with higher mortality. Overt HE is a clinical diagnosis while Covert HE, needs specialized diagnostic strategies. Mainstay of treatment of HE is nonabsorbable disaccharides such as lactulose as well as rifaximin; however, investigational therapies are discussed in this review. Better tools are needed to prognosticate which patients will go on to develop HE but microbiome and metabolomic-driven strategies are promising. Here we review methods to prevent the HE development and admissions.

Alcoholic hepatitis (AH) is a unique clinical syndrome on the spectrum of alcohol-associated liver disease (ALD). It constitutes a rising epidemic with increasing incidence and major public health implications. In severe AH, 30-day mortality approaches 30%, yet therapeutic options remain limited. Survival benefit from corticosteroids, the mainstay of medical treatment, is short-lived. Among corticosteroid nonresponders, the use of early liver transplantation is heterogeneous across centers and remains limited by significant barriers. Long-term prognosis is largely dictated by abstinence; however, comorbid alcohol use disorder remains undertreated. Efforts to address these challenges are required to curb the AH epidemic.

Cirrhosis is the end-stage of chronic liver disease and constitutes a leading cause of potential years of working life lost, especially in the Americas and Europe. Its natural history is characterized by an asymptomatic phase called compensated cirrhosis, followed by a rapidly progressive phase characterized by liver-related complications termed decompensated cirrhosis. Complications could be related to portal hypertension and/or liver dysfunction, including ascites, portal hypertensive gastrointestinal bleeding, encephalopathy, and jaundice. This review will discuss some of the most important precipitants of hepatic decompensation, including acute variceal bleeding, spontaneous bacterial peritonitis, and hepatic encephalopathy.

Patients with cirrhosis frequently require admission to the intensive care unit (ICU). Common indications for admission to ICU include one or more reasons of sepsis, shock due to any cause, acute gastrointestinal bleeding, and altered mentation either due to hepatic encephalopathy, alcohol withdrawal/intoxication, or metabolic encephalopathy. The appropriate critical care of an individual can determine the outcomes of these sick patients. The Airway, Breathing, Circulation, Disability (ABCD) approach to a patient admitted to ICU includes airway, breathing, circulation, and disability management. In this review, the authors discuss the common indications for ICU admission in a patient with cirrhosis and also their management.

Sarcopenia and frailty are frequent in cirrhosis, and both contribute to increased morbidity and mortality. The complex pathogenesis of sarcopenia in cirrhosis is mainly determined by hyperammonemia and malnutrition. Sarcopenia/frailty screening and reevaluation should be undertaken in all cirrhotic patients. Frailty tests are useful in the ambulatory setting, whereas the computed tomography scan is the diagnostic gold standard for sarcopenia. To manage sarcopenia/frailty, a multidisciplinary team should develop a personalized comprehensive care plan that includes patient education, protein/calorie intake goals, late evening meals, exercise programs, and micronutrient replenishment. In selected patients, branched-chain amino acids and testosterone supplements may also be beneficial.

Liver transplantation (LT) is a life-saving and evidence-based intervention for patients with acute liver failure and chronic end-stage liver disease. Significant progress has been made in advancing pre-LT management, transplant techniques, post-LT long-term care, and immunosuppression regimes. However, as rates of DC continue to increase, causes of liver disease and indications for LT continue to be investigated to ensure equity and further improve liver allocation models, waitlist outcomes, and post-LT outcomes for all patient populations.

Biological agents have in the last two decades become very important therapeutic agents, particularly for the treatment of various autoimmune disorders. The most widely used biologics are the tumor necrosis factor-α (TNF-α) receptor antagonists: infliximab, adalimumab, and etanercept. Other commonly used biological agents are interleukin (IL)-1 receptor antagonist (Anakinra), interleukin (IL)-6 receptor antagonist (tocilizumab), and CD20 surface antigen antagonist (rituximab). The current review will however focus on TNF-α receptor antagonists.

Foreword

Mnemonics Got Us Through

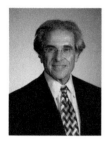

Jack Ende, MD, MACP
Consulting Editor

If your medical school experience was like mine, you may still recall your concerns (or in my case, nervous anxiety) about mastering the art of differential diagnosis. Life before medical school had not prepared us to consider that a single event might have so many causes. Then, we arrived in medical school, where X may have been caused by Y, but we were expected to also consider that X also might have been caused by A through Z.

Our introduction to liver disease was a case in point. What might be the cause of this patient's jaundice? What might be the etiology of that patient's cirrhosis? It was not that other areas of medicine were more straightforward, but, somehow, hepatology seemed to challenge us at every turn to consider multiple causes of single abnormalities.

Enter the mnemonic—"a device," according to the *Oxford English Dictionary* (OED), "such as a pattern of letters, ideas or associations that assist in remembering something." The OED continues, "for example, Richard Of York Gave Battle In Vain, for the colors of the spectrum (red, orange, yellow, green, blue, indigo, and violet)."

We have many mnemonics in medicine, although admittedly not all are as classic as *Richard Of York*. The one that worked best for me and enabled me to appear at least somewhat intelligent when I was asked, for example, what might be the cause of my patient's ascites, was VINDICATE. VINDICATE prompts medical students to consider that their patient's presentation might be caused by vascular, infectious, degenerative, iatrogenic/intoxications, congenital, autoimmune, traumatic, or endocrine causes. Mnemonics got us through rounds and stressful situations at conferences, such as Resident Report.

Truth be told, experienced clinicians rarely use mnemonics. Instead, they mostly rely on experience and make diagnoses based upon the repertoire of similar cases they have handled in the past. But they also have available knowledge of pathophysiology, epidemiology, and probability, enabling them to identify the actual cause of the

---

Med Clin N Am 107 (2023) xv–xvi
https://doi.org/10.1016/j.mcna.2023.02.002
0025-7125/23/© 2023 Published by Elsevier Inc.

patient's disease. And that takes us to this outstanding issue of *Medical Clinics of North America*, "Hepatology: An Update." Crafted by our two guest editors, Drs Kulkarni and Reddy, this issue brings together a team of experienced hepatologists who share their wisdom in a manner that will aid practicing clinicians. If you care for patients with liver disease, this issue is a "must read." If you wonder if your time invested in this issue will be well spent, you will be VINDICATED, I'm sure.

Jack Ende, MD, MACP
Perelman School of Medicine of the
University of Pennsylvania
Philadelphia, PA 19104, USA

E-mail address:
jack.ende@pennmedicine.upenn.edu

Preface

Hepatology Update for Clinicians

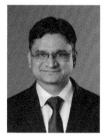 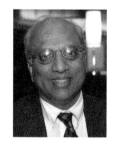

Anand V. Kulkarni, MD, DM   K. Rajender Reddy, MD
Editors

The discipline of Hepatology encompasses a broad spectrum of acute and chronic liver diseases with ultimately some patients requiring and benefiting from liver transplantation. While a remarkable achievement has been of the development of safe and effective chronic hepatitis C therapies, there has been a steady increase in disease burden due to nonalcoholic fatty liver disease and cirrhosis. The rate of hospitalization in those with cirrhosis has steadily increased, and this has led to enormous resource utilization and health care costs. As such, several specialists and nonspecialists, such as Gastroenterologists, Hepatologists, Internists, Hospitalists, Advance Practice Providers, and Nurses, have varying types and degrees of health care contact with those with liver disease.

Over the past decade or two, several clinical diagnostic and therapeutic advances have been made in Hepatology, while robust research has complemented clinical care. There are several guidelines for each disease that are frequently updated, but these may be difficult to follow in a busy clinical practice. To that end, in this update, experts across the globe discuss the current state-of-the-art diagnosis and management of a spectrum of liver disease in a clinically relevant, simple, but comprehensive manner. The topics included are broad and range from diseases presenting to the outpatient clinic to critical care of end-stage liver disease patients to liver transplantation. The health care provider in the outpatient clinic comes across nonalcoholic fatty liver disease and chronic hepatitis B virus, and an understanding of the screening, diagnostic, and therapeutic algorithm should help in an efficient and cost-effective care. There has been a rising burden of alcoholic hepatitis, and an article with the most current information addresses it. The physician on the inpatient side encounters complications of cirrhosis, such as ascites, variceal bleeding, and hepatic encephalopathy, and timely and important contributions to address them are part of this issue. The intensivist is often called upon to take care of a patient with cirrhosis, and an understanding of the relevant issues and their care in the intensive care unit is critical for

Med Clin N Am 107 (2023) xvii–xviii
https://doi.org/10.1016/j.mcna.2023.01.007
0025-7125/23/© 2023 Published by Elsevier Inc.

medical.theclinics.com

proper critical care; this topic has been covered in great detail. Other important and practical and clinically relevant topics covered include inpatient hepatology consults, the assessment and management of sarcopenia and frailty in cirrhosis, and hepatic involvement in systemic disease. In addition, the readers can understand the mechanisms and management of drug-induced liver injury due to biologics and immune check point inhibitors, drugs that recently are more frequently being used in clinical practice. In the patient with end-stage liver disease, liver transplantation is a consideration in select patients, and an overview on the current status of liver transplantation is presented.

To summarize, this issue provides comprehensive and practically relevant clinical updates on a variety of chronic liver diseases and their complications, by renowned experts in the field. The topics are easy to read and follow, and they provide practical guidance. We certainly enjoyed reading them, and we hope you find them useful in your clinical practice.

Anand V. Kulkarni, MD, DM
Department of Hepatology, AIG Hospitals
Hyderabad, India-500032.

K. Rajender Reddy, MD
University of Pennsylvania
Philadelphia, PA 19104, USA

E-mail addresses:
anandvk90@gmail.com (A.V. Kulkarni)
ReddyR@PennMedicine.upenn.edu (K.R. Reddy)

The Past, Present, and Future of Noninvasive Test in Chronic Liver Diseases

Douglas Chee, MBBS (S'pore)[a,1], Cheng Han Ng[a,1], Kai En Chan[a],
Daniel Q. Huang, MBBS (S'pore), MRCP (UK), MMED (S'pore)[a,b,c],
Margaret Teng, MBBS (S'pore), MRCP (UK), MMED (S'pore)[a,b,c],
Mark Muthiah, MBBS (S'pore), MRCP (UK), MMED (S'pore)[a,b,c,*]

KEYWORDS

- Chronic liver disease • Noninvasive test • Fibrosis • Steatosis

KEY POINTS

- Noninvasive tests (NITs) for the assessment of hepatic steatosis and fibrosis have gained significant traction in recent years in an attempt to tackle chronic liver diseases.
- NITs can be categorized broadly into serologic and imaging-based markers with varied accuracy and utility.
- Future developments in NITs may potentially improve diagnostic and prognostic practices in the field of hepatology.

INTRODUCTION

Chronic liver disease (CLD) is a major global health threat and is the 11th leading cause of death globally. CLD affects an estimated 1.5 billion people worldwide[1] and accounted for 1.32 million deaths globally in 2017.[2] CLD refers to an umbrella of liver conditions but is primarily caused by viral hepatitis, alcohol (ALD), and nonalcoholic fatty liver disease (NAFLD).[1] However, the advent of antivirals and substantial progress in the accessibility of hepatitis B (HBV) vaccines has since reduced the prevalence of viral hepatitis, and NAFLD has become the leading cause of CLD. Globally, NAFLD is thought to affect 32.4% of the global population[3] and has increased in

[a] Division of Gastroenterology and Hepatology, Department of Medicine, National University Hospital, Tower Block Level 10, 1E Kent Ridge Road, Singapore 119228, Singapore; [b] Yong Loo Lin School of Medicine, National University of Singapore, Tower Block Level 10, 1E Kent Ridge Road, Singapore 119228, Singapore; [c] National University Centre for Organ Transplantation, National University Health System, Tower Block Level 10, 1E Kent Ridge Road, Singapore 119228, Singapore
[1] These authors contributed equally to this work and share first authorship.
* Corresponding author.
E-mail address: mdcmdm@nus.edu.sg

Med Clin N Am 107 (2023) 397–421
https://doi.org/10.1016/j.mcna.2022.12.001
0025-7125/23/© 2023 Elsevier Inc. All rights reserved.

conjunction with the growing obesity and metabolic dysfunction that perpetuated the global crisis of fatty liver (FL). The identification of steatosis and fibrosis is important in the diagnosis and prognostication of CLD[4] and a liver biopsy (LB) has traditionally been considered the gold standard for the diagnosis of CLD. Importantly, the stage of fibrosis is closely tied to adverse outcomes. A recent meta-analysis of 17,301 NAFLD individuals found a stepwise increase in mortality with each increase in fibrosis stage, with an estimated 10-year all-cause mortality of 7.7% for stage F0-2 and 41.5% for F4 fibrosis.[5]

In HCV, the presence of high-grade fibrosis resulted in a significant risk of the development of cirrhosis (hazard ratio [HR] 9.07, 95% CI: 3.68 to 22.13).[6] The presence of advanced fibrosis in ALD is also associated with an elevated 10-year mortality (F3/4: 45% vs F0-2: 0%, $P < .001$).[7] Increasing stages of fibrosis and cirrhosis are in turn associated with a higher incidence of hepatocellular carcinoma (HCC).[8] However, LB has many shortcomings, including sampling variability[9] and inter-operator variation in reporting,[10] resulting in serious adverse events including puncture site hematoma, large intraabdominal bleed or hemopneumothorax, making sequential biopsies for longitudinal follow-up impractical.[11] As a result, noninvasive tests (NITs) for CLD have gained significant traction in recent years as an alternative to LB. Broadly, NITs can include serologic biomarkers and imaging techniques. Although initial serologic tests were often indirect measures of fibrosis or steatosis using a combination of liver enzymes with patient characteristics, more specific imaging and serologic markers for architectural fibrosis have been developed in recent years. Herein, we seek to review the current era of NITs commonly used in CLD on the role of identifying steatosis, fibrosis, risk stratification, and prognostication of CLD.

Identification of Hepatic Steatosis

Hepatic steatosis is defined by the presence of abnormal fat accumulation of >5% in hepatocytes on histology. It is most commonly associated with NAFLD but can also be caused by alcohol liver disease and viral hepatitis. In a recent meta-analysis of 54 studies (28,648 patients), an estimated 32.8% of individuals with chronic HBV had FL.[12] Among patients with HCV, an estimated 55% to 80% had FL.[13,14] However, the impact of FL on viral hepatitis remains debatable. Although the presence of FL was not associated with an increased prevalence of fibrosis in HBV,[12] hepatic steatosis has been shown to reduce virologic response to antiviral treatment[15] and worsen the progression of fibrosis[16] in HCV. There is also an emerging debate between the overlapping fields of NAFLD and ALD. The presence of FL in ALD has been shown to have similar risk factors to NAFLD by which metabolic dysregulation and PNPLA3 mutations result in more severe fibrosis in ALD.[17] Broadly, common assessment methods of hepatic steatosis can be divided into blood-based and imaging-based markers and an overview of the various tests can be found in **Table 1**.

The Fatty Liver Index (FLI) developed by Begdoni and colleagues[18] is commonly used for liver fat estimation at the population level, consisting of triglycerides (TG), body mass index (BMI), gamma-glutamyl transferase (GGT), and waist circumference (WC). It was developed against ultrasonography (USG) evidence of steatosis with a receiver-operating characteristic (AUROC) of 0.85. Similarly, the Hepatic Steatosis Index (HSI) (BMI, diabetes [DM], female sex, aspartate aminotransferase [AST], alanine aminotransferase [ALT]) was developed with ultrasound detected steatosis and has an AUROC of 0.81.[19] With reference to magnetic resonance spectroscopy (MRS), the NAFLD fat score (NFS) consisting of the presence of metabolic syndrome (MetS), DM, fasting serum insulin, AST, and ALT was found to have an AUROC of 0.86 to 0.87 among 460 subjects.[20] However, the use of fasting serum insulin limits its

Table 1
Noninvasive tests for the assessment of hepatic steatosis

Test	Details	Accuracy	Limitations	Feasibility
Biological Biomarkers and Serologic Tests				
Fatty Liver Index (FLI)	BMI, WC, TG, GGT	AUROC 0.83 for steatosis on histology • Sn 76% • Sp 87%	• Cannot differentiate steatosis grades	High–components readily accessible, cost-effective, good accuracy
Hepatic Steatosis Index (HSI)	BMI, DM, female Sex, AST:ALT	AUROC 0.81 for steatosis on histology • Sn 62% • Sp 93%	• Cannot differentiate steatosis grades • Inaccurate in patients with high BMI (will be positive if BMI >30)	High–components readily accessible, cost-effective, good accuracy
SteatoTest	Six components of FibroTest–ActiTest, BMI, TG, Cholesterol, glucose adjusted for age and sex	AUROC 0.72 to 0.86 for > S2 on histology • Sn 85% to 100% • Sp 83% to 100%	• High Cost and low availability of FibroTest-ActiTest • Cannot differentiate steatosis grades	Intermediate–due to proprietary nature of panel
NAFLD Liver Fat Score	T2DM, MetS, AST:ALT, fS-insulin, fS-AST	AUROC 0.80 for steatosis on histology • Sn 65% • Sp 87%	• Limited availability of serum fasting insulin • Cannot differentiate steatosis grades	Intermediate–serum fasting insulin required
US-FLI	FLI and B-more USG	AUROC 0.88 for Steatosis on histology AUROC 0.763 for NASH and 0.796 for severe NASH • NPV 94% for NASH Differential AUROC for identification of steatosis on histology vs FLI • >S1 0.231 • >S2 0.242	–	Intermediate–not used on its own, but supplements FLI in discriminating severity of steatosis and identification of NASH

(continued on next page)

Table 1
(continued)

Imaging Biomarkers

Test	Details	Accuracy	Limitations	Feasibility
B-mode USG	Increased scatter by intrahepatic lipid droplets results in a hyperechoic appearance of a steatotic liver	AUROC 0.93 for steatosis on histology • Sn 69.7% • Sp 79.6%	• Inter- and intraobserver variability • low sensitivity in mild steatosis and obesity, advanced fibrosis	High–low cost, widespread availability, safe, no radiation
Hamaguchi Score (USG)	Based on USG with the following scoring domains • bright liver and hepatorenal echo contrast (0 to 3) • deep attenuation (0 to 2) • vessel blurring (0 to 1)	AUROC 0.98 for steatosis on histology • Sn 91.7% • Sp 100%	• Not validated in large cohort	High–simple and effective supplement to USG
CAP via VCTE	Dissipation of USG waves occurs more rapidly in a steatotic liver	AUROC 0.82 for steatosis on histology • Sn 69% • Sp 82%	• Cannot differentiate steatosis grades • High failure rate in patients with obesity or MetS	High–rapid assessment tool, widespread availability, safe, no radiation
CT	Liver Attenuation measured in HU, in both absolute terms as well as in relation to the spleen	AUROC 0.95 for >10% steatosis on histology • Sn 81% • Sp 94%	• Poor performance in picking up mild steatosis or quantifying steatosis • multiple confounding factors (iron, copper, fibrosis, edema) • Radiation	Intermediate–rapid assessment tool, widespread availability, however, has radiation
MRS	Provides a spectrum of signals for fat fraction estimation	AUROC 0.97 for steatosis on histology	• High cost and limited availability	Low–high cost and very limited availability

MRI-PDFF	Picks up proton signals from unbound molecules such as triglycerides	AUROC 0.96 for steatosis on histology • Sn 85% • Sp 100%	• high technical difficulty in operating • High cost and limited availability • Time-consuming • less accurate with inflammation/iron overload	Intermediate–high cost and limited availability
QUS	Based on Raw data on parameters such as speed, sound, backscatter,	AUROC 0.886 for steatosis on histology • Sn 86.5% • Sp 89.8%	• Poor performance in severe obesity • limited validating studies	Intermediate–not adequately validated

Abbreviations: fS, fasting serum; MetS, metabolic syndrome; Sn, Sensitivity; Sp, Specificity.

widespread use. A study of 324 individuals undergoing liver biopsies found FLI, NFS, and HSI detected steatosis with an AUROC of 0.83, 0.80, and 0.81, respectively.[21] However, these tests have relatively low sensitivities (<80%) and the ability to quantify the severity of steatosis. The HSI also has a major flaw in those patients with a BMI ≥30 who would register a positive test.[22] Augmentation of FLI with USG (US-FLI) improved its discriminating power between steatosis grades (differential AUROC of 0.23 for > S1 [5% to 33% steatosis], and 0.24 for > S2 [34% to 66% steatosis]),[23] allowing the identification of NASH with an AUROC of 0.76 and NPV of 94%,[24] guiding the need for LB. Less commonly used tests include the SteatoTest, NAFL risk score, NAFL screening score, and NAFL ridge score. The routine applicability of the SteatoTest importantly has been limited by the proprietary nature.

Brightness-mode (B-mode) USG is the most widely used imaging tool in the assessment of steatosis due to its availability and low cost. Increased scatter by intrahepatic lipid droplets results in a hyperechoic appearance of a steatotic liver. In a study of 120 patients with biopsy-proven steatosis, USG identified steatosis with an AUROC of 0.761.[25] However, USG is less adept at identifying mild steatosis and quantifying the degree of steatosis. It is also impaired by the presence of inflammation, fibrosis,[26] and obesity (AUROC 0.82)[27,28] and is susceptible to interobserver and intraobserver variability.[29] The Hamaguchi scoring system[30] although rarely used may improve the accuracy of B-mode USG. The Quantitative ultrasound (QUS) uses parameters such as the speed of sound, attenuation, and backscatter coefficient (BSC) to quantify the tissue microstructure,[31] which was found to be more accurate at quantifying liver steatosis than B-mode USG and have been found to have an AUROC of 0.886.[32]

Vibration-controlled transient elastography (VCTE) reflects the increased rate of ultrasound energy dissipation in a steatotic liver via controlled attenuation parameter (CAP). In a meta-analysis of 2735 patients with CLD, CAP detected steatosis with an AUROC of 0.82[33] with thresholds of 248, 268, and 280 dB/m for S1-3, respectively, with good inter and intraobserver consistency with a concordance correlation coefficient (CCC) of 0.82.[34] However, it is less accurate in obese individuals, females, and individuals with MetS.[35] The development of the XL probe improved CAP measurements in obese individuals,[35] maintaining comparable accuracy to the M probe.[36–38] Notably, CAP thresholds vary significantly between different etiologies of CLD[39] and discriminates poorly between steatosis grades.

Computed Tomography (CT) characterizes the attenuation of the liver and identifies steatosis when the liver attenuation is < 40 Hounsfield units (HU), >10 HU less than spleen attenuation, or has a liver-to-spleen attenuation ratio <1. A meta-analysis of 1782 patients found CT to detect >10% steatosis with an AUROC of 0.80, with a significant improvement to 0.95 for diagnosing steatosis of >10%,[40] demonstrating poor performance in diagnosing mild steatosis. It also performs poorly in the quantification of steatosis.[41] Its performance is also confounded by presence of iron, copper, glycogen, fibrosis, or edema.[42] Although there has been interest in using dual-energy computed tomography (DECT)[43,44] to remove some of such confounders, it remains to be properly validated.

Proton magnetic resonance spectroscopy (H-MRS) detects nuclear resonance signals to produce spectral data depicting the chemical composition within specific regions of interest. It is highly accurate at detecting steatosis (AUROC 0.97).[45] However, it is technically challenging to perform, and not widely available, thus limiting its clinical utility and remaining largely a research tool. MRI-PDFF, unlike conventional MRI, can pick up proton signals from unbound molecules such as triglycerides and has near complete concordance with H-MRS. In a study involving 89 adults with biopsy-confirmed NAFLD, MRI-PDFF detected steatosis with an AUROC of 0.92 to 0.96.[46] With a much higher accuracy than CAP (AUROC 0.99 vs 0.85).[47] MRI-PDFF is also more sensitive to the degree of steatosis than CAP[48] making it a potentially suitable choice for longitudinal monitoring of steatosis. Despite the promise of MRI-PDFF, its high cost and limited availability remain a significant barrier to its use in routine evaluation, particularly among the lower income countries.

Identification of Hepatic Fibrosis

Fibrosis is a regenerative process in response to insults to the liver. Worsening fibrosis portends a poorer prognosis that results in cirrhosis, decompensation, and HCC.[49,50] Broadly, common assessment methods of hepatic fibrosis can be divided into blood-based and imaging-based markers and an overview of the various tests can be found in **Table 2**.

Serologic markers used in the identification of fibrosis include both non-proprietary and proprietary markers. Non-proprietary markers often reflect hepatic dysfunction and injury [for example, platelet count, prothrombin time (PT), liver enzymes] and are often combined with other clinical parameters. The AST/ALT ratio (AAR) and the AST/platelet ratio (APRI) were initially developed for use in HCV and later adapted for use with other etiologies. Although they reliably excluded advanced fibrosis (negative predictive value (NPV) 0.93 and 0.84, respectively),[51] a study involving 162 NAFLD patients found that they performed only modestly at detecting advanced fibrosis (AUROC 0.66 to 0.74 and AUROC 0.74, respectively)[52] due to poor sensitivities of 40% and 66%, respectively, resulting in many false negatives. The Fibrosis-4 (FIB-4) index was initially developed in 2006 for patients with HCV/Human Immunodeficiency Virus (HIV) coinfection and comprises age, AST, ALT, and platelets.[53] Given the simplicity of FIB-4, it has been widely used for the identification of advanced fibrosis. In a meta-analysis of 13,046 NAFLD patients, FIB-4 identified advanced fibrosis with an AUROC of 0.84.[54] However, the use of FIB-4 in younger adults below the age of 35 is limited by poor diagnostic accuracy (AUROC 0.6)[55] due to low sensitivity. The NAFLD Fibrosis Score (NFS) was developed in NAFLD patients and comprises age, BMI, DM, AAR, platelet count, and serum albumin levels. In the same study as above, NFS had a similar accuracy to FIB-4 in identifying advanced fibrosis (AUROC 0.84).[54] Similar to FIB-4, NFS also performed poorly in younger adults below 35 years old (AUROC 0.52),[55] similarly due to poor sensitivity. A more recent individual patient data meta-analysis comprising NAFLD patients with paired liver histology and VCTE reported AAR and APRI had a modest performance with AUROC≤0.70, whereas FIB-4 and NFS had AUROC of 0.76 and 0.73, respectively, for identification of advanced fibrosis.[56] NFS however, is more resource intensive due to the need for diabetes testing, and has only been designed and validated in NAFLD, thus FIB-4 remains the more practical tool. Another study done in the general population found both FIB-4 and NFS to be suboptimal screening tools as almost 1/3 were false positives, with a larger proportion of false negatives in at-risk patients compared with the general population.[57] The BARD Score, consisting of BMI, AAR and the presence of DM has an NPV 96%[51] for advanced fibrosis but has modest accuracy for the identification of advanced fibrosis (AUROC 0.76).[54]

Hyaluronic acid (HA) plays a key role in the formation of extracellular matrix (ECM) in fibrosis[58] and detects advanced fibrosis with AUROC of 0.89.[59] Procollagen III amino-terminal peptide (PIIINP) is generated during the synthesis of type III collagen and can detect advanced fibrosis with an AUROC of 0.82.[60] PRO-C3 is a collagen neo-epitope enzyme-linked immunosorbent assay (ELISA) of PIIINP generated during formation of type III collagen[61] which is specific to liver collagen. However, a meta-analysis of 2058

Table 2
Noninvasive tests for the assessment of hepatic fibrosis

Test	Details	Accuracy	Limitations	Feasibility
Non-proprietary Serlogic Markers				
ALT/AST Ratio	AST, ALT	AUROC 0.66 to 0.74 for advanced fibrosis • Sn 40% • Sp 80%	• Modest accuracy with low sensitivity in picking up fibrosis • fluctuation of transaminases over time	High–components readily accessible, cost-effective, good accuracy
AST/Platelet Ratio (APRI)	ASR, Platelet count	AUROC 0.74 for advanced fibrosis • Sn 66% • Sp 72%	• Modest Accuracy • fluctuation of transaminases over time	High–components readily accessible, cost-effective, good accuracy, high NPV for advanced fibrosis and cirrhosis
FIB-4	Age, AST, ALT Platelet count	AUROC 0.84 for advanced fibrosis • Sn 82% • Sp 93%	• Poor performance in patients <35 and >65 • fluctuation of transaminases over time	High–components readily accessible, cost-effective, good accuracy
NAFLD Fibrosis Score	Age, BMI, DM, AST, ALT, Platelet count, Albumin	AUROC 0.82 for advanced fibrosis • Sn 73% to 82% • Sp 96% to 98%	• Poor performance in patients <35 • differing BMI interpretation in various ethnic groups • fluctuation of transaminases over time	High–components readily accessible, cost-effective, good accuracy
BARD	AST, ALT, BMI, Diabetes	AUROC 0.69 to 0.81 for advanced fibrosis • Sn 62% • Sp 66%	• differing BMI interpretation in various ethnic groups • fluctuation of transaminases over time	High–components readily accessible, cost-effective, good accuracy
Proprietary Serologic Markers				

Hyaluronic Acid	Plays key role in ECM formation in fibrosis	AUROC 0.89 for advanced fibrosis • Sn 85% • Sp 80%	• Not recommended for use in isolation	Intermediate–limited availability
PIIINP	Generated during synthesis of type III collagen	AUROC 0.82 for advanced fibrosis • Sn 48.1% • Sp 79.7%	• Not recommended for use in isolation	Intermediate–limited availability
PRO-C3	Neo-epitope ELISA of PIIINP specific to liver collagen	AUROC 0.82 for advanced fibrosis • Sn 68% • Sp 79%	• Not recommended for use in isolation • Not well validated outside of NAFLD	Intermediate–limited availability
TIMP1	Regulates matrix metalloproeinases	AUROC 0.97 for advanced fibrosis in NASH • Sn 97% • Sp 100%	• Not recommended for use in isolation • Limited availability • Not well validated outside of NASH	Intermediate–limited availability
ELF	PIIINP, Hyaluronic acid, and TIMP1	AUROC 0.83 for advanced fibrosis • Sn 65% • Sp 86%	• Less sensitive for early fibrosis	Intermediate–limited availability and costly
Fibrotest	Age, Gender, α2-macroglobulin, Haptoglobin, Apolipoprotein A1, Bilirubin, GGT	AUROC 0.88 for advanced fibrosis • Sn 95% • Sp 71%	• Less sensitive for early fibrosis • Less validated outside of viral hepatitis	Intermediate–limited availability and costly
FibroMeter NAFLD	Age, Body weight, AST, ALT, Platelet Count, Glucose, Ferritin	AUROC 0.94 for advanced fibrosis • Sn 78.5% • Sp 95.9%	—	Intermediate–limited availability and costly

(continued on next page)

Table 2
(continued)

Test	Details	Accuracy	Limitations	Feasibility
FibroMeter VCTE	FibroMeter NAFLD and LSM via VCTE	AUROC 0.94 for advanced fibrosis • Sn 70% • Sp 93%	–	Intermediate–limited availability and costly
ADAPT	Age, DM, Pro-C3, and Platelet count	AUROC 0.86 to 0.87 for advanced fibrosis • Sn 58% • Sp 97%	–	Intermediate–limited availability and costly
FIBC3	Age, BMI, T2DM, platelet count, PRO-C3	AUROC 0.85 for advanced fibrosis • Sn 75% • Sp 75%	–	Intermediate–limited availability and costly
ABC3D	Simplified version of the FIBC3 with similar components	AUROC 0.83 for advanced fibrosis • Sn 66% • Sp 75%	–	Intermediate–limited availability and costly
Imaging Biomarkers				
LSM via VCTE	Generation of mechanical shear waves to measure liver stiffness	AUROC 0.88 for advanced fibrosis for M probe • Sn 88.9% • Sp 77.2% AUROC of 0.88 for advanced fibrosis for XL probe • Sn 75.3% • Sp 74%	• Poor performance in obesity with high failure rate • Confounded by many factors such as fluid status, adequate fasting, ongoing transaminitis and inflammation	High–low cost, widespread availability, safe, no radiation

	Description	Performance	Limitations	Safety/availability
p-SWE	Generation of an acoustic impulse to measure liver stiffness at a single point	AUROC 0.91 for advanced fibrosis • Sn 73% • Sp 92%	• Quality criteria not well defined • Technically steeper learning curve than VCTE	High–safe, no radiation, can be performed on commercial ultrasound machines
2D-SWE	Generation of an acoustic impulse to measure liver stiffness in a larger area	AUROC 0.92 for advanced fibrosis • Sn 71.4% • Sp 94.4%	• Quality criteria not well defined • Technically steeper learning curve than VCTE	High–safe, no radiation, can be performed on commercial ultrasound machines
MRE	Utilizes a modified phase-contrast for imaging a sheer wave propagation through the liver	AUROC 0.89 to 0.96 for advanced fibrosis • Sn 85.7% • Sp 90.8%	—	Intermediate–safe, no radiation, but costly and with lower availability

NAFLD patients found that PRO-C3 was only modestly accurate in identifying advanced fibrosis with AUROC of 0.79.[62] Tissue inhibitor of metalloproteinases 1 (TIMP1) regulates matrix metalloproteinases and accounts for the ECM composition.[63] It can accurately identify NASH in obese individuals.[64]

The Enhanced Liver Fibrosis (ELF) Test comprises three components: PIIINP, HA, and TIMP1. In a meta-analysis of 11 studies, it identified advanced fibrosis with an AUROC of 0.83.[65] However, it has a varying performance depending on the etiology of CLD.[66,67] The Fibrotest comprising total bilirubin, $\alpha 2m$, serum levels of GGT, haptoglobin, and apolipoprotein was initially developed in HCV[68] before being validated in CLD of other etiologies.[69] It detects fibrosis with a greater accuracy (AUROC 0.88) than FIB-4.[70] FibroMeter NAFLD comprises body weight, fasting glucose, prothrombin index, ferritin, ALT, and AST. In a study of 235 NAFLD patients, it detected advanced fibrosis with an AUROC of 0.937. Combining it with VCTE also improved its diagnostic accuracy, improving its positive predictive value (PPV) from 0.8 to 0.89.[71] Various algorithms developed with PRO-C3 such as the ADAPT (age, AM, Pro-C3, and platelet count), FIBC3 (Age, BMI, T2DM, platelet count, PRO-C3), and its simplified form ABC3D have also been found to significantly outperform FIB-4 at identifying advanced fibrosis (AUROC 0.87,[72] 0.89 and 0.88, respectively[73]).

VCTE generates a mechanical shear wave to assess liver stiffness measurement (LSM) measured in kilopascals (kPa). A meta-analysis of 13,046 NAFLD individuals found that LSM was able to diagnose advanced fibrosis with an AUROC of 0.88 and 0.85 for the M and XL probes, respectively.[54] LSM has also been validated in NASH,[74] with cut-off values of 8.8, 11.7 and 14 kPa for F2-4 fibrosis, respectively. It should be noted that there is a range of published cut-offs based on various study populations, and there is heterogeneity in clinical practice regarding exact cut-offs used.[75] Similar to the CAP score, LSM has a high failure rate in obese patients.[76] It is also confounded by factors like congestive cardiac disease, acute hepatitis, and cholestasis.[77]

Acoustic radiation force impulse (ARFI) is a similar technique but uses short-duration acoustic pulses instead to generate the shear wave. It can be further divided into point-shear wave elastography (p-SWE) and two-dimension shear wave elastography (2D-SWE). p-SWE allows the operator to select a fixed region of interest (ROI) whereas 2D-SWE allows adjustment to the size of the ROI. Unlike VCTE, ARFI allows direct visualization of the ROI resulting in a much lower failure rate compared with VCTE (0.7% vs 14.4%).[78] ARFI can also be performed on a normal ultrasound machine, whereas VCTE requires a separate machine. A meta-analysis of 11,345 patients revealed comparable diagnostic capabilities of ARFI techniques and VCTE[79] with 2D-SWE having a slightly higher sensitivity than p-SWE (0.84 vs 0.76). Despite its advantages, ARFI remains less well-validated across various populations compared with VCTE and has a technically steeper learning curve for operators.

Magnetic resonance elastography (MRE) adopts a modified phase-contrast for imaging of a shear wave propagation that images the whole liver and reduces sampling error.[47,80] It is also less susceptible to confounding factors such as obesity, congestive cardiac failure, and acute hepatitis[81] and has a very low failure rate of <5%[82] with smaller inter and intra-reporter variability compared with VCTE and ARFI.[83] A meta-analysis of 14,609 patients with NAFLD found MRE to be not only more accurate than VCTE and ARFI for identifying advanced fibrosis (AUROC 0.91, 0.85, and 0.86, respectively), but also highly discriminatory between different fibrosis stages with an AUROC of >90%[47] The cut-off values for F1-4 fibrosis are 6.2, 7.6, 8.8, and 11.8 kPa, respectively.[84] However, utility of MRE is limited by availability and cost, limiting routine use of this modality.

Prognostication and Predicting Outcomes

The progression of liver fibrosis has been shown to be associated with an increase in mortality as well as liver-related morbidity.[5-7] Fibrosis stage is also the strongest predictor of mortality in NAFLD (HR 3.3 [95% CI 2.27 to 4.76, P < .001] in patients with F3-4 vs F0-2[85]). By extension, there has thus been an increasing interest in the prognosticating abilities of NITs for liver-related events and mortality.[86-89] An increase in liver stiffness on VCTE or MRE is associated with an increased risk of both liver-related and cardiovascular events.[90,91] A retrospective longitudinal analysis of 265 patients found each 1-kPa increase in LSM on MRE was associated with a 2.20-fold increase in odds of developing hepatic decompensation and HCC. In another longitudinal study of 2373 patients with CLD, the aHR (95% CI) for patients with MRE >4.7 kPa vs MRE <3 kPa for liver decompensation, HCC, extrahepatic cancers, major adverse cardiovascular events (MACE), and all-cause mortality were 67.5 (9.2 to 492), 4.20 (2.2 to 8.2), 0.90 (0.5 to 1.7), 0.83 (0.4 to 1.7), and 2.90 (1.6 to 5.4), respectively.[92] Similarly, an LSM >8.2 kPa on VCTE has been shown to be associated with multiple cardiovascular and metabolic risk factors.[93] In a study of 2052 patients with CLD of various causes, an increase in LSM of 1 kPa on VCTE was associated with a 5% increased risk of mortality or liver complications.[94] This was corroborated in another study of 400 patients with type 2 DM and NAFLD, where an increased LSM of 1 kPa on VCTE was associated with a 5% increased risk of MACE and a 4% increase in mortality.[95]

FIB-4 and NFS have been shown to predict liver and cardiovascular outcomes at a population level. A Swedish population study of more than 100,000 individuals found FIB-4 predicted the development of severe liver disease at 10 years with AUROC of 0.702, outperforming the NFS (AUROC 0.624).[96] Another Israeli population study found individuals with FIB-4 >2.67 to have a higher risk of developing CVD (HR: 1.69, 95% CI: 1.21 to 2.35), with the NFS performing similarly albeit with limited statistical power in that study.[97] Similarly, FIB-4 and NFS have also been shown to predict mortality among NAFLD patients at the tertiary level. In a recent meta-analysis of 12,380 NAFLD patients, an FIB-4 score of >2.67 was associated with an increased risk of both CVD mortality (SHR: 1.421, CI: 1.040 to 1.942, P = .027) and MACE (OR: 1.554, CI: 1.211 to 1.997, P < .001).[98] NFS also predicted increased odds of MACE with an OR: 1.202 (CI: 1.073 to 1.347, P = .002) for −1.455< NFS <0.675 and OR: 1.761 (CI: 1.515 to 2.046, P < .001) for NFS ≥0.675.[98] Another study involving 5033 NAFLD patients found that patients with NFS >0.675 had a relative risk (RR) of 4.54 (95%CI: 1.85 to 11.17) of mortality.[99] This was also corroborated by another study of 320 NAFLD patients, where FIB-4 predicted liver-related events and mortality with an AUROC of 0.81 and 0.67, respectively, and NFS predicted them with an AUROC of 0.86 and 0.70, respectively.[100] The ELF was also found to predict liver-related morbidity and death in patients. A study of 457 patients over 7 years found a unit change of in ELF to be associated with doubling the risk of liver-related outcomes; compared with patients with an ELF <8.34, patients with an ELF of 8.34 to 10.4, 10.4 to 12.5, and 12.5 to 16.7 had an HR of 5, 10 and 75, respectively.[101]

Screening and Risk Stratification

Compensated advanced CLD (cACLD) was conceptualized at the Baveno VII conference to better reflect the spectrum of fibrosis and compensated liver cirrhosis in asymptomatic patients[102] with the goal of simplifying the risk stratification process for clinically significant portal hypertension (CSPH) and hepatic decompensation and avoiding unnecessary endoscopy (**Fig. 1**). LSM measurement by VCTE was recommended to screen for cACLD, with LSM <10 kPa effectively ruling out, 10 to 15 kPa

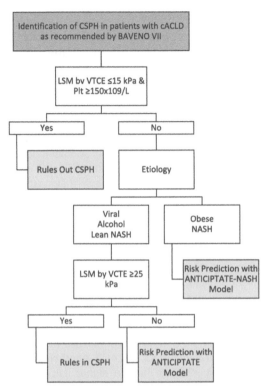

Fig. 1. Identification of CSPH in patients with compensated advanced chronic liver disease (CaCLD) as recommended by BAVENO VII.

being suggestive of and >15 kPa being highly suggestive of cACLD. For LSM 10 to 15 kPa, additional serum-based NITs can be used to complement the suspicion of cACLD (FIB-4 ≥2.67, ELF ≥9.8, FibroTest ≥0.58 for ALD/viral hepatitis, FibroTest ≥0.48 for NAFLD).[103] However, a real-world multicenter study involving 5,648 patients with CLD of various etiologies found these cut-offs to have suboptimal sensitivity of 75% and 96% specificity to exclude and diagnose cACLD, proposing lower cutoffs of <8 kPa (<7 kPa for viral hepatitis) and >12 kPa which improved sensitivities and ensured lower likelihood of false negatives.[74] Yearly screening with VCTE is recommended in patients with established cACLD; a significant decrease in LSM of ≥20% with an LSM <20kPa or a decrease to <10kPa is associated with decreased risk of decompensation and liver-related mortality.[74]

The development of portal hypertension in cirrhotic patients is a key mechanism through which liver-related complications such as esophageal or gastric varices, ascites, and hepatorenal syndrome (HRS) develop.[104] Although clinically significant portal hypertension (CSPH) is classically defined as hepatic venous pressure gradient (HPVG) ≥10mm Hg, there is an increasing drive to use NITs to predict the likelihood of CSPH. A study of 150 patients found LSM of >21kPa to predict CSPH with an AUROC of 0.945. This was corroborated by a Korean study of 59 patients with cirrhosis in which LSM of >21.95kPa predicted CSPH with an AUROC of 0.851.[105] LSM measurement of >20 to 25 kPa by VCTE has been shown to correlate with CSPH and HVPG.[106] Guidelines hence support using VCTE for noninvasive diagnosis of CSPH for risk stratification, ideally in combination with platelet count or spleen size.[103,107] An improved accuracy in identifying CPSH with the addition of platelet count resulted in the Baveno VI conference's recommendation for patients with LSM ≤20kPa and a platelet count of ≥150,000 to avoid endoscopic screening in view of low risk of varices, the adoption of which reduce endoscopies by 20%, missing only <4% of high-risk varices.[108,109] However, a meta-analysis of 1399 patients found that lowering the recommended screening threshold of 21 to 25 kPa to 13.6 to 18kPa resulted in significantly improved sensitivity and AUROC (71.2% vs 91.7% and 0.769 vs 0.921, respectively).[110] The Baveno VII consensus subsequently tightened the threshold to LSM ≤15 kPa with a platelet count of ≥150,000 for ruling out CSPH[103] which was validated in a study of 76 patients to have a sensitivity of 100% and a specificity of 95%.[111] In addition, Baveno VII proposes the 'rule of five' for LSM by VCTE (10 to 15 to 20 to 25 kPa), indicating increasing risks of hepatic decompensation and liver-related mortality with increasing LSM, independent of etiology of CLD.

In NAFLD, the American Gastroenterological Association (AGA) recommends the use of FIB-4 and VCTE for routine screening[112] Patients with intermediate risk (FIB-4 1.3 to 2.67 and LSM 8 to 12 kPa) or high risk (FIB-4 >2.67 or FIB-4 1.3 to 2.67 and LSM >12kPa) should be managed by a multidisciplinary team led by a hepatologist. The American Association of Clinical Endocrinology (AACE) recommends screening of patients with obesity, features of MetS or type 2 DM for NAFLD and advanced fibrosis.[113] Patients with indeterminate risk (FIB-4 1.3 to 2.67; ELF 7.7 to 9.8; LSM 8 to 12 kPa) or high risk (FIB-4 >2.67; ELF >9.8; LSM >12 kPa) are recommended to be referred to a hepatologist for management.

Latest Developments in Novel NITs

In light of the promise of NITs, various new panels have been developed. AGILE 3+ comprising AAR, platelet count, DM, sex, age, and LSM by VCTE was developed by echosens for detecting advanced fibrosis in NAFLD patients and outperformed FIB-4 and NFS in detecting advanced fibrosis (AUROC of 0.89, 0.7 and 0.74, respectively)[114] and LSM via VCTE in predicting liver-related events at 96 months (AUROC 0.97 vs 0.95; P = .001).[115] The AGILE 4 which was developed with similar parameters as the AGILE 3+ (excluding sex) for detecting cirrhosis in NAFLD patients, however, has yet to be conclusively validated.

The FAST score (comprising LSM and CAP via VCTE and AST identifies high-risk NASH that may necessitate treatment (NASH + NAFLD activity score [NAS] ≥4 + F ≥ 2) with an AUROC of 0.85.[116] It was further validated (AUROC 0.81) in another study of 585 NAFLD patients.[117] The MAST score (comprising MRE, MRI-PDFF, and AST) was developed for the same purpose and validated more recently in 2022 to outperform FAST, NFS and FIB-4 (AUROC 0.929, 0.868, 0.689, and 0.711, respectively).[118] The MEFIB index combines MRE and FIB-4 to improve the identification of high-risk NASH (AUROC 0.9 vs 0.87 and 0.72, respectively).[119] A meta-analysis of 2018 patients also found a positive MEFIB (MRE ≥3.3 kPa and FIB-4 ≥1.6) to be strongly associated (HR 20.6, 95% CI: 10.4 to 40.8, P < .001) with portal hypertensive complications (EV requiring treatment, ascites and hepatic encephalopathy), with a negative MEFIB to effectively ruling them out (NPV 99.1%) at 5 years.[120] A recent study of 563 NAFLD patients comparing the above three NITs found MEFIB to outperform both MAST and FAST (AUROC 0.768 vs 0.719 vs 0.687) for diagnosing high-risk NASH, with a better PPV (95.3% vs 90.0% vs 83.5%) and NPV (90.1% vs 69.6% vs 71.7%) for significant fibrosis.[121] Most recently, the Fibrosis-5 (FIB-5) score was developed through machine learning (combining FIB-4 and LSM measurement via VCTE) to predict incident complications of portal hypertension in patients with CaCLD and was found to be superior to FIB-4 or LSM alone (AUROC 0.845 to 0.868 vs 0.672 vs 0.688).[122]

Impact of Noninvasive Tests on Treatment Decisions and Clinical Trials

NIT assessment of fibrosis before initiation of antiviral therapy in viral hepatitis is recommended in various international guidelines.[123–126] In HBV, the presence of cirrhosis affects both the decision to treat as well as the decision to stop nucleoside/nucleotide analogs (NAs) upon hepatitis B surface antigen loss.[126] Consequently, all HBV patients not actively on treatment should undergo fibrosis monitoring to determine if an indication for treatment has arisen. Conversely, HCV should always be treated until a sustained virologic response (SVR) is attained; however, the presence of fibrosis necessitates adjustments in certain direct acting antiviral (DAA) regimens[125] and patients with F3-4 fibrosis pretreatment require continued HCC surveillance even after completion of therapy.[127] Fibrosis monitoring is not routinely recommended in HCV after completion of antiviral treatment. Patients with HCV post-SVR experience improvements in fibrosis, liver-related outcomes, and mortality.[128–130] However, risk stratification after the achievement of SVR is challenging. Studies have found that after HCV cure, NITs such as posttreatment follow-up LSM or von Willebrand factor/platelet count ratio (VITRO) may predict posttreatment hepatic decompensation in patients with pretreatment cACLD,[131] and posttreatment LSM <12 kPa with platelet >150 was able to exclude CSPH with high sensitivity of 99.2%.[132]

As per AGA and AACE guidelines, NAFLD patients identified as indeterminate or high risk should be referred to a hepatologist for management with an emphasis on weight loss, CVD management and optimizing cardiometabolic risk factors. Specifically, due to increased mortality risk,[133] the United States Food and Drug Administration (FDA) and the European Medicines Agency (EMA) recommend for patients with high-risk NASH to be considered for enrollment into Phase III trials for pharmacologic therapy.[134] There is much promise in the utility of the newer NITs discussed above in identifying such patients. Due to the limitations of an LB, both FDA and EMA have encouraged the development of NITs to replace an LB in clinical trials.[135,136] Given its high diagnostic accuracy, MRE has been shown to be suitable for use as inclusion criteria and primary endpoint measurement in NASH trials.[137,138] MRI-PDFF response ($\geq$30% relative reduction in steatosis) shows promise in its utility as an end-point measurement in NASH trials, correlating well with the histologic improvement of steatosis in non-alcoholic steatohepatitis (NASH).[139,140]

SUMMARY

As a result, a joint meeting between members of the American Association for the study of liver diseases (AASLD) and the European Association for the Study of the Liver (EASL) is considering an all-encompassing definition to increase awareness of FL in ALD and viral hepatitis beyond NAFLD. With more recent evidence, the growth in the role of NITs in the diagnosis, prognostication, and management of CLDs has become increasingly evident. The development of novel NITs also shows great promise in improving diagnostic accuracies. Several markers, such as MRI-based markers have been adopted in clinical trials to great effect. Moving forward, further developments in NITs may potentially change the practice of hepatology.

CLINICS CARE POINTS

- The preliminary assessment of liver steatosis and fibrosis with noninvasive tests (NITs) has been increasingly recommended by various international guidelines in the management of liver diseases as effective measures for risk stratification

- While promising, the clinical utility of NITs remains to be conclusively validated in future clinical trials assessing diagnostic and prognostic accuracies

FUNDING

This work is funded in part by an IAF-PP grant (H18/01/a0/017) from the Agency for Science, Technology and Research (Singapore) on Ensemble of Multi-disciplinary Systems and Integrated Omics for NAFLD (EMULSION) diagnostic and therapeutic discovery.

DISCLOSURE

All authors do not have any commercial or financial conflicts of interest or any funding sources to disclose.

REFERENCES

1. Moon AM, Singal AG, Tapper EB. Contemporary Epidemiology of Chronic Liver Disease and Cirrhosis. Clin Gastroenterol Hepatol 2020;18(12):2650–66.
2. Sepanlou SG, Safiri S, Bisignano C, et al. The global, regional, and national burden of cirrhosis by cause in 195 countries and territories, 1990–2017: a systematic analysis for the Global Burden of Disease Study 2017. Lancet Gastroenterol Hepatol 2020;5(3):245–66.
3. Riazi K, Azhari H, Charette JH, et al. The prevalence and incidence of NAFLD worldwide: a systematic review and meta-analysis. Lancet Gastroenterol Hepatol 2022;7(9):851–61.
4. Fazel Y, Koenig AB, Sayiner M, et al. Epidemiology and natural history of non-alcoholic fatty liver disease. Metabolism 2016;65(8):1017–25.
5. Ng CH, Lim WH, Lim GEH, et al. Mortality Outcomes by Fibrosis Stage in Nonalcoholic Fatty Liver Disease: A Systematic Review and Meta-analysis. Clin Gastroenterol Hepatol 2022;0(0). https://doi.org/10.1016/J.CGH.2022.04.014.
6. Yano M, Kumada H, Kage M, et al. The long-term pathological evolution of chronic hepatitis C. Hepatology 1996;23(6):1334–40.
7. Lackner C, Spindelboeck W, Haybaeck J, et al. Histological parameters and alcohol abstinence determine long-term prognosis in patients with alcoholic liver disease. J Hepatol 2017;66(3):610–8.
8. Kim NJ, Vutien P, Cleveland E, et al. Fibrosis Stage-specific Incidence of Hepatocellular Cancer After Hepatitis C Cure With Direct-acting Antivirals: A Systematic Review and Meta-analysis. Clin Gastroenterol Hepatol 2022. https://doi.org/10.1016/J.CGH.2022.04.013.
9. Bedossa P, Dargère D, Paradis V. Sampling Variability of Liver Fibrosis in Chronic Hepatitis C. Hepatology 2003;38(6):1449–57.
10. Davison BA, Harrison SA, Cotter G, et al. Suboptimal reliability of liver biopsy evaluation has implications for randomized clinical trials. J Hepatol 2020;73(6):1322–32.
11. Muthiah MD, Sanyal AJ. Burden of Disease due to Nonalcoholic Fatty Liver Disease. Gastroenterol Clin North Am 2020;49(1):1–23.
12. Zheng Q, Zou B, Wu Y, et al. Systematic review with meta-analysis: prevalence of hepatic steatosis, fibrosis and associated factors in chronic hepatitis B. Aliment Pharmacol Ther 2021;54(9):1100–9.

13. Modaresi Esfeh J, Ansari-Gilani K. Steatosis and hepatitis C. Gastroenterol Rep (Oxf) 2015;gov040. https://doi.org/10.1093/gastro/gov040.

14. Asselah T, Rubbia-Brandt L, Marcellin P, et al. Steatosis in chronic hepatitis C: Why does it really matter? Gut 2006;55(1):123–30.

15. Siphepho PY, Liu YT, Shabangu CS, et al. The impact of steatosis on chronic hepatitis c progression and response to antiviral treatments. Biomedicines 2021;9(10). https://doi.org/10.3390/biomedicines9101491.

16. Negro F. Mechanisms and significance of liver steatosis in hepatitis C virus infection. World J Gastroenterol : WJG 2006;12(42):6756.

17. Israelsen M, Juel HB, Detlefsen S, et al. Metabolic and Genetic Risk Factors Are the Strongest Predictors of Severity of Alcohol-Related Liver Fibrosis. Clin Gastroenterol Hepatol 2021. https://doi.org/10.1016/j.cgh.2020.11.038.

18. Bedogni G, Bellentani S, Miglioli L, et al. The fatty liver index: A simple and accurate predictor of hepatic steatosis in the general population. BMC Gastroenterol 2006;6. https://doi.org/10.1186/1471-230X-6-33.

19. Lee JH, Kim D, Kim HJ, et al. Hepatic steatosis index: A simple screening tool reflecting nonalcoholic fatty liver disease. Dig Liver Dis 2010;42(7):503–8.

20. Kotronen A, Peltonen M, Hakkarainen A, et al. Prediction of Non-Alcoholic Fatty Liver Disease and Liver Fat Using Metabolic and Genetic Factors. Gastroenterology 2009;137(3):865–72.

21. Fedchuk L, Nascimbeni F, Pais R, et al. Performance and limitations of steatosis biomarkers in patients with nonalcoholic fatty liver disease. Aliment Pharmacol Ther 2014;40(10):1209–22.

22. Wanless IR, Lentz JS. Fatty liver hepatitis (steatohepatitis) and obesity: an autopsy study with analysis of risk factors. Hepatology 1990;12(5):1106–10.

23. Xavier SA, Monteiro SO, Arieira CM, et al. US-FLI score – Is it possible to predict the steatosis grade with an ultrasonographic score? Mol Genet Metab 2021;132(3):204–9.

24. Ballestri S, Lonardo A, Romagnoli D, et al. Ultrasonographic fatty liver indicator, a novel score which rules out NASH and is correlated with metabolic parameters in NAFLD. Liver Int 2012;32(8):1242–52.

25. Bae JS, Lee DH, Suh KS, et al. Noninvasive assessment of hepatic steatosis using a pathologic reference standard: comparison of CT, MRI, and US-based techniques. Ultrasonography 2021;41(2):344–54.

26. Hannah WN, Harrison SA. Noninvasive imaging methods to determine severity of nonalcoholic fatty liver disease and nonalcoholic steatohepatitis. Hepatology 2016;64(6):2234–43.

27. de Moura Almeida A, Cotrim HP, Barbosa DBV, et al. Fatty liver disease in severe obese patients: Diagnostic value of abdominal ultrasound. World J Gastroenterol 2008;14(9):1415–8.

28. Bril F, Ortiz-Lopez C, Lomonaco R, et al. Clinical value of liver ultrasound for the diagnosis of nonalcoholic fatty liver disease in overweight and obese patients. Liver Int 2015;35(9):2139–46.

29. Strauss S, Gavish E, Gottlieb P, et al. Interobserver and intraobserver variability in the sonographic assessment of fatty liver. Am J Roentgenol 2007;189(6):1449.

30. Hamaguchi M, Kojima T, Itoh Y, et al. The severity of ultrasonographic findings in nonalcoholic fatty liver disease reflects the metabolic syndrome and visceral fat accumulation. Am J Gastroenterol 2007;102(12):2708–15.

31. Cloutier G, Destrempes F, Yu F, et al. Quantitative ultrasound imaging of soft biological tissues: a primer for radiologists and medical physicists. Insights Imaging 2021;12(1). https://doi.org/10.1186/s13244-021-01071-w.
32. Gao F, He Q, Li G, et al. A novel quantitative ultrasound technique for identifying non-alcoholic steatohepatitis. Liver Int 2022;42(1):80–91.
33. Karlas T, Petroff D, Sasso M, et al. Individual patient data meta-analysis of controlled attenuation parameter (CAP) technology for assessing steatosis. J Hepatol 2017;66(5):1022–30.
34. Ferraioli G, Tinelli C, Lissandrin R, et al. Interobserver reproducibility of the controlled attenuation parameter (CAP) for quantifying liver steatosis. Hepatol Int 2014;8(4):576–81.
35. Wong VWS, Petta S, Hiriart JB, et al. Validity criteria for the diagnosis of fatty liver by M probe-based controlled attenuation parameter. J Hepatol 2017;67(3): 577–84.
36. Eddowes PJ, Sasso M, Allison M, et al. Accuracy of FibroScan Controlled Attenuation Parameter and Liver Stiffness Measurement in Assessing Steatosis and Fibrosis in Patients With Nonalcoholic Fatty Liver Disease. Gastroenterology 2019;156(6):1717–30.
37. Oeda S, Takahashi H, Imajo K, et al. Accuracy of liver stiffness measurement and controlled attenuation parameter using FibroScan® M/XL probes to diagnose liver fibrosis and steatosis in patients with nonalcoholic fatty liver disease: a multicenter prospective study. J Gastroenterol 2020;55(4):428–40.
38. Petroff D, Blank V, Newsome PN, et al. Assessment of hepatic steatosis by controlled attenuation parameter using the M and XL probes: an individual patient data meta-analysis. Lancet Gastroenterol Hepatol 2021;6(3):185–98.
39. Caussy C, Alquiraish MH, Nguyen P, et al. Optimal threshold of controlled attenuation parameter with MRI-PDFF as the gold standard for the detection of hepatic steatosis. Hepatology 2018;67(4):1348–59.
40. Zheng D, Tian W, Zheng Z, et al. Accuracy of computed tomography for detecting hepatic steatosis in donors for liver transplantation: A meta-analysis. Clin Transpl 2017;31(8):e13013.
41. Park SH, Kim PN, Kim KW, et al. Macrovesicular Hepatic Steatosis in Living Liver Donors: Use of CT for Quantitative and Qualitative Assessment1. Radiology 2006;239(1):105–12.
42. Limanond P, Raman SS, Lassman C, et al. Macrovesicular Hepatic Steatosis in Living Related Liver Donors: Correlation between CT and Histologic Findings1. Radiology 2004;230(1):276–80.
43. Ma J, Song ZQ, Yan FH. Separation of Hepatic Iron and Fat by Dual-Source Dual-Energy Computed Tomography Based on Material Decomposition: An Animal Study. PLoS One 2014;9(10):e110964.
44. Fischer MA, Gnannt R, Raptis D, et al. Quantification of liver fat in the presence of iron and iodine: An ex-vivo dual-energy CT study. Invest Radiol 2011;46(6): 351–8.
45. van Werven JR, Marsman HA, Nederveen AJ, et al. Assessment of Hepatic Steatosis in Patients Undergoing Liver Resection: Comparison of US, CT, T1-weighted Dual-Echo MR Imaging, and Point-resolved 1H MR Spectroscopy1. Radiology 2010;256(1):159–68.
46. Tang A, Desai A, Hamilton G, et al. Accuracy of MR imaging-estimated proton density fat fraction for classification of dichotomized histologic steatosis grades in nonalcoholic fatty liver disease. Radiology 2015;274(2):416–25.

47. Park CC, Nguyen P, Hernandez C, et al. Magnetic Resonance Elastography vs Transient Elastography in Detection of Fibrosis and Noninvasive Measurement of Steatosis in Patients With Biopsy-Proven Nonalcoholic Fatty Liver Disease. Gastroenterology 2017;152(3):598–607, e2.

48. Bannas P, Kramer H, Hernando D, et al. Quantitative magnetic resonance imaging of hepatic steatosis: Validation in ex vivo human livers. Hepatology 2015; 62(5):1444–55.

49. Yano M, Kumada H, Kage M, et al. The Long-Term Pathological Evolution of Chronic Hepatitis C. Hepatology 1996;23(6):1334–40.

50. Younossi ZM, Stepanova M, Rafiq N, et al. Pathologic criteria for nonalcoholic steatohepatitis: Interprotocol agreement and ability to predict liver-related mortality. Hepatology 2011;53(6):1874–82.

51. McPherson S, Stewart SF, Henderson E, et al. Simple noninvasive fibrosis scoring systems can reliably exclude advanced fibrosis in patients with nonalcoholic fatty liver disease. Gut 2010;59(9):1265–9.

52. Wong VWS, Wong GLH, Chim AML, et al. Validation of the NAFLD fibrosis score in a Chinese population with low prevalence of advanced fibrosis. Am J Gastroenterol 2008;103(7):1682–8.

53. Sterling RK, Lissen E, Clumeck N, et al. Development of a simple noninvasive index to predict significant fibrosis in patients with HIV/HCV coinfection. Hepatology 2006;43(6):1317–25.

54. Xiao G, Zhu S, Xiao X, et al. Comparison of laboratory tests, ultrasound, or magnetic resonance elastography to detect fibrosis in patients with nonalcoholic fatty liver disease: A meta-analysis. Hepatology 2017;66(5):1486–501.

55. McPherson S, Hardy T, Dufour JF, et al. Age as a Confounding Factor for the Accurate Noninvasive Diagnosis of Advanced NAFLD Fibrosis. Am J Gastroenterol 2017;112(5):740.

56. Mózes FE, Lee JA, Selvaraj EA, et al. Diagnostic accuracy of noninvasive tests for advanced fibrosis in patients with NAFLD: an individual patient data meta-analysis. Gut 2022;71(5). https://doi.org/10.1136/GUTJNL-2021-324243.

57. Graupera I, Thiele M, Serra-Burriel M, et al. Low Accuracy of FIB-4 and NAFLD Fibrosis Scores for Screening for Liver Fibrosis in the Population. Clin Gastroenterol Hepatol 2021. https://doi.org/10.1016/J.CGH.2021.12.034.

58. Gudowska M, Gruszewska E, Panasiuk A, et al. Hyaluronic acid concentration in liver diseases. Clin Exp Med 2016;16(4):523–8.

59. Suzuki A, Angulo P, Lymp J, et al. Hyaluronic acid, an accurate serum marker for severe hepatic fibrosis in patients with non-alcoholic fatty liver disease. Liver Int 2005;25(4):779–86.

60. Wang Y, Pan W, Zhao D, et al. Diagnostic Value of Serum Procollagen III N-Terminal Peptide for Liver Fibrosis in Infantile Cholestasis. Front Pediatr 2020;8. https://doi.org/10.3389/fped.2020.00131.

61. Nielsen MJ, Nedergaard AF, Sun S, et al. The Neo-Epitope Specific PRO-C3 ELISA Measures True Formation of Type III Collagen Associated with Liver and Muscle Parameters. Am J Transl Res 2013;5(3):303–15. Available at: www.ajtr.org.

62. Mak AL, Lee J, van Dijk AM, et al. Systematic review with meta-analysis: Diagnostic accuracy of pro-c3 for hepatic fibrosis in patients with non-alcoholic fatty liver disease. Biomedicines 2021;9(12). https://doi.org/10.3390/biomedicines9121920.

63. Hemmann S, Graf J, Roderfeld M, et al. Expression of MMPs and TIMPs in liver fibrosis - a systematic review with special emphasis on anti-fibrotic strategies. J Hepatol 2007;46(5):955–75.

64. Abdelaziz R, Elbasel M, Esmat S, et al. Tissue inhibitors of metalloproteinase-1 and 2 and obesity related non-alcoholic fatty liver disease: Is there a relationship? Digestion 2015;92(3):130–7.

65. Vali Y, Lee J, Boursier J, et al. Enhanced liver fibrosis test for the noninvasive diagnosis of fibrosis in patients with NAFLD: A systematic review and meta-analysis. J Hepatol 2020;73(2):252–62.

66. Lichtinghagen R, Pietsch D, Bantel H, et al. The Enhanced Liver Fibrosis (ELF) score: Normal values, influence factors and proposed cut-off values. J Hepatol 2013;59(2):236–42.

67. Younossi ZM, Felix S, Jeffers T, et al. Performance of the Enhanced Liver Fibrosis Test to Estimate Advanced Fibrosis among Patients with Nonalcoholic Fatty Liver Disease. JAMA Netw Open 2021;4(9). https://doi.org/10.1001/jamanetworkopen.2021.23923.

68. Imbert-Bismut F, Ratziu V, Pieroni L, et al. Biochemical markers of liver fibrosis in patients with hepatitis C virus infection: a prospective study. Lancet 2001; 357(9262):1069–75.

69. Ratziu V, Massard J, Charlotte F, et al. Diagnostic value of biochemical markers (Fibro Test-FibroSURE) for the prediction of liver fibrosis in patients with non-alcoholic fatty liver disease. BMC Gastroenterol 2006;6. https://doi.org/10.1186/1471-230X-6-6.

70. Munteanu M, Tiniakos D, Anstee Q, et al. Diagnostic performance of FibroTest, SteatoTest and ActiTest in patients with NAFLD using the SAF score as histological reference. Aliment Pharmacol Ther 2016;44(8):877–89.

71. Loong TCW, Wei JL, Leung JCF, et al. Application of the combined FibroMeter vibration-controlled transient elastography algorithm in Chinese patients with non-alcoholic fatty liver disease. J Gastroenterol Hepatol (Australia) 2017; 32(7):1363–9.

72. Daniels SJ, Leeming DJ, Eslam M, et al. ADAPT: An Algorithm Incorporating PRO-C3 Accurately Identifies Patients With NAFLD and Advanced Fibrosis. Hepatology 2019;69(3):1075–86.

73. Boyle M, Tiniakos D, Schattenberg JM, et al. Performance of the PRO-C3 collagen neo-epitope biomarker in non-alcoholic fatty liver disease. JHEP Rep 2019;1(3):188–98.

74. Papatheodoridi M, Hiriart JB, Lupsor-Platon M, et al. Refining the Baveno VI elastography criteria for the definition of compensated advanced chronic liver disease. J Hepatol 2021;74(5):1109–16.

75. Lazarus Jv, Castera L, Mark HE, et al. Real-world evidence on noninvasive tests and associated cut-offs used to assess fibrosis in routine clinical practice. JHEP Rep 2022;22:100596.

76. Wong GLH, Chan HLY, Choi PCL, et al. Association Between Anthropometric Parameters and Measurements of Liver Stiffness by Transient Elastography. Clin Gastroenterol Hepatol 2013;11(3). https://doi.org/10.1016/j.cgh.2012.09.025.

77. Castera L, Foucher J, Bernard PH, et al. Pitfalls of liver stiffness measurement: A 5-year prospective study of 13,369 examinations. Hepatology 2010;51(3): 828–35.

78. Cassinotto C, Erome Boursier J, de L Edinghen V, et al. Liver Stiffness in Nonalcoholic Fatty Liver Disease: A Comparison of Supersonic Shear Imaging, Fibro-Scan, and ARFI With Liver Biopsy a he study of liver diseases t american association for. Hepatology 2016;63(6):1817–27.

79. Zhou X, Rao J, Wu X, et al. Comparison of 2-D Shear Wave Elastography and Point Shear Wave Elastography for Assessing Liver Fibrosis. Ultrasound Med Biol 2021;47(3):408–27.

80. Imajo K, Kessoku T, Honda Y, et al. Magnetic Resonance Imaging More Accurately Classifies Steatosis and Fibrosis in Patients with Nonalcoholic Fatty Liver Disease Than Transient Elastography. Gastroenterology 2016;150(3): 626–37, e7.

81. Caussy C, Chen J, Alquiraish MH, et al. Association Between Obesity and Discordance in Fibrosis Stage Determination by Magnetic Resonance vs Transient Elastography in Patients With Nonalcoholic Liver Disease. Clin Gastroenterol Hepatol 2018;16(12):1974–82, e7.

82. Loomba R, Adams LA. Advances in noninvasive assessment of hepatic fibrosis. Gut 2020;69(7):1343–52.

83. Imajo K, Honda Y, Kobayashi T, et al. Direct Comparison of US and MR Elastography for Staging Liver Fibrosis in Patients With Nonalcoholic Fatty Liver Disease. Clin Gastroenterol Hepatol 2022;20(4):908–17, e11.

84. Hsu C, Caussy C, Imajo K, et al. Magnetic Resonance vs Transient Elastography Analysis of Patients With Nonalcoholic Fatty Liver Disease: A Systematic Review and Pooled Analysis of Individual Participants. Clin Gastroenterol Hepatol 2019; 17(4):630–7, e8.

85. Ekstedt M, Hagström H, Nasr P, et al. Fibrosis stage is the strongest predictor for disease-specific mortality in NAFLD after up to 33 years of follow-up. Hepatology 2015;61(5):1547–54.

86. Gidener T, Yin M, Dierkhising RA, et al. Magnetic resonance elastography for prediction of long-term progression and outcome in chronic liver disease: A retrospective study. Hepatology 2022;75(2):379–90.

87. Matsui N, Imajo K, Yoneda M, et al. Magnetic resonance elastography increases usefulness and safety of noninvasive screening for esophageal varices. J Gastroenterol Hepatol 2018;33(12):2022–8.

88. Tamaki N, Kurosaki M, Higuchi M, et al. Validation of albumin, bilirubin, and platelet criteria for avoiding screening endoscopy in patients with advanced fibrosis. Hepatol Res 2020;50(8):996–9.

89. Unalp-Arida A, Ruhl CE. Noninvasive fatty liver markers predict liver disease mortality in the U.S. population. Hepatology 2016;63(4):1170–83.

90. Shili-Masmoudi S, Wong GLH, Hiriart JB, et al. Liver stiffness measurement predicts long-term survival and complications in non-alcoholic fatty liver disease. Liver Int 2020;40(3):581–9.

91. Tamaki N, Higuchi M, Kurosaki M, et al. Risk Difference of Liver-Related and Cardiovascular Events by Liver Fibrosis Status in Nonalcoholic Fatty Liver Disease. Clin Gastroenterol Hepatol 2022;20(5):1171–3, e2.

92. Higuchi M, Tamaki N, Kurosaki M, et al. Longitudinal association of magnetic resonance elastography-associated liver stiffness with complications and mortality. Aliment Pharmacol Ther 2022;55(3):292–301.

93. Long MT, Zhang X, Xu H, et al. Hepatic Fibrosis Associates With Multiple Cardiometabolic Disease Risk Factors: The Framingham Heart Study. Hepatology 2021;73(2):548–59.

94. Pang JXQ, Zimmer S, Niu S, et al. Liver Stiffness by Transient Elastography Predicts Liver-Related Complications and Mortality in Patients with Chronic Liver Disease. PLoS One 2014;9(4). https://doi.org/10.1371/JOURNAL.PONE.0095776.

95. Cardoso CRL, Villela-Nogueira CA, Leite NC, et al. Prognostic impact of liver fibrosis and steatosis by transient elastography for cardiovascular and mortality outcomes in individuals with nonalcoholic fatty liver disease and type 2 diabetes: the Rio de Janeiro Cohort Study. Cardiovasc Diabetol 2021;20(1). https://doi.org/10.1186/S12933-021-01388-2.

96. Hagström H, Talbäck M, Andreasson A, et al. Ability of Noninvasive Scoring Systems to Identify Individuals in the Population at Risk for Severe Liver Disease. Gastroenterology 2020;158(1):200–14.

97. Schonmann Y, Yeshua H, Bentov I, et al. Liver fibrosis marker is an independent predictor of cardiovascular morbidity and mortality in the general population. Dig Liver Dis 2021;53(1):79–85.

98. Chew NWS, Ng CH, Chan KE, et al. The Fibrosis-4 (FIB-4) Index Predicts Cardiovascular Major Adverse Events and Mortality in Patients with Non-alcoholic Fatty Liver Disease. Can J Cardiol 2022;0(0).

99. Jaruvongvanich V, Wijarnpreecha K, Ungprasert P. The utility of NAFLD fibrosis score for prediction of mortality among patients with nonalcoholic fatty liver disease: A systematic review and meta-analysis of cohort study. Clin Res Hepatol Gastroenterol 2017;41(6):629–34.

100. Angulo P, Bugianesi E, Bjornsson ES, et al. Simple Noninvasive Systems Predict Long-term Outcomes of Patients With Nonalcoholic Fatty Liver Disease. Gastroenterology 2013;145(4):782–9, e4.

101. Parkes J, Roderick P, Harris S, et al. Enhanced liver fibrosis test can predict clinical outcomes in patients with chronic liver disease. Gut 2010;59(9):1245–51.

102. Kamath PS, Mookerjee RP. Expanding consensus in portal hypertension: Report of the Baveno VI Consensus Workshop: Stratifying risk and individualizing care for portal hypertension. J Hepatol 2015;63(3):743–52.

103. de Franchis R, Bosch J, Garcia-Tsao G, et al. Baveno VII – Renewing consensus in portal hypertension. J Hepatol 2022;76(4):959–74.

104. Castéra L, García-Tsao G. When the spleen gets tough, the varices get going. Gastroenterology 2013;144(1):19–22.

105. Hong WK, Kim MY, Baik SK, et al. The usefulness of noninvasive liver stiffness measurements in predicting clinically significant portal hypertension in cirrhotic patients: Korean data. Clin Mol Hepatol 2013;19(4):370.

106. Reiberger T. The Value of Liver and Spleen Stiffness for Evaluation of Portal Hypertension in Compensated Cirrhosis. Hepatol Commun 2022;6(5):950–64.

107. Berzigotti A, Tsochatzis E, Boursier J, et al. EASL Clinical Practice Guidelines on noninvasive tests for evaluation of liver disease severity and prognosis – 2021 update. J Hepatol 2021;75(3):659–89.

108. Stafylidou M, Paschos P, Katsoula A, et al. Performance of Baveno VI and Expanded Baveno VI Criteria for Excluding High-Risk Varices in Patients With Chronic Liver Diseases: A Systematic Review and Meta-analysis. Clin Gastroenterol Hepatol 2019;17(9):1744–55, e11.

109. Szakács Z, Erőss B, Soós A, et al. Baveno criteria safely identify patients with compensated advanced chronic liver disease who can avoid variceal screening endoscopy: A diagnostic test accuracy meta-analysis. Front Physiol 2019; 10(AUG):1028.

110. You MW, Kim KW, Pyo J, et al. A Meta-analysis for the Diagnostic Performance of Transient Elastography for Clinically Significant Portal Hypertension. Ultrasound Med Biol 2017;43(1):59–68.

111. Podrug K, Trkulja V, Zelenika M, et al. Validation of the New Diagnostic Criteria for Clinically Significant Portal Hypertension by Platelets and Elastography. Dig Dis Sci 2022;67(7):3327.

112. Kanwal F, Shubrook JH, Adams LA, et al. Clinical Care Pathway for the Risk Stratification and Management of Patients With Nonalcoholic Fatty Liver Disease. Gastroenterology 2021;161(5):1657–69.

113. Cusi K, Isaacs S, Barb D, et al. American Association of Clinical Endocrinology Clinical Practice Guideline for the Diagnosis and Management of Nonalcoholic Fatty Liver Disease in Primary Care and Endocrinology Clinical Settings: Co-Sponsored by the American Association for the Study of Liver Diseases (AASLD). Endocr Pract 2022;28(5):528–62.

114. De A, Duseja A, Mehta M, et al. AGILE 3+ Score for Assessing Hepatic Fibrosis in Patients with Non-Alcoholic Fatty Liver Disease (NAFLD) – Validation in an Indian Cohort. J Clin Exp Hepatol 2022;12:S65.

115. Pennisi G, Enea M, Pandolfo A, et al. AGILE 3+ Score for the Diagnosis of Advanced Fibrosis and for Predicting Liver-related Events in NAFLD. Clin Gastroenterol Hepatol 2022. https://doi.org/10.1016/J.CGH.2022.06.013.

116. Newsome PN, Sasso M, Deeks JJ, et al. FibroScan-AST (FAST) score for the noninvasive identification of patients with non-alcoholic steatohepatitis with significant activity and fibrosis: a prospective derivation and global validation study. Lancet Gastroenterol Hepatol 2020;5(4):362.

117. Woreta TA, van Natta ML, Lazo M, et al. Validation of the accuracy of the FAST™ score for detecting patients with at-risk nonalcoholic steatohepatitis (NASH) in a North American cohort and comparison to other noninvasive algorithms. PLoS One 2022;17(4):e0266859.

118. Noureddin M, Truong E, Gornbein JA, et al. MRI-based (MAST) score accurately identifies patients with NASH and significant fibrosis. J Hepatol 2022;76(4):781–7.

119. Jung J, Loomba RR, Imajo K, et al. MRE combined with FIB-4 (MEFIB) Index in detection of candidates for pharmacologic treatment of NASH related fibrosis. Gut 2021;70(10):1946.

120. Ajmera V, Kim BK, Yang K, et al. Liver Stiffness on Magnetic Resonance Elastography and the MEFIB Index and Liver-Related Outcomes in Nonalcoholic Fatty Liver Disease: A Systematic Review and Meta-Analysis of Individual Participants. Gastroenterology 2022. https://doi.org/10.1053/J.GASTRO.2022.06.073.

121. Kim BK, Tamaki N, Imajo K, et al. Head to head comparison between MEFIB, MAST, and FAST for detecting stage 2 fibrosis or higher among patients with NAFLD. J Hepatol 2022;13. https://doi.org/10.1016/J.JHEP.2022.07.020.

122. Vutien P, Berry K, Feng Z, et al. Combining FIB-4 and liver stiffness into the FIB-5, a single model that accurately predicts complications of portal hypertension. Am J Gastroenterol 2022. https://doi.org/10.14309/AJG.0000000000001906.

123. Terrault NA, Lok ASF, McMahon BJ, et al. Update on Prevention, Diagnosis, and Treatment and of Chronic Hepatitis B: AASLD 2018 Hepatitis B Guidance. Hepatology 2018;67(4):1560.

124. Ghany MG, Morgan TR. Hepatitis C Guidance 2019 Update: American Association for the Study of Liver Diseases–Infectious Diseases Society of America Recommendations for Testing, Managing, and Treating Hepatitis C Virus Infection. Hepatology 2020;71(2):686–721.

125. Pawlotsky JM, Negro F, Aghemo A, et al. EASL recommendations on treatment of hepatitis C: Final update of the series. J Hepatol 2020;73(5):1170–218.

126. Lampertico P, Agarwal K, Berg T, et al. EASL 2017 Clinical Practice Guidelines on the management of hepatitis B virus infection. J Hepatol 2017;67(2):370–98.
127. Ioannou GN. HCC surveillance after SVR in patients with F3/F4 fibrosis. J Hepatol 2021;74(2):458–65.
128. Carrat F, Fontaine H, Dorival C, et al. Clinical outcomes in patients with chronic hepatitis C after direct-acting antiviral treatment: a prospective cohort study. The Lancet 2019;393(10179):1453–64.
129. D'Ambrosio R, Degasperi E, Anolli MP, et al. Incidence of liver- and non-liver-related outcomes in patients with HCV-cirrhosis after SVR. J Hepatol 2022; 76(2):302–10.
130. D'Ambrosio R, Aghemo A, Rumi MG, et al. A morphometric and immunohisto-chemical study to assess the benefit of a sustained virological response in hepatitis C virus patients with cirrhosis. Hepatology 2012;56(2):532–43.
131. Semmler G, Binter T, Kozbial K, et al. Noninvasive Risk Stratification After HCV Eradication in Patients With Advanced Chronic Liver Disease. Hepatology 2021; 73(4):1275–89.
132. Semmler G, Lens S, Meyer EL, et al. Noninvasive tests for clinically significant portal hypertension after HCV cure. J Hepatol 2022;0(0). https://doi.org/10.1016/J.JHEP.2022.08.025.
133. Dulai PS, Singh S, Patel J, et al. Increased risk of mortality by fibrosis stage in nonalcoholic fatty liver disease: Systematic review and meta-analysis. Hepatology 2017;65(5):1557–65.
134. Loomba R, Ratziu V, Harrison SA, et al. Expert Panel Review to Compare FDA and EMA Guidance on Drug Development and Endpoints in Nonalcoholic Steatohepatitis. Gastroenterology 2022;162(3):680–8.
135. Noncirrhotic Nonalcoholic Steatohepatitis With Liver Fibrosis: Developing Drugs for Treatment | FDA. Available at: https://www.fda.gov/regulatory-information/search-fda-guidance-documents/noncirrhotic-nonalcoholic-steatohepatitis-liver-fibrosis-developing-drugs-treatment. Accessed August 21, 2022.
136. Draft reflection paper on regulatory requirements for the development of medicinal products for chronic non-infectious liver diseases (PBC, PSC, NASH) | European Medicines Agency. Available at: https://www.ema.europa.eu/en/draft-reflection-paper-regulatory-requirements-development-medicinal-products-chronic-non-infectious. Accessed August 21, 2022.
137. Nakajima A, Eguchi Y, Yoneda M, et al. Randomised clinical trial: Pemafibrate, a novel selective peroxisome proliferator-activated receptor α modulator (SPPARMα), versus placebo in patients with non-alcoholic fatty liver disease. Aliment Pharmacol Ther 2021;54(10):1263.
138. Flint A, Andersen G, Hockings P, et al. Randomised clinical trial: semaglutide versus placebo reduced liver steatosis but not liver stiffness in subjects with non-alcoholic fatty liver disease assessed by magnetic resonance imaging. Aliment Pharmacol Ther 2021;54(9):1150.
139. Tamaki N, Munaganuru N, Jung J, et al. Clinical utility of 30% relative decline in MRI-PDFF in predicting fibrosis regression in non-alcoholic fatty liver disease. Gut 2022;71(5):983–90.
140. Stine JG, Munaganuru N, Barnard A, et al. Change in MRI-PDFF and Histologic Response in Patients With Nonalcoholic Steatohepatitis: A Systematic Review and Meta-Analysis. Clin Gastroenterol Hepatol 2021;19(11):2274–83, e5.

Chronic Hepatitis C
Advances in Therapy and the Remaining Challenges

Saleh A. Alqahtani, MD[a,b], Mark S. Sulkowski, MD[c],*

KEYWORDS

- Hepatitis C • Direct-acting antiviral agents • Protease inhibitors • HCV elimination
- NS5A inhibitors

KEY POINTS

- Introducing direct-acting antiviral agents (DAAs) has revolutionized treatment of hepatitis C virus (HCV) infection.
- Several clinically significant issues remain unresolved after successful HCV eradication by DAAs, including hepatocellular carcinoma (HCC) occurrence after achieving sustained virological response in patients with cirrhosis.
- Although initial concerns about DAAs and HCC were raised, multiple studies have confirmed a 50% to 70% reduction in HCC risk in patients who achieved HCV cure with DAAs.
- Substantial investment and large-scale screening and treatment implementation programs are needed to realize the benefits of DAA therapy at the population level.
- The World Health Organization endorsed a plan to eliminate HCV as a public health threat by 2030 through increased diagnosis, treatment, and prevention. Although research continues, effective HCV vaccines are unavailable to prevent HCV infection and reinfection after treatment.

INTRODUCTION

It is estimated that 58 million people suffer from chronic hepatitis C virus (HCV) infection worldwide, which significantly contributes to chronic liver disease and liver-related mortality.[1] Chronic HCV infection can lead to liver cirrhosis and hepatocellular carcinoma (HCC), often requiring liver transplantation (LT).[2] HCV is an enveloped, positive-strand RNA virus classified in the Hepacivirus genus of the Flaviviridae.[3]

[a] Liver Transplant Centre, King Faisal Specialist Hospital & Research Centre, Riyadh, Saudi Arabia; [b] Division of Gastroenterology and Hepatology, Johns Hopkins University, Baltimore, MD, USA; [c] Department of Medicine, Johns Hopkins University School of Medicine, Baltimore, MD, USA
* Corresponding author.
E-mail address: msulkowski@jhmi.edu

Med Clin N Am 107 (2023) 423–433
https://doi.org/10.1016/j.mcna.2023.01.001

During the viral life cycle, the translation of HCV RNA produces a polyprotein that is cleaved into 3 structural proteins (E1, E2, and core) and 7 nonstructural (NS) proteins (NS2, NS3, NS4A and B, NS5A and B, as well as p7, **Fig. 1**).[4] HCV is genetically diverse. There are 6 major genotypes of hepatitis C, known as genotypes 1 to 6.[5] More than 50% of all cases worldwide are caused by genotype 1. About 20% of all cases are classified as genotype 3, whereas around 25% are classified as genotypes 2, 4, and 6.[6] The remainder of less than 5% is accounted for by genotype 5.[6] To understand the development of direct-acting antiviral agents (DAAs), we need to understand the HCV life cycle. HCV-encoded proteins are vital to the replication of the virus and are the prime targets of recent HCV treatments.[7,8]

After HCV RNA enters the hepatocyte, it is translated into a polyprotein and cleaved into mature viral proteins, including the critical NS proteins.[9] NS3 and NS4A proteases are involved in this posttranslational processing.[10] The replication complex synthesizes new viral RNA composed of the NS3, NS4A, NS4B, NS5A, and NS5B proteins.[11] Antiviral therapies target these proteins, blocking viral replication. The antiviral treatment outcome for clinical trials and care is the achievement of sustained virological response (SVR), defined as the absence of HCV 12 weeks or more after the treatment completion.

Several revolutionary antivirals have been developed in recent years that promise cure rates never before thought possible for HCV.[12] This review highlights the current state-of-the-art of antiviral treatment of HCV and gives an outlook for upcoming therapies.

A BRIEF HISTORY OF HEPATITIS C VIRUS AND ITS THERAPY

The discovery of the hepatitis B virus (HBV) by Blumberg and colleagues in 1965 was followed by the hepatitis A virus (HAV) in 1973, leading to the recognition that these pathogens were not the cause of posttransfusion hepatitis in some patients. Until the discovery of HCV in 1989, patients with posttransfusion hepatitis in the absence of HAV or HBV were designated as having non-A, non-B hepatitis (NANBH).[13–15]

Interferon-Alpha

NANBH was treated with interferon (IFN)-alpha in the mid-1980s before the discovery of HCV.[16,17] IFN-alpha stimulates antiviral and immunologic response mechanisms to inhibit viral replication and eliminate infected cells.[18,19] In the NANBH era, IFN led to serum alanine aminotransferase (ALT) normalization in some patients, which subsequently was demonstrated to be the result of HCV RNA reduction in the blood.[17] From the early 1990s, IFN monotherapy was the standard of care for treating patients with chronic HCV infection, leading to low SVR in the range of 6% to 19% and associated with significant adverse events, including influenza-like symptoms and cytopenias.[20]

Ribavirin

The next significant advance for treating patients with chronic HCV infection was ribavirin (RBV), a guanosine nucleoside analog, in 1998.[21] In an early pilot study of RBV monotherapy, treatment was associated with a decline in ALT but not the virus levels, demonstrating limited efficacy in patients with HCV infection.[21] However, in randomized, controlled trials, the combination of RBV plus INF significantly increased the SVR rate (31%–43%) compared with IFN alone, primarily by reducing the rate of viral relapse after stopping therapy.[20,22] The mechanism of RBV remains incompletely understood, with evidence that RBV may induce an immune response and inhibit

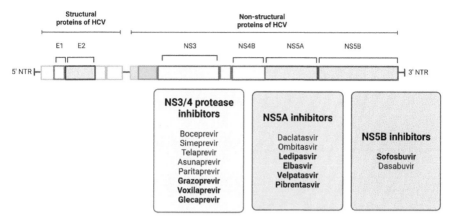

Fig. 1. Targets for HCV therapy marked in the HCV genome structure. (*Adapted from* Lohmann V. Hepatitis C virus cell culture models: an encomium on basic research paving the road to therapy development. Med Microbiol Immunol (Berl). 2019;208(1):3-24. https://doi.org/10.1007/s00430-018-0566-x.)

inosine monophosphate dehydrogenase and HCV replication by increasing viral mutagenesis.[23]

Pegylated Interferon-Alpha

HCV therapy reached another milestone, adding polyethylene glycol to INF-alpha, creating a longer acting pegylated IFN (Peg-IFN). Compared with standard IFN, Peg-IFN led to sustained antiviral activity during 1 week, leading to improved adherence with once-weekly dosing and higher SVR rates.[24,25] Until 2015, Peg-IFN and RBV were the backbones of HCV treatment (**Fig. 2**). However, this regimen was associated with significant adverse effects, sometimes treatment-limiting, and many patients were not eligible or elected to defer treatment with PEG-IFN plus RBV.[26–28] Further, SVR rates for HCV genotype 1 remained relatively low due partly to heterogeneity of IFN responses because of polymorphisms near the interleukin-28b gene.

Hepatitis C Virus NS3/4A Protease Inhibitors

The first DAAs targeted the HCV NS3/4A protease (see **Fig. 1**), thus preventing polyprotein cleavage and inhibiting HCV viral replication.[29] Not unexpectedly, monotherapy with first-generation HCV protease inhibitors rapidly selected for HCV variants that were resistant to the drugs, leading to studies of these DAAs in combination with PEG-IFN/RBV. In 2011, the first NS3/4A protease inhibitors, telaprevir, and boceprevir were approved in combination with PEG-IFN plus RBV, improving SVR rates in patients with HCV genotype 1 infection (SVR: 60%–88%).[30–32] However, combination therapy with telaprevir or boceprevir plus PEG-IFN/RBV was poorly tolerated with more severe side effects than PEG-IFN/RBV, including severe anemia and, with telaprevir, severe rash. Although beneficial for some patients, their adverse effect profile limited the overall impact of these first-generation agents. In 2013, simeprevir (SIM) was the next HCV NS3/4A protease inhibitor approved in combination with PEG-IFN/RBV.[29,33] The once-daily dosing schedule and improved safety profile, including the absence of anemia and rash, made it superior to the first 2 protease inhibitors, although SVR rates were similar.[34,35] However, the off-label use of SIM plus sofosbuvir (SOF) was the primary contribution of this agent to the HCV treatment landscape. In

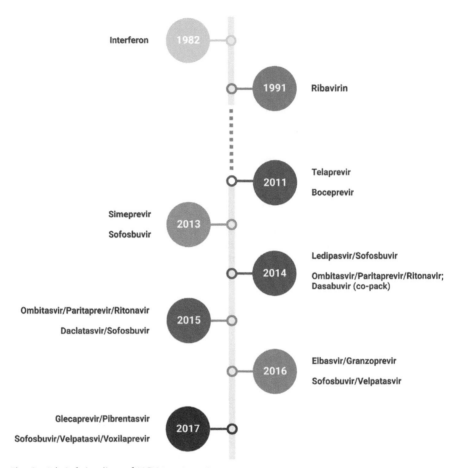

Fig. 2. A brief timeline of HCV treatments.

the phase 2 COSMOS trial, SIM plus the oral NS5B polymerase inhibitor SOF achieved high SVR rates in HCV genotype 1 infection (>90%). Based on the HCV guideline recommendations from the American Association for the Study of Liver Disease (AASLD) and the Infectious Diseases Society of America (IDSA) in 2014, SIM plus SOF was the first highly effective, IFN-free DAA regimen mainly used in patients who were ineligible for IFN.[36]

Sofosbuvir, a Nucleotide Analog Inhibitor of Hepatitis C Virus NS5B Polymerase

SOF acts as a defective substrate for the HCV NS5B RNA-dependent RNA polymerase, which is essential for HCV RNA transcription. In clinical trials, SOF demonstrated potent antiviral activity against all HCV genotypes with a high barrier to viral resistance and minimal adverse effects.[37,38] In 2013, the United States Food and Drug Administration (FDA) approved SOF in combination with RBV for HCV genotype 2 and 3 infections and with PEG-IFN/RBV for HCV genotype 1 infection. Although high SVR rates were observed with 12 weeks of SOF plus PEG-IFN/RBV (70%–80%), SOF also replaced PEG-IFN/RBV as the backbone of therapy with the NS3/4A protease inhibitor, SIM.[39] As discussed above, SIM, also approved in late 2013, enabled the off-label combination of SIM plus SOF to treat HCV genotype 1 infection.

NS5A Inhibitors

NS5A inhibitors exert antiviral activity by binding the NS5A NS protein, preventing RNA replication and virion assembly.[40,41] In 2015, the FDA approved the pan-genotypic NS5A inhibitor daclatasvir for use with SOF to treat HCV genotype 1 and 3 infections. This combination represented the first oral, highly effective DAA regimen for patients with genotype 3 infection, including those with cirrhosis with an excellent safety profile in patients with renal and hepatic impairments.[42–44] Ledipasvir (LED), which has antiviral activity against HCV genotypes 1 and 4, was also approved in 2015 as a once-daily single-tablet regimen, leading to SVR in more than 95% of patients treated for 12 weeks.[39] Similarly, the combination of grazoprevir, an NS3/4A protease inhibitor, plus elbasvir, an NS5A inhibitor, was highly effective for treating patients with HCV genotype 1 and 4 infections.[45] These high SVR rates, coupled with minimal side effects, led to substantial increases in HCV treatment rates in the United States and other regions beginning in 2015.

Pan-Genotypic Direct-Acting Antiviral Agent Regimens and Simplified Treatment Guidelines

In 2016 and 2017, the FDA approved 2 pan-genotypic DAA regimens with excellent safety, tolerability, and efficacy rates across diverse patient populations, launching the era of simplified HCV treatment.[46,47] SOF plus velpatasvir (VEL), a pan-genotypic NS5A inhibitor, was approved in 2016, taken as a single tablet once daily for 12 weeks for patients with HCV genotype 1 to 6 infections.[48] The combination of the pan-genotypic NS3/4A protease inhibitor glecaprevir (GLE) and NS5A inhibitor pibrentasvir (PIB) was approved in 2017, taken as 3 tablets once daily for 8 or 12 weeks for patients with HCV genotype 1 to 6 infections.[49] Both regimens, SOF/VEL and GLE/PIB, are well-tolerated, leading to SVR in most patients treated (97%–99%) including those with compensated cirrhosis. The availability of these highly effective, safe DAA regimens led the AASLD/IDSA guidelines panel to publish simplified HCV treatment recommendations with treatment-naive adults without cirrhosis, removing the need for assessing HCV genotype before treatment and for measuring laboratory tests during treatment (see **Fig. 1**).[36]

SPECIAL SUBGROUPS

With DAA regimens, most patient populations considered "difficult to treat" with IFN-based therapies achieved high SVR rates, including patients with compensated and decompensated cirrhosis and those with chronic kidney disease.[50]

Patients with decompensated cirrhosis

HCV treatment is prioritized for patients with cirrhosis since SVR decreases the incidence of complications of liver disease, including decompensation and HCC, in this population.[51,52] HCV treatment of decompensated liver disease (Child-Pugh B or C) is complicated by the inability to use HCV NS3/4A protease inhibitors such as GLE due to decreased liver metabolism and increased risk of liver injury. In the ASTRAL-4 trial, SOF/VEL was well tolerated in patients with decompensated cirrhosis, leading to an SVR rate of 78% to 100%, with higher rates in those treated with RBV.[52] In the SOLAR-1 and SOLAR-2 trials, 117 patients with Child-Pugh class B or C cirrhosis received SOF/LED plus RBV, achieving relatively high SVR rates.[53,54] Based on these and other trials, professional societies recommend using SOF/LED or VEL plus RBV to treat patients with decompensated liver disease.[55] Despite all this progress, finding the optimal treatment regimen for patients with decompensated cirrhosis may still be a challenge, and some experts recommend deferring HCV treatment until after LT.[56]

Patients with end-stage kidney disease

Patients with chronic kidney disease, particularly those requiring renal replacement therapy, were not treated with RBV due to the risk of severe hemolytic anemia. Hemodialysis patients are candidates for treatment with GLE/PIB, which includes drugs metabolized by the liver or SOF/VEL, which has been studied extensively in this population.[57–59] In clinical trials, both regimens were safe and effective, with SVR rates similar to other patient populations (98%).[58,59]

UNRESOLVED CHALLENGES

In the era of DAAs, resistant-associated substitution (RAS) and HCC during or after treatment have emerged as clinical concerns.[60] Although SVR is associated with improved survival and decreased HCC incidence, patients with cirrhosis before treatment remain at risk of HCC after achieving SVR.[61]

Resistant-Associated Substitutions and Treatment Failure

Virologic nonresponse following DAA treatment is relatively uncommon (1%–2%) in the setting of adherence and persistence to the recommended treatment course. Among those who do not achieve SVR, NS5A inhibitor RAS conferring decreased susceptibility to the drug class are typically present and persist. In contrast, NS5B inhibitor (SOF) RASs are uncommon, reflecting the high barrier to resistance with this agent.[62,63] For patients who do not respond to first-line treatment, retreatment with the 3-DAA combination of SOF/VEL plus the NS3/4A inhibitor voxilaprevir (VOX) leads to SVR in 96% of patients despite the presence of RASs.[64] As such, the number of patients adherent to therapy who fail to achieve SVR following first-line DAA treatment and rescue treatment with SOF/VEL/VOX is remarkably low. Expert guidelines recommend the treatment of these patients with a 24-week course of SOF plus GLE/PIB with or without RBV because more extended therapy and the inclusion of PIB may increase the likelihood of SVR.[50,65]

Hepatocellular Carcinoma

For patients with preexisting cirrhosis, SVR reduces but does not eliminate the risk of HCC.[66] In a recent study, SVR was associated with low rates of hepatic failure and complications of portal hypertension; HCC was the most frequent liver-related complication after HCV cure.[67] However, SVR reduces the risk of HCC in the medium to long term.[68] One study estimated the incidence of HCC to be 1.45/100 person-year follow in patients with cirrhosis and SVR with lower risk among those with bridging fibrosis (F3).[69] Among patients with cirrhosis, the HCC incidence is higher with advanced age, persistently elevated liver stiffness and alfa fetoprotein (AFP), and ongoing alcohol consumption.[61] For patients with cirrhosis who achieve SVR, expert guidelines recommend HCC surveillance with liver ultrasound with or without AFP to detect liver cancer early when the patient may be a candidate for curative treatments, such as tumor ablation/resection or LT.[70]

Hepatitis C as a Public Health Threat: Need for Global Elimination

In 2020, Harvey J. Alter, Michael Houghton, and Charles M. Rice received the Nobel prize for discovering the HCV that "made possible blood tests and new medicines that have saved millions of lives."[71] In 2016, the World Health Organization (WHO) set the goal of eliminating HCV as a public health threat by 2030, with a 65% reduction in HCV-related mortality and a 90% reduction in incident HCV infection. The WHO established targets required to achieve elimination: diagnosis of 90% of people with HCV and treatment of 80% of those infected, along with harm reduction to reduce the incidence of infection in persons at high risk, such as persons who inject drugs.[72] Many countries are not on track to achieve HCV elimination by 2030.[73] To realize the benefits of DAAs at the population level, substantial investments and large-scale screening and treatment implementation programs are needed.[74] Simplified HCV care models,[75] access to affordable DAAs,[76] and reducing stigma associated with HCV[77] are also crucial elements of elimination programs.

Hepatitis C Vaccine

Despite highly effective treatments, HCV elimination without an effective vaccine will be challenging.[78] Since its discovery in 1989, efforts to develop an effective HCV vaccine have fallen short.[3] In contrast, within 1 year of its emergence as a global pathogen, effective vaccines have been developed against SARS-CoV-2.[79] Several factors complicate the development of an HCV vaccine complex, including extensive viral heterogeneity.[62] HCV is also capable of evading the host immune response.[78] Yet, spontaneous clearance is observed in 25% to 50% of people with acute hepatitis C, giving rise to the expectation that an effective HCV vaccine is within reach with the commitment of adequate resources.[80]

DISCLOSURE

Authors declare no competing or conflicting interests.

FUNDING

Authors did not receive any financial support from any organization for this study.

REFERENCES

1. Basit H, Tyagi I, Koirala J. Hepatitis C. [Updated 2022 Nov 26]. In: StatPearls [Internet]. Treasure Island (FL): StatPearls Publishing; 2022. Available at: https://www.ncbi.nlm.nih.gov/books/NBK430897/. Accessed December 4, 2022.
2. Maasoumy B, Wedemeyer H. Natural history of acute and chronic hepatitis C. Best Pract Res Clin Gastroenterol 2012;26(4):401–12.
3. Alter HJ, Holland PV, Purcell RH, et al. Transmissible agent in non-a, non-b hepatitis. The Lancet 1978;311(8062):459–63.
4. Kumar A, Hossain RA, Yost SA, et al. Structural insights into hepatitis C virus receptor binding and entry. Nature 2021;598(7881):521–5.
5. Simmonds P. Genetic diversity and evolution of hepatitis C virus - 15 years on. J Gen Virol 2004;85(11):3173–88.
6. Petruzziello A, Marigliano S, Loquercio G, et al. Global epidemiology of hepatitis C virus infection: An up-date of the distribution and circulation of hepatitis C virus genotypes. World J Gastroenterol 2016;22(34):7824–40.
7. Bukh J. The history of hepatitis C virus (HCV): Basic research reveals unique features in phylogeny, evolution and the viral life cycle with new perspectives for epidemic control. J Hepatol 2016;65(1 Suppl):S2–21.
8. Lohmann V. Hepatitis C virus cell culture models: an encomium on basic research paving the road to therapy development. Med Microbiol Immunol (Berl) 2019; 208(1):3–24.

9. Grakoui A, Wychowski C, Lin C, et al. Expression and identification of hepatitis C virus polyprotein cleavage products. J Virol 1993;67(3):1385–95.
10. Bartenschlager R, Ahlborn-Laake L, Mous J, et al. Nonstructural protein 3 of the hepatitis C virus encodes a serine-type proteinase required for cleavage at the NS3/4 and NS4/5 junctions. J Virol 1993;67(7):3835–44.
11. Tomei L, Failla C, Santolini E, et al. NS3 is a serine protease required for processing of hepatitis C virus polyprotein. J Virol 1993;67(7):4017–26.
12. Ng V, Saab S. Effects of a Sustained Virologic Response on Outcomes of Patients With Chronic Hepatitis C. Clin Gastroenterol Hepatol 2011;9(11):923–30.
13. Senior JR. Post-transfusion hepatitis. Gastroenterology 1965;49(3):315–20.
14. Prince A, Grady G, Hazzi C, et al. Long-incubation post-transfusion hepatitis without serological evidence of exposure to hepatitis-b virus. The Lancet 1974; 304(7875):241–6.
15. Koziol DE, Holland PV, Alling DW, et al. Antibody to hepatitis B core antigen as a paradoxical marker for non-A, non-B hepatitis agents in donated blood. Ann Intern Med 1986;104(4):488–95.
16. Levin S, Hahn T. Interferon system in acute viral hepatitis. Lancet Lond Engl 1982; 1(8272):592–4.
17. Hoofnagle JH, Mullen KD, Jones DB, et al. Treatment of Chronic Non-A, Non-B Hepatitis with Recombinant Human Alpha Interferon. N Engl J Med 1986; 315(25):1575–8.
18. Der SD, Zhou A, Williams BRG, et al. Identification of genes differentially regulated by interferon α, β, or γ using oligonucleotide arrays. Proc Natl Acad Sci 1998;95(26):15623–8.
19. Guo JT, Sohn JA, Zhu Q, et al. Mechanism of the interferon alpha response against hepatitis C virus replicons. Virology 2004;325(1):71–81.
20. McHutchison JG, Gordon SC, Schiff ER, et al. Interferon alfa-2b alone or in combination with ribavirin as initial treatment for chronic hepatitis C. Hepatitis Interventional Therapy Group. N Engl J Med 1998;339(21):1485–92.
21. Reichard O, Andersson J, Schvarcz R, et al. Ribavirin treatment for chronic hepatitis C. The Lancet 1991;337(8749):1058–61.
22. Poynard T, Marcellin P, Lee SS, et al. Randomised trial of interferon alpha2b plus ribavirin for 48 weeks or for 24 weeks versus interferon alpha2b plus placebo for 48 weeks for treatment of chronic infection with hepatitis C virus. International Hepatitis Interventional Therapy Group (IHIT). Lancet Lond Engl 1998; 352(9138):1426–32.
23. Feld JJ, Hoofnagle JH. Mechanism of action of interferon and ribavirin in treatment of hepatitis C. Nature 2005;436(7053):967–72.
24. McHutchison JG, Manns M, Patel K, et al. Adherence to combination therapy enhances sustained response in genotype-1-infected patients with chronic hepatitis C. Gastroenterology 2002;123(4):1061–9.
25. Wills RJ, Dennis S, Spiegel HE, et al. Interferon kinetics and adverse reactions after intravenous, intramuscular, and subcutaneous injection. Clin Pharmacol Ther 1984;35(5):722–7.
26. Tosone G, Borgia G, Gentile I, et al. A case of pegylated interferon alpha-related diabetic ketoacidosis: can this complication be avoided? Acta Diabetol 2007; 44(3):167–9.
27. Hegade VS, Sood R, Saralaya D, et al. Pulmonary complications of treatment with pegylated interferon for hepatitis C infection-two case reports. Ann Hepatol 2013; 12(4):629–33.

28. Gentile I, Viola C, Reynaud L, et al. Hemolytic anemia during pegylated IFN-alpha2b plus ribavirin treatment for chronic hepatitis C: ribavirin is not always the culprit. J Interferon Cytokine Res Off J Int Soc Interferon Cytokine Res 2005;25(5):283–5.
29. Manns M, Marcellin P, Poordad F, et al. Simeprevir with pegylated interferon alfa 2a or 2b plus ribavirin in treatment-naive patients with chronic hepatitis C virus genotype 1 infection (QUEST-2): a randomised, double-blind, placebo-controlled phase 3 trial. Lancet Lond Engl 2014;384(9941):414–26.
30. Bacon BR, Gordon SC, Lawitz E, et al. Boceprevir for previously treated chronic HCV genotype 1 infection. N Engl J Med 2011;364(13):1207–17.
31. Jacobson IM, McHutchison JG, Dusheiko G, et al. Telaprevir for previously untreated chronic hepatitis C virus infection. N Engl J Med 2011;364(25):2405–16.
32. Ezat AA, Elshemey WM. A comparative study of the efficiency of HCV NS3/4A protease drugs against different HCV genotypes using in silico approaches. Life Sci 2019;217:176–84.
33. Jacobson IM, Dore GJ, Foster GR, et al. Simeprevir with pegylated interferon alfa 2a plus ribavirin in treatment-naive patients with chronic hepatitis C virus genotype 1 infection (QUEST-1): a phase 3, randomised, double-blind, placebo-controlled trial. Lancet Lond Engl 2014;384(9941):403–13.
34. Vaidya A, Perry CM. Simeprevir: first global approval. Drugs 2013;73(18):2093–106.
35. Reddy KR, Zeuzem S, Zoulim F, et al. Simeprevir versus telaprevir with peginterferon and ribavirin in previous null or partial responders with chronic hepatitis C virus genotype 1 infection (ATTAIN): a randomised, double-blind, non-inferiority phase 3 trial. Lancet Infect Dis 2015;15(1):27–35.
36. Lawitz E, Sulkowski MS, Ghalib R, et al. Simeprevir plus sofosbuvir, with or without ribavirin, to treat chronic infection with hepatitis C virus genotype 1 in non-responders to pegylated interferon and ribavirin and treatment-naive patients: the COSMOS randomised study. Lancet Lond Engl 2014;384(9956):1756–65.
37. Soriano V, Vispo E, de Mendoza C, et al. Hepatitis C therapy with HCV NS5B polymerase inhibitors. Expert Opin Pharmacother 2013;14(9):1161–70.
38. Bhatia HK, Singh H, Grewal N, et al. Sofosbuvir: A novel treatment option for chronic hepatitis C infection. J Pharmacol Pharmacother 2014;5(4):278–84.
39. Abraham GM, Spooner LM. Sofosbuvir in the treatment of chronic hepatitis C: new dog, new tricks. Clin Infect Dis Off Publ Infect Dis Soc Am 2014;59(3):411–5.
40. Gao M, Nettles RE, Belema M, et al. Chemical genetics strategy identifies an HCV NS5A inhibitor with a potent clinical effect. Nature 2010;465(7294):96–100.
41. Gitto S, Gamal N, Andreone P. NS5A inhibitors for the treatment of hepatitis C infection. J Viral Hepat 2017;24(3):180–6.
42. Pawlotsky JM. NS5A inhibitors in the treatment of hepatitis C. J Hepatol 2013;59(2):375–82.
43. Lee C. Discovery of hepatitis C virus NS5A inhibitors as a new class of anti-HCV therapy. Arch Pharm Res 2011;34(9):1403–7.
44. Nelson DR, Cooper JN, Lalezari JP, et al. All-oral 12-week treatment with daclatasvir plus sofosbuvir in patients with hepatitis C virus genotype 3 infection: ALLY-3 phase III study. Hepatol Baltim Md 2015;61(4):1127–35.
45. Gane EJ, Pianko S, Roberts SK, et al. Safety and efficacy of an 8-week regimen of grazoprevir plus ruzasvir plus uprifosbuvir compared with grazoprevir plus elbasvir plus uprifosbuvir in participants without Cirrhosis infected with hepatitis C virus genotypes 1, 2, or 3 (C-CREST-1 and C-CREST-2, part A): two randomised, phase 2, open-label trials. Lancet Gastroenterol Hepatol 2017;2(11):805–13.

46. Rodríguez-Torres M. Sofosbuvir (GS-7977), a pan-genotype, direct-acting anti-viral for hepatitis C virus infection. Expert Rev Anti Infect Ther 2013;11(12):1269–79.
47. Hézode C. Pan-genotypic treatment regimens for hepatitis C virus: Advantages and disadvantages in high- and low-income regions. J Viral Hepat 2017;24(2):92–101.
48. Feld JJ, Jacobson IM, Hézode C, et al. Sofosbuvir and Velpatasvir for HCV Genotype 1, 2, 4, 5, and 6 Infection. N Engl J Med 2015;373(27):2599–607.
49. Puoti M, Foster GR, Wang S, et al. High SVR12 with 8-week and 12-week glecaprevir/pibrentasvir therapy: An integrated analysis of HCV genotype 1-6 patients without Cirrhosis. J Hepatol 2018;69(2):293–300.
50. Manns MP, Maasoumy B. Breakthroughs in hepatitis C research: from discovery to cure. Nat Rev Gastroenterol Hepatol 2022;19(8):533–50.
51. Rincon D, Ripoll C, Iacono OL, et al. Antiviral Therapy Decreases Hepatic Venous Pressure Gradient in Patients with Chronic Hepatitis C and Advanced Fibrosis. Off J Am Coll Gastroenterol ACG 2006;101(10):2269–74.
52. Curry MP, O'Leary JG, Bzowej N, et al. Sofosbuvir and Velpatasvir for HCV in Patients with Decompensated Cirrhosis. N Engl J Med 2015;373(27):2618–28.
53. Charlton M, Everson GT, Flamm SL, et al. Ledipasvir and Sofosbuvir Plus Ribavirin for Treatment of HCV Infection in Patients With Advanced Liver Disease. Gastroenterology 2015;149(3):649–59.
54. Manns M, Samuel D, Gane EJ, et al. Ledipasvir and sofosbuvir plus ribavirin in patients with genotype 1 or 4 hepatitis C virus infection and advanced liver disease: a multicentre, open-label, randomised, phase 2 trial. Lancet Infect Dis 2016;16(6):685–97.
55. Pawlotsky JM, Negro F, Aghemo A, et al. EASL recommendations on treatment of hepatitis C: Final update of the series. J Hepatol 2020;73(5):1170–218.
56. Navasa M, Forns X. Antiviral therapy in HCV decompensated Cirrhosis: to treat or not to treat? J Hepatol 2007;46(2):185–8.
57. Bruchfeld A. HCV eradication in chronic kidney disease: ready for prime time? Lancet Gastroenterol Hepatol 2020;5(10):880–2.
58. Gane E, Lawitz E, Pugatch D, et al. Glecaprevir and Pibrentasvir in Patients with HCV and Severe Renal Impairment. N Engl J Med 2017;377(15):1448–55.
59. Borgia SM, Dearden J, Yoshida EM, et al. Sofosbuvir/velpatasvir for 12 weeks in hepatitis C virus-infected patients with end-stage renal disease undergoing dialysis. J Hepatol 2019;71(4):660–5.
60. Dietz J, Müllhaupt B, Buggisch P, et al. Long-term persistence of HCV resistance-associated substitutions after DAA treatment failure. J Hepatol 2022;S0168-8278(22):03016–21.
61. Semmler G, Meyer EL, Kozbial K, et al. HCC risk stratification after cure of hepatitis C in patients with compensated advanced chronic liver disease. J Hepatol 2022;76(4):812–21.
62. Abdelrahman T, Hughes J, Main J, et al. Next-generation sequencing sheds light on the natural history of hepatitis C infection in patients who fail treatment. Hepatol Baltim Md 2015;61(1):88–97.
63. Dietz J, Susser S, Vermehren J, et al. Patterns of Resistance-Associated Substitutions in Patients With Chronic HCV Infection Following Treatment With Direct-Acting Antivirals. Gastroenterology 2018;154(4):976–88, e4.
64. Bourlière M, Gordon SC, Flamm SL, et al. Sofosbuvir, Velpatasvir, and Voxilaprevir for Previously Treated HCV Infection. N Engl J Med 2017;376(22):2134–46.

65. Reau N, Kwo PY, Rhee S, et al. Glecaprevir/Pibrentasvir Treatment in Liver or Kidney Transplant Patients With Hepatitis C Virus Infection. Hepatol Baltim Md 2018; 68(4):1298–307.
66. De Mitri MS, Poussin K, Baccarini P, et al. HCV-associated liver cancer without Cirrhosis. Lancet Lond Engl 1995;345(8947):413–5.
67. D'Ambrosio R, Degasperi E, Anolli MP, et al. Incidence of liver- and non-liver-related outcomes in patients with HCV-cirrhosis after SVR. J Hepatol 2022; 76(2):302–10.
68. Piscaglia F, Granito A, Bolondi L. DAAs for HCV and risk of hepatocellular carcinoma: current standpoint. Lancet Gastroenterol Hepatol 2018;3(11):736–8.
69. Sanduzzi-Zamparelli M, Mariño Z, Lens S, et al. Liver cancer risk after HCV cure in patients with advanced liver disease without non-characterized nodules. J Hepatol 2022;76(4):874–82.
70. Mueller PP, Chen Q, Ayer T, et al. Duration and cost-effectiveness of hepatocellular carcinoma surveillance in hepatitis C patients after viral eradication. J Hepatol 2022;77(1):55–62.
71. Ward JW. The Nobel Prize for discovery of HCV is a call to end hepatitis. Lancet Lond Engl 2020;396(10264):1733.
72. World Health Organization. Combating hepatitis B and C to reach elimination by 2030: advocacy brief. World Health Organization; 2016. Available at: https://apps.who.int/iris/handle/10665/206453. Accessed November 17, 2022.
73. Polaris Observatory HCV Collaborators. Global change in hepatitis C virus prevalence and cascade of care between 2015 and 2020: a modelling study. Lancet Gastroenterol Hepatol 2022;7(5):396–415.
74. Wiktor S. How feasible is the global elimination of HCV infection? Lancet Lond Engl 2019;393(10178):1265–7.
75. Marshall AD, Matthews GV. Simplifying hepatitis C care models: a crucial step towards hepatitis C elimination. Lancet Gastroenterol Hepatol 2022;7(12):1066–8.
76. The Lancet Gastroenterology Hepatology null. Drug pricing: still a barrier to elimination of HCV. Lancet Gastroenterol Hepatol 2018;3(12):813.
77. Buti M, Craxi A, Foster GR, et al. Viral hepatitis elimination: Towards a hepatitis-free world. J Hepatol 2022;77(5):1444–7.
78. Neumann-Haefelin C, Thimme R. Another important step toward a prophylactic vaccine against hepatitis C. Hepatol Baltim Md 2022;76(4):917–9.
79. El Sahly HM, Baden LR, Essink B, et al. Efficacy of the mRNA-1273 SARS-CoV-2 Vaccine at Completion of Blinded Phase. N Engl J Med 2021;385(19):1774–85.
80. Donnison T, McGregor J, Chinnakannan S, et al. A pan-genotype hepatitis C virus viral vector vaccine generates T cells and neutralizing antibodies in mice. Hepatol Baltim Md 2022;76(4):1190–202.

Chronic Hepatitis B Virus: What an Internist Needs to Know

Serologic Diagnosis, Treatment Options, and Hepatitis B Virus Reactivation

Peter D. Block, MD[a], Joseph K. Lim, MD[b],*

KEYWORDS

- Hepatitis B • Epidemiology • Diagnosis • Treatment • Drug therapy • Reactivation

KEY POINTS

- Chronic hepatitis B infection remains a global public health burden associated with significant morbidity and mortality due to cirrhosis and hepatocellular carcinoma.
- Patients with chronic hepatitis B require regular laboratory monitoring and screening for liver cancer based on the assessment of individual risk.
- Antiviral therapy with oral nucleos(t)ide analogs or pegylated interferon is indicated in patients with immunoactive disease based on HBeAg status, hepatitis B virus (HBV) DNA, serum ALT, and stage of liver fibrosis.
- Current therapies are not associated with the virologic cure but are aimed at virologic suppression, which is associated with a decreased risk for cirrhosis, liver failure, hepatocellular carcinoma, and liver-related mortality.
- HBV reactivation may occur in hepatitis B surface antigen (HBsAg) positive or HBsAg negative/HBcAb positive individuals (with or without anti-HBsAb) in the context of immunosuppressive drug therapy and may be associated with hepatitis flare and liver failure.

INTRODUCTION

Hepatitis B virus (HBV) remains a challenge for primary care providers on a global scale. Current estimates place the worldwide prevalence of chronic HBV infection (CHB) approximately 292 million individuals.[1] Among those living with HBV, 15% to 40% may develop HBV-related complications including cirrhosis, liver failure, and hepatocellular carcinoma (HCC).[2] (**Figs. 1 and 2**)

[a] Section of Digestive Diseases, Yale School of Medicine, New Haven, CT, USA; [b] Section of Digestive Diseases and Yale Liver Center, Yale School of Medicine, 333 Cedar Street, LMP 1080, New Haven, CT 06520, USA
* Corresponding author.
E-mail address: joseph.lim@yale.edu

Med Clin N Am 107 (2023) 435–447
https://doi.org/10.1016/j.mcna.2022.12.002
0025-7125/23/© 2022 Elsevier Inc. All rights reserved.

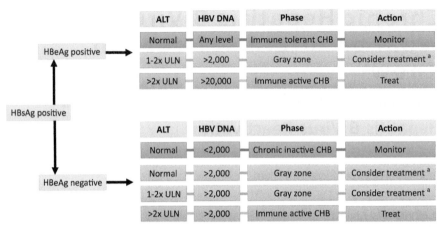

Fig. 1. Approach to treatment of chronic hepatitis B infection. Chronic infection is established by persistently positive HBsAg, then stratified by the presence or absence of HBeAg. The decision to start antiviral therapy is then determined by mainly by the ALT level, HBV DNA level, and degree of liver fibrosis. If patients fall within a "gray zone" for treatment, then other patient factors are weighed in the decision process. ^aTreat if advanced fibrosis or cirrhosis is present. Consider treatment if >40 years old, family history of HCC, or abnormal ALT without alternate cause.

Despite the availability of effective vaccines and antiviral therapies, an inadequate cascade of care has limited efforts by the health care community to detect, monitor, and treat those with HBV. In the United States, only 15% of the nearly 1 million individuals with CHB are aware of their infection, and only 4.5% are receiving antiviral

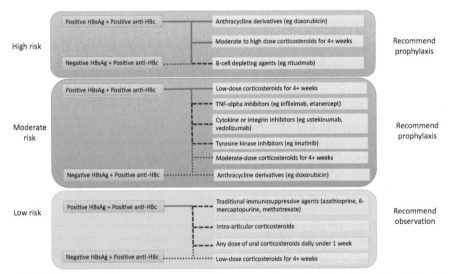

Fig. 2. Risk stratification to guide prevention management of HBV reactivation. Patients' risk of HBV reactivation is determined by their serology, namely HBsAg and anti-HBC, and the type of immunosuppression. Patients stratified into a moderate or high-risk group are recommended to receive antiviral prophylaxis. Low-risk patients can be observed with surveillance lab work to monitor for HBV reactivation.

therapy.[3] Gaps in care are attributable to both patient and provider factors. Patient-related barriers include a confluence of social, economic, cultural, and educational factors.[4–6] On the other hand, surveys of both primary care providers and subspecialty clinicians have consistently illustrated gaps in the knowledge and application of guideline recommendations for HBV management.[7–12]

This article provides a concise review of the fundamentals of CHB management with the purpose to serve as a touchstone for primary care clinicians overseeing the care of patients with CHB in their clinic.

DIAGNOSIS AND CLINICAL EVALUATION

Diagnosis of HBV infection is based on the interpretation of multiple viral antigens and antibodies. These markers can indicate the presence of acute, chronic, or past infection with or without protective immunity. Important HBV blood tests and interpretation of common serological patterns are outlined in **Tables 1** and **2**.

Chronic hepatitis B infection (CHB) is defined by the presence of Hepatitis B surface antigen (HBsAg) over 6 months. Loss of HBsAg with or without the development of antibodies against HBsAg (anti-HBs) is termed seroclearance and is considered a functional cure.[13–15] Protective immunity is regarded as anti-HBs levels >10 IU/mL.[16]

If CHB is established, a comprehensive assessment of the patients' history, exam, serological data, and radiographic imaging should be collated to determine the phase of HBV infection, degree of underlying liver fibrosis, and presence of co-existing causes of chronic liver disease. This includes assessing patients' alcohol use, the

Table 1
Overview of hepatitis B virus tests

HBV Tests	Clinical Relevance
HBsAg	Primary marker for infection. Positive HBsAg over 6 months defines chronic HBV
Anti-HBs	Defines immunity against HBV. Antibody levels above 10 IU/mL is protective
HBeAg	Marker of viral replication and infectivity in CHB
Anti-HBe	Loss of HBeAg and gain of anti-HBe is termed "seroconversion". Seroconversion after age 40 is associated with increased risk of HCC, whereas seroconversion before age 30 is a good prognostic sign
Anti-HBc IgM	Marker of acute infection. May be present before other viral markers are detected
Anti-HBc (total or IgG)	Indicates an active or past infection. Other viral markers (eg, HBsAg, anti-HBs, and HBV DNA) are needed to interpret anti-HBc IgG
HBV DNA	Important in determining phase of infection and carries prognostic value. Higher DNA levels are associated with a higher risk of developing cirrhosis or HCC
ALT	Used to determine the presence of hepatic necroinflammation in CHB. Elevations of ALT above ULN signify a proportionally elevated level of inflammation within the liver

Summary of clinically relevant blood tests for diagnosis, evaluation, prognostication, and management of hepatitis B.

Abbreviations: Anti-HBc, IgG or all antibodies against hepatitis B core antigen; anti-HBc IgM, IgM antibodies against hepatitis B core antigen; anti-HBe, antibody against HBeAg; anti-HBs, antibody against HBsAg; HBeAg, hepatitis e antigen; HBsAg, hepatitis B surface antigen; HCC, hepatocellular carcinoma; ULN, upper limit of normal.

Table 2
Summary of hepatitis B virus serological patterns commonly encountered in screening for hepatitis B virus

HBsAg	Anti-HBc	Anti-HBs	Interpretation
–	+	–	Chronic hepatitis B
–	+	+	Past infection, now immune. Risk of reactivation if immunocompromised
–	+	–	Past infection, occult HBV infection, or false positive test. Risk of reactivation if immunocompromised
–	–	+	Immune from vaccination
–	–	–	Naïve to HBV (not immune, not exposed). Susceptible to infection

Abbreviations: anti-HBc, HBV core antibody; anti-HBs, HBV surface antibody; HBsAg, HBV surface antigen.

presence of metabolic risk factors (obesity, diabetes), and family history of HCC. Co-existing infections, including hepatitis A virus (HAV), human immunodeficiency virus (HIV), hepatitis C virus (HCV), and hepatitis D virus (HDV) should be evaluated. Immunization for HAV should also be provided for patients who do not show immunity.

Notably, laboratory values at a single time point are unreliable in characterizing a patient's disease status given the inherently variable clinical course of CHB. Regular monitoring of HBV DNA and liver enzymes is therefore of paramount importance to determine a patients' phase of infection and guide the potential initiation of antiviral therapy. Determining the degree of underlying hepatic inflammation and liver fibrosis will also inform the decision to treat patients with anti-viral therapy, and requires either liver biopsy or noninvasive fibrosis testing.

ASSESSMENT OF FIBROSIS

Assessment of liver fibrosis is an important step in the evaluation of those with CHB. The gold standard diagnostic intervention to assess for fibrosis is liver biopsy.[17,18] However, its use in routine clinical practice is limited given the inherent invasiveness and potentially severe complications associated with the technique.[18] Noninvasive tools to assess liver fibrosis have become increasingly used within clinical practice. These tools include both novel imaging modalities and serum assays.

Imaging tests to assess fibrosis include transient elastography (TE), shear wave elastography (SWE), and magnetic resonance elastography (MRE). TE and SWE are ultrasound-based techniques in which a probe transmits a wave through the liver parenchyma to quantify liver stiffness in kPa units, termed "liver stiffness measurement (LSM)".[19] The LSM is used to determine the presence of severe fibrosis, cirrhosis, or normal liver parenchyma.[20] In those with CHB, an LSM of 11.0 kPa or above is the recommended cutoff to diagnose cirrhosis.[21] Perhaps the most common example is FibroScan, which is a commercially available type of transient elastography.[19]

Serum-based tools include the aspartate aminotransferase (AST)-to-platelet ratio index (APRI), Fibrosis-4 test (FIB-4), as well as biochemical markers that predict the degree of hepatic fibrosis.[22] One of the most commonly used serum biomarker tests is the FibroTest.[22] Finally, some studies have suggested that using both elastography and serum biomarker tests in patients can improve the accuracy of fibrosis assessment, decreasing the potential need for liver biopsy.

NATURAL HISTORY OF INFECTION

The natural history of HBV infection reflects the dynamic interplay between host and viral factors, carrying clinical consequences in the management of CHB. Although those exposed to HBV in adulthood will often spontaneously eliminate the virus from serological detection, most infections occur perinatally and result in CHB.

In those with CHB, four phases of infection have been described and are defined with similar terms across the major hepatology professional societies.[13–15,23] Determining a patient's phase of infection sheds insight on the patient's disease status and guides treatment decisions.

The four phases of CHB include an immune tolerant phase, an immune active phase with positive HBeAg, an inactive carrier state, and an immune (re)activated phase with negative HBeAg.[23] Although typically sequential, the duration of each phase can vary between patients. Moreover, patients may not pass through all four phases during their course of infection. In turn, characterizing a patient's phase of infection requires serial monitoring of patients' virological markers and liver chemistries. These phases are outlined in **Table 3**.

SCREENING

Initial screening for HBV should include an assessment of HBsAg, anti-HBc, and anti-HBs. According to the US Preventive Services Task Force (USPSTF) 2020 guidelines, screening for HBV should include HBsAg testing in all high-risk populations. This includes all persons from endemic countries (HBsAg seroprevalence of 2% or greater), pregnant women, men who have sex with men, persons with a history of intravenous drug use, and those with end-stage renal disease.[24] However, the CDC published new draft guidance in April 2022 which recommends universal screening of all US adults age 18 or older with one-time serologic testing of HBsAg, anti-HBc, and anti-HBs, and is expected to be implemented in 2023.[25]

TREATMENT

In the United States, treatment of CHB includes two broad categories: nucleoside/nucleotide analogs (NAs) and interferon (IFN) therapy. NAs are well tolerated, effective, and carry an excellent safety profile.[26] IFN therapy has more side effects and is less well tolerated than NAs, but has the advantage of a time-limited treatment course. Guidelines are in general agreement that entecavir, tenofovir, or pegylated IFN should be used as initial therapy for CHB.[14,15,23]

CHB cannot be cured with currently available antiviral therapies. The viral template that establishes chronic infection, covalently closed circular DNA (cccDNA), can persist within hepatocytes irrespective of therapy, thereby posing a lifelong risk of HBV-related complications. Nevertheless, antiviral therapies are effective at suppressing viral replication to undetectable HBV DNA levels in greater than 90% of patients, which in turn is associated with a decreased risk of cirrhosis, hepatic decompensation, and hepatocellular carcinoma, and a decrease in liver-related mortality.[27]

Once therapy is started, regular monitoring of patients' HBV DNA, viral serology, and ALT should be performed to track the response to therapy. Although the overall side effect profile for NAs is excellent, rare side effects have been identified. All NAs carry an FDA black box warning of lactic acidosis, though this is a rare adverse event.[26] Tenofovir disoproxil fumarate (TDF) has also been associated with acute and chronic kidney injury, as well as reduced bone density, though the overall incidence of TDF-associated renal or bone dysfunction is low.[26] Moreover, renal and

Table 3
Phases of chronic hepatitis B virus infection

	Immune Tolerant	Immune Active–HBeAg Positive	Inactive	Immune Active–HBeAg Negative
HBsAg	High	High/intermediate	Low	Negative
HBeAg	Positive	Positive	Negative	Negative
HBV DNA	High (>106 IU/mL)	104 to 107 IU/mL)	<2000 IU/mL	<2000 IU/mL
ALT	Normal	Elevated	Normal	Elevated
Histology	Normal	Inflammation	Minimal inflammation	Moderate/severe inflammation
Clinical characteristics	Typically seen in children and young adults infected perinatally	ALT fluctuates, representing flares of immune-mediated inflammation	HBeAg seroconversion occurs in this phase. Seroconversion >40 years old is associated with higher HCC risk	Variable ALT and DNA. Older population and higher rate of cirrhosis

Serological patterns, typical histology on liver biopsy, and characteristic clinical features are highlighted.

bone side effects are rare with the newest formulation of tenofovir, and tenofovir ala-fenamide (TAF).[23]

INDICATIONS FOR TREATMENT

There are two main indications for the treatment of CHB. First, treatment is indicated for those with immuneactive CHB. This is defined as an ALT >2 ULN plus HBV DNA >20,000 IU/mL (HBeAg positive) or >2000 IU/mL (HBeAg negative). The second indication is in those with CHB and underlying cirrhosis. In patients with decompensated cirrhosis, antiviral therapy should be started irrespective of ALT level or HBV DNA level, as antiviral therapy has been shown to improve liver function and liver-related mortality.[28] In patients with compensated cirrhosis, all patients with detectable HBV DNA should be treated with antivirals, irrespective of ALT level.[23] IFN therapy is contraindicated in patients with decompensated cirrhosis due to the risk of hepatotoxicity and hepatic decompensation.[23] Thus, NAs are the agents of choice in patients with HBV-related cirrhosis.

INDICATIONS FOR OBSERVATION

In those with immune-tolerant CHB or chronic inactive CHB, observation is generally recommended over treatment. Immune-tolerant CHB is defined as normal ALT (<35 U/L in males, <25 U/L in females) with high HBV DNA levels (>10^6 IU/mL). Similarly, chronic inactive CHB is defined as normal ALT levels with low-level viremia (HBV DNA <2000 IU/mL) and negative HBeAg. This recommendation is based on prior studies which have not shown a reduction in liver-related complications in patients with immune-tolerant CHB treated with antivirals.[13] In turn, the potential harms of prolonged antiviral therapy (eg, side effects, cost, development of viral resistance) are considered to outweigh potential benefits by society guidelines.[13–15] Thus, regular monitoring of serum ALT and HBV DNA is recommended at 6-month intervals to monitor for transition to the immune active phase, at which time antiviral therapy would be indicated.[13]

GRAY AREAS FOR TREATMENT

Patients commonly are observed to have ALT and HBV DNA profiles that do not neatly fall within established phases of infection to determine treatment eligibility. This includes two common scenarios, such as the patient with borderline elevated HBV DNA (2000 to 20,000 IU/mL) and ALT (1 to 2x ULN but not 2x ULN, defined as <70 U/L for men, <50 U/L for women) and the patient with very high HBV DNA (>1,000,000 IU/mL) but persistently normal ALT (defined as <35 U/L for men, <25 U/L for women). In these cases, it is important to weigh other risk factors in determining whether to initiate treatment or actively monitor, including the presence of significant fibrosis (F2 fibrosis or greater on biopsy or noninvasive testing), older age (>40 years old), genotype C HBV, or family history of HCC.[13] The presence of any of one of these risk factors could strengthen consideration to initiate treatment. Indeed, the AASLD recommends that treatment be considered in older age individuals (>40 years old) with normal ALT, high HBV DNA levels (>1,000,000 IU/mL), and liver biopsy with moderate-to-severe necroinflammation or fibrosis.[23]

DURATION OF THERAPY

Treatment duration with NAs is typically considered "long-term," as such medications do not eliminate cccDNA or viral DNA integrated into host genomes. Long-term NA therapy is generally well-tolerated given the excellent safety profile, high threshold for drug resistance, and strong long-term efficacy in suppressing HBV DNA replication.[26] On the other hand, indefinite therapy is challenging for patients to sustain, exposes patients to rare side effects, may be associated with financial burden due to specialty prescription drugs, and uncommonly may result in drug resistance due to treatment interruptions and nonadherence.[13]

Cessation of therapy can therefore be considered in select patient populations without cirrhosis who achieve HBeAg seroconversion (among patients with HBeAg positive infection at baseline), which occurs in approximately 20% to 40% of patients within 5 years of NA therapy, and/or HBsAg loss, which occurs in fewer than 5% of patients within 5 years of NA therapy.[23] In those who may qualify for treatment cessation, the potential risks should be discussed frankly with the patient. These risks include virological reactivation, hepatic decompensation, and death. If discontinuation of anti-viral therapy is planned, then it is recommended that treatment be continued for an additional 6 to 12 months after the above criteria are met.[13] This period of "consolidation therapy" has been shown to decrease the likelihood of virological relapse once therapy is stopped.[29] Following consolidation therapy, patients' lab work (eg HBV DNA and ALT levels) should be monitored regularly during the first 12 months off therapy to assess for viral recurrence and hepatitis flares.[13]

COMPLICATIONS OF CHRONIC HEPATITIS B VIRUS INFECTION

The two major liver-related complications related to CHB are cirrhosis and HCC. The risk of developing these complications is influenced by viral, host, and environmental factors. The most important viral determinants for progression to cirrhosis are HBV DNA level, ALT, and HBeAg status. Similarly, viral and host factors most strongly associated with the onset of HBV-related HCC include the presence of cirrhosis, HBV DNA level, HBeAg status, genotype, HDV coinfection, and family history of HCC. Of note, unlike other etiologies of chronic liver disease, HBV-associated HCC can develop at any stage of liver fibrosis and does not require advanced fibrosis/cirrhosis.

HEPATOCELLULAR CARCINOMA MONITORING

CHB is a major cause of HCC, accounting for the majority of cases worldwide. The oncogenic nature of the virus is reflected in its ability to lead to HCC even in the absence of cirrhosis, although the presence of cirrhosis significantly raises the risk of HCC in those with CHB.[30] High levels of HBV DNA have also been linked to a higher likelihood of HCC.[31] Suppression of viral replication with antiviral therapy reduces but does not eliminate, the risk of HCC.[32]

For these reasons, surveillance for HCC with an abdominal ultrasound every 6 months is recommended in those with CHB and additional risk factors. Measurement of AFP alone is insufficient for HCC surveillance but can be used as an adjunct surveillance test with ultrasound. Screening should be done whether or not patients are receiving antiviral therapy.

All patients with CHB and cirrhosis should be screened for HCC every 6 months. In those without cirrhosis, high-risk groups in whom twice annual HCC surveillance should be performed: black men or women > age 20 years, Asian men > age 40 years, Asian women >50 years old, family history of HCC, or HDV coinfection.[23,33–36]

REACTIVATION OF HEPATITIS B VIRUS

HBV reactivation (HBVr) is defined as the re-emergence of infection in those with previously resolved HBV infection or chronically inactive CHB.[37] The key pathophysiological factors are cccDNA and host immune suppression, where cccDNA serves as a reservoir for rapid viral propagation in an immunocompromised host.[38]

HBVr has three different clinical phenotypes.[38] In the first phenotypic presentation, HBVr can be a silent event in which HBV DNA rises without aberrations in liver tests. Alternatively, HBVr can manifest with acute hepatitis illustrated by abnormal liver tests. Finally, HBVr can present with fulminant liver failure, represented by elevated HBV DNA in the setting of acute encephalopathy and hepatic synthetic dysfunction.

Initiation of immunosuppressive or immunomodulatory therapy is the main risk factor for HBVr.[39] The type of immunosuppressive regimen and serological pattern of HBV both influence the risk of reactivation. Reactivation rates have been reported as high as 41% to 53% in patients receiving anti-neoplastic therapies with positive anti-HBc and positive HBsAg levels.[40] Reactivation also occurs in those with positive anti-HBc and negative HBsAg levels, though at lower rates of occurrence (8%–18%).[41]

Although historical data have shown the risk of HBVr with conventional chemotherapies and immunosuppressive medications (eg, B-cell depleting agents), emerging evidence indicates that varying degrees of risk are also present with newer classes of both immunosuppressive and immunomodulatory therapies. Whereas antiviral prophylaxis is not recommended for patients undergoing therapies associated with low HBVr risk (tyrosine kinase inhibitors, T-cell depleting agents, and immune checkpoint inhibitors), antiviral therapy may be considered for patients undergoing treatment associated with high (B-cell depleting therapies, Janus kinase inhibitors) or intermediate HBV risk (cytokine inhibitors, CAR-T cell immunotherapy, and calcineurin inhibitors).[42]

HBVr can be prevented by screening those about to receive immunosuppression, stratifying their risk of reactivation, and then tailoring management based on their risk. In terms of screening, HBsAg and anti-HBc levels should be obtained. If either test is positive, then HBV DNA should be measured to establish a baseline level. Guidelines vary on whether anti-HBs should be included in HBVr screening, as data are limited on its clinical utility in risk stratification of HBV.[14,15,23,37,43] Whether anti-HBs influence the clinical severity of viral reactivation or if quantitatively high levels of anti-HBs lower the risk of HBVr are two scenarios without evidence-based answers.[37] Importantly, HBVr can still occur in those with positive anti-HBs level, where reactivation occurs at an estimated rate of 4.3% in those with positive levels of anti-HBc and anti-HBs.[37] Thus, checking HBsAg and anti-HBc with or without anti-HBs are the consensus serological tests that should be obtained for HBVr screening purposes.

HBV testing is recommended before initiation of immunosuppressive therapy,[14,15] although clinical practice patterns to date suggest low rates of adherence.[38,39,44] If screening tests are positive, then patients should be stratified based on their serological HBV pattern and immunosuppressive regimen. The AGA HBVr guideline categorizes patients into three risk groups: high (>10%), moderate (1%–10%), and low risk (<1%) for HBVr.[37] Determining a patients' risk category will guide their HBV management plan while on immunosuppression.

If patients fall within the high-risk group, then they should receive antiviral prophylaxis.[37] Similarly, patients with moderate risk of HBVr are recommended to receive antiviral prophylaxis, although active monitoring off therapy is an alternative option if the patient prefers avoiding antiviral medications.[37] Low-risk patients do not typically need antiviral prophylaxis, but should be monitored with interval blood work with antiviral therapy available "on-demand" if HBVr is identified.[37] Tenofovir or entecavir are first-line agents for antiviral prophylaxis, as prior studies have shown that these medications result in a decreased incidence of HBVr, hepatitis flares, and mortality in comparison to prophylaxis with lamivudine.[23]

Antiviral prophylaxis should be started before initiation of immunosuppressive therapy when possible, but chemotherapy should not be delayed. This treatment should be continued throughout the duration of immunosuppressive therapy and then continued for an additional 6 to 12 months after the immunosuppressive regimen is completed.[37] Routine blood work should be obtained to monitor for HBVr (HBV DNA, liver tests) in patients receiving immunosuppressive therapy, preferably every 1 to 3 months, and for an additional 12 months after cessation of immunosuppressive therapy.[23]

SUMMARY

Although HBV infection remains a public health challenge worldwide, there are effective tools available to the primary care provider to mitigate its impact. This includes an armory of serological and radiographic tools to screen, stage, and prognosticate infection. Oral medications that are well-tolerated and reduce the risk of HBV-related complications are also available for the treatment of chronic infection, as well as evidence-based guidelines that can provide insights into the nuanced management of CHB. However, effective and appropriate employment of these tools can be daunting, especially given the often silent, yet pernicious and complex, course of chronic infection. This review article has provided a concise overview of CHB management to serve as a resource for the primary care provider to guide decision-making through the complex care cascade faced by patients and providers.

CLINICS CARE POINTS

- Chronic hepatitis B infection remains a global public health burden associated with significant morbidity and mortality due to cirrhosis and hepatocellular carcinoma
- Chronic hepatitis B infection is defined by positive hepatitis B surface antigen (HBsAg) and/or positive hepatitis B virus (HBV) DNA of 6 months duration or longer
- Patients with chronic hepatitis B require regular laboratory monitoring and screening for liver cancer based on the assessment of individual risk
- Antiviral therapy with oral nucleos(t)ide analogs or pegylated interferon is indicated in patients with immunoactive disease based on HBeAg status, HBV DNA, serum ALT, and stage of liver fibrosis
- Current therapies are not associated with the virologic cure but are aimed at virologic suppression, which is associated with a decreased risk for cirrhosis, liver failure, hepatocellular carcinoma, and liver-related mortality
- HBV reactivation may occur in HBsAg positive or HBsAg negative/HBcAb positive individuals (with or without anti-HBsAb) in the context of immunosuppressive drug therapy, and may be associated with hepatitis flare and liver failure
- Antiviral prophylaxis may be indicated in patients identified as moderate or high risk of HBV reactivation based on HBsAg/HBcAb status and immunosuppressive drug class

---

DISCLOSURE

P.D. Block reports no disclosures. J.K. Lim reports research contracts (to institution) from: Allergan, Celgene, Eiger, Gilead, Intercept, Pfizer, Viking.

REFERENCES

1. Polaris Observatory Collaborators. Global prevalence, treatment, and prevention of hepatitis B virus infection in 2016: a modelling study. Lancet Gastroenterol Hepatol 2018;3(6):383–403.
2. Lok ASF, McMahon BJ. Chronic hepatitis B. Hepatology 2007;45(2):507–39.
3. Le MH, Yeo YH, Cheung R, et al. Chronic hepatitis B prevalence among foreign-born and U.S.-born adults in the United States, 1999-2016. Hepatology 2020; 71(2):431–43.
4. Xu JJ, Tien C, Chang M, et al. Demographic and serological characteristics of Asian Americans with hepatitis B infection diagnosed at community screenings. J Viral Hepat 2013;20(8):575–81.
5. Hu KQ, Pan CQ, Goodwin D. Barriers to screening for hepatitis B virus infection in Asian Americans. Dig Dis Sci 2011;56(11):3163–71.
6. Hyun S, Ko O, Kim S, et al. Sociocultural barriers to hepatitis B health literacy in an immigrant population: a focus group study in Korean Americans. BMC Public Health 2021;21(1):404.
7. Kallman JB, Arsalla A, Park V, et al. Screening for hepatitis B, C and non-alcoholic fatty liver disease: a survey of community-based physicians. Aliment Pharmacol Ther 2009;29(9):1019–24.
8. Foster T, Hon H, Kanwal F, et al. Screening high risk individuals for hepatitis B: physician knowledge, attitudes, and beliefs. Dig Dis Sci 2011;56(12):3471–87.
9. Ku KC, Li J, Ha NB, et al. Chronic hepatitis B management based on standard guidelines in community primary care and specialty clinics. Dig Dis Sci 2013; 58(12):3626–33.
10. Nguyen NH, Nguyen V, Trinh HN, et al. Treatment eligibility of patients with chronic hepatitis B initially ineligible for therapy. Clin Gastroenterol Hepatol 2013;11(5):565–71.
11. Zhang S, Ristau JT, Trinh HN, et al. Undertreatment of Asian chronic hepatitis B patients on the basis of standard guidelines: a community-based study. Dig Dis Sci 2012;57(5):1373–83.
12. Kim LH, Nguyen VG, Trinh HN, et al. Low treatment rates in patients meeting guideline criteria in diverse practice settings. Dig Dis Sci 2014;59(9):2091–9.
13. Terrault NA, Bzowej NH, Chang KM, et al. AASLD guidelines for treatment of chronic hepatitis B. Hepatology 2016;63(1):261–83.
14. European Association for the Study of the Liver. EASL 2017 clinical practice guidelines on the management of hepatitis B virus infection. J Hepatol 2017; 67(2):370–98.
15. Sarin SK, Kumar M, Lau GK, et al. Asian-Pacific clinical practice guidelines on the management of hepatitis B: a 2015 update. Hepatol Int 2016;10(1):1–98.
16. Nguyen MH, Wong G, Gane E, et al. Hepatitis B virus: advances in prevention, diagnosis, and therapy. Clin Microbiol Rev 2020;33(2):000466-19.
17. Goodman ZD. Grading and staging systems for inflammation and fibrosis in chronic liver diseases. J Hepatol 2007;47(4):598–607.
18. Amarapurkar D, Amarapurkar A. Indications of liver biopsy in the era of noninvasive assessment of liver fibrosis. J Clin Exp Hepatol 2015;5(4):314–9.
19. Wong GLH. Update of liver fibrosis and steatosis with transient elastography (Fibroscan). Gastroenterol Rep (Oxf) 2013;1(1):19–26.
20. Barr G, Ferraioli G, Palmeri M, et al. Elastography assessment of liver fibrosis: society of radiologists in ultrasound consensus conference statement. Ultrasound Q 2016;32(2):94–107.

21. Lim JK, Flamm SL, Singh S, et al. Clinical guidelines committee of the american gastroenterological association. american gastroenterological association institute guideline on the role of elastography in the evaluation of liver fibrosis. Gastroenterology 2017;152(6):1536–43.

22. EASL-ALEH Clinical Practice Guidelines. Non-invasive tests for evaluation of liver disease severity and prognosis. J Hepatol 2015;63(1):237–64.

23. Terrault NA, Lok ASF, McMahon BJ, et al. Update on prevention, diagnosis, and treatment of chronic hepatitis B: AASLD 2018 hepatitis B guidance. Hepatology 2018;67(4):1560–99.

24. US Preventive Services Task Force, Krist AH, Davidson KW, Barry MJ, et al. Screening for hepatitis B virus infection in adolescents and adults: US preventive services task force recommendation statement. JAMA 2020;324(23):2415–22.

25. Centers for Disease Control and Prevention. Federal register notice #CDC-2022-07050 for Hepatitis B screening and testing. 2022. Available at: https://www.cdc.gov/hepatitis/policy/isireview/HepBFederalRegisterNotice.htm.   Accessed November 30, 2022.

26. Fung J, Lai CL, Seto WK, et al. Nucleoside/nucleotide analogues in the treatment of chronic hepatitis B. J Antimicrob Chemother 2011;66(12):2715–25.

27. Lok ASF, McMahon BJ, Brown RS Jr, et al. Antiviral therapy for chronic hepatitis B viral infection in adults: A systematic review and meta-analysis. Hepatology 2016; 63(1):284–306.

28. Jang JW, Choi JY, Kim YS, et al. Long-term effect of antiviral therapy on disease course after decompensation in patients with hepatitis B virus-related cirrhosis. Hepatology 2015;61(6):1809–20.

29. Chien RN, Yeh CT, Tsai SL, et al. Determinants for sustained HBeAg response to lamivudine therapy. Hepatology 2003;38(5):1267–73.

30. Fattovich G, Stroffolini T, Zagni I, et al. Hepatocellular carcinoma in cirrhosis: incidence and risk factors. Gastroenterology 2004;127(5 Suppl 1):S35–50.

31. Chen CJ, Yang HI, Su J, et al. Risk of hepatocellular carcinoma across a biological gradient of serum hepatitis B virus DNA level. JAMA 2006;295(1):65–73.

32. Lok A. Does antiviral therapy for hepatitis B and C prevent hepatocellular carcinoma? J Gastroenterol Hepatol 2011;26(2):221–7.

33. Yu M, Lin C, Lin C, et al. Influence of metabolic risk factors on risk of hepatocellular carcinoma and liver-related death in men with chronic hepatitis B: a large cohort study. Gastroenterology 2017;153(4):1006–17.e5.

34. Chan A, Wong G, Chan H, et al. Concurrent fatty liver increases risk of hepatocellular carcinoma among patients with chronic hepatitis B. J Gastroenterol Hepatol 2017;32(3):667–76.

35. Huang Y, Yang H, Liu J, et al. Mediation analysis of hepatitis B and C in relation to hepatocellular carcinoma risk. Epidemiology 2016;27(1):14–20.

36. Ioannou G, Bryson C, Weiss N, et al. The prevalence of cirrhosis and hepatocellular carcinoma in patients with human immunodeficiency virus infection. Hepatology 2013;57(1):249–57.

37. Reddy KR, Beavers KL, Hammond SP, et al. American gastroenterological association institute guideline on the prevention and treatment of hepatitis B virus reactivation during immunosuppressive drug therapy. Gastroenterology 2015; 148(1):215–9.

38. Myint A, Tong MJ, Beaven SW. Reactivation of hepatitis B virus: a review of clinical guidelines. Clin Liver Dis 2020;15(4):162–7.

39. Su J, Lim JK. Hepatitis B virus reactivation in the setting of immunosuppressive drug therapy. Gastroenterol Hepatol 2019;15(11):585–92.

40. Lau GKK, Yiu HHY, Fong DYT, et al. Early is superior to deferred preemptive lam-ivudine therapy for hepatitis B patients undergoing chemotherapy. Gastroenter-ology 2003;125(6):1742–9.

41. Huang YH, Hsiao LT, Hong YC, et al. Randomized controlled trial of entecavir pro-phylaxis for rituximab-associated hepatitis B virus reactivation in patients with lymphoma and resolved hepatitis B. J Clin Oncol 2013;31(22):2765–72.

42. Papatheodoridis GV, Lekakis V, Voulgaris T, et al. Hepatitis B virus reactivation associated with new classes of immunosuppressants and immunomodulators: a systematic review, meta-analysis, and expert opinion. J Hepatol 2022;77(6): 1670–89.

43. Hwang JP, Feld JJ, Hammond SP, et al. Hepatitis B virus screening and manage-ment for patients with cancer prior to therapy: ASCO provisional clinical opinion update. J Clin Oncol 2020;38(31):3698–715.

44. Kwak YE, Stein SM, Lim JK. Practice patterns in hepatitis B virus screening before cancer chemotherapy in a major US hospital network. Dig Dis Sci 2018; 63(1):61–71.

Nonalcoholic Fatty Liver Disease

A Unique Entity or Part of the Metabolic Syndrome or Both

Terry Cheuk-Fung Yip, PhD[a,b,c], Grace Lai-Hung Wong, MD[a,b,c],
Vincent Wai-Sun Wong, MD[a,b,c],
George Boon-Bee Goh, MBBS (UK), MRCP (UK), M Med (Int Med), FAMS (Singapore)[d,e,*],
Wah-Kheong Chan, MBBS (UM), MRCP (UK), PhD (Malaya), AM[f,*]

KEYWORDS

• Dyslipidemia • Hypertension • Obesity • Type 2 diabetes • Malignancies

KEY POINTS

- Nonalcoholic fatty liver disease (NAFLD) is bidirectionally related to metabolic syndrome, which has led to a heated debate on updating the nomenclature to metabolic dysfunction-associated fatty liver disease.
- Coexistence of NAFLD and metabolic syndrome results in more adverse clinical outcomes such as cardiovascular diseases, extrahepatic malignancies, liver-related complications, and mortality.
- Multidisciplinary care pathways are crucial to identify patients with NAFLD at risk of liver and non-liver complications and provide necessary lifestyle modifications, control of metabolic risk factors, and potentially beneficial treatments.

[a] Department of Medicine and Therapeutics, 9/F Prince of Wales Hospital, 30-32 Ngan Shing Street, Shatin, Hong Kong; [b] Medical Data Analytics Centre (MDAC), The Chinese University of Hong Kong, Hong Kong; [c] Institute of Digestive Disease, The Chinese University of Hong Kong, Hong Kong; [d] Department of Gastroenterology and Hepatology, Singapore General Hospital, 20 College Road, Academia, Singapore 169856; [e] Duke-NUS Medical School, Singapore; [f] Gastroenterology and Hepatology Unit, Department of Medicine, Faculty of Medicine, University of Malaya, 50603 Kuala Lumpur, Malaysia
* Corresponding authors. George Boon-Bee Goh, Department of Gastroenterology and Hepatology, Singapore General Hospital, 20 College Road, Academia, Singapore 169856; Wah-Kheong Chan, Gastroenterology and Hepatology Unit, Department of Medicine, Faculty of Medicine, University of Malaya, 50603 Kuala Lumpur, Malaysia.
E-mail addresses: goh.boon.bee@singhealth.com.sg (G.B.-B.G.); wahkheong2003@hotmail.com (W.-K.C.)

Med Clin N Am 107 (2023) 449–463
https://doi.org/10.1016/j.mcna.2022.12.003
0025-7125/23/© 2022 Elsevier Inc. All rights reserved.
medical.theclinics.com

INTRODUCTION

Nonalcoholic fatty liver disease (NAFLD) encompasses a spectrum of liver conditions that are characterized by excess accumulation of fat in the liver.[1] It is closely associated with obesity and metabolic syndrome but is also seen among nonobese persons with increased visceral adiposity.[2] The prevalence of NAFLD has been increasing rapidly alongside the increasing prevalence of obesity worldwide. NAFLD is the most common cause of chronic liver disease, with its prevalence increasing from 21.9% to 37.3% between 1991 and 2019.[3] Nonalcoholic fatty liver (NAFL) is characterized by more than 5% hepatic steatosis with no or only minimal lobular inflammation, whereas nonalcoholic steatohepatitis (NASH) is the more severe form of NAFLD defined histologically by the presence of lobular inflammation and hepatocyte ballooning (**Fig. 1**). Fibrosis progression occurs more rapidly in patients with NASH compared with patients with NAFL.[4] The risk of liver-related complications and mortality increases exponentially with increasing fibrosis stage, so patients with NASH-related cirrhosis are over 40 times more likely to die of liver-related complications compared with patients with NAFLD without liver fibrosis.[5] In patients with NASH-related cirrhosis, hepatocellular carcinoma (HCC) develops at an annual rate of 0.5% to 2.6%.[6] NASH is already recognized as the most rapidly increasing indication and one of the leading indications for liver transplantation among waitlist registrants as well as for HCC in the United States.[7,8] Besides liver-related complications, patients with NAFLD are at increased risk of cardiovascular disease due to the close relationship between NAFLD and metabolic syndrome. In fact, cardiovascular disease is the leading cause of death in patients with NAFLD. This review focuses on the interplay between NAFLD and metabolic syndrome and how the increasing understanding of this intricate relationship may help improve the management and outcome of patients with NAFLD.

METABOLIC SYNDROME

The term metabolic syndrome refers to a constellation of risk factors for cardiovascular disease.[9,10] The first description of clustering of these risk factors dated back to the early twentieth century when scientists observed the frequent coexistence of hypertension and diabetes mellitus, and subsequently gout, obesity, and coronary artery disease. In 1981, the term metabolic syndrome was described, which included type 2 diabetes (T2DM), hyperinsulinemia, obesity, hypertension, hyperlipidemia, gout,

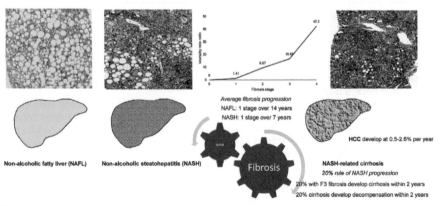

Fig. 1. Natural history of NAFLD.

Box 1
Definitions of metabolic syndrome

World Health Organization (WHO)
Insulin resistance plus at least two of the following criteria:
- Hypertension,
- Elevated triglycerides,
- Low high-density lipoprotein (HDL) cholesterol,
- Obesity (increased body mass index or waist-to-hip ratio), and
- Microalbuminuria.

European Group for the Study of Insulin Resistance (EGIR)
Insulin resistance plus at least two of the following criteria:
- Central obesity,
- Dyslipidemia (high triglycerides or low HDL cholesterol),
- Hypertension, and
- Fasting plasma glucose $\geq$6.1 mmol/L.

National Cholesterol Education Program/Adult Treatment Panel III (NCEP/ATP III)
At least three of the following criteria:
- Abdominal obesity,
- Elevated triglycerides,
- Low HDL cholesterol,
- Blood pressure (BP) $\geq$130/85 mm Hg, and
- Fasting glucose $\geq$6.1 mmol/L.

International Diabetes Federation (IDF)
Central obesity (waist circumference $\geq$94 cm for Europid men, and $\geq$80 cm for Europid women, with ethnicity-specific values for other groups) plus at least two of the following criteria:
- Raised triglyceride level ($\geq$1.7 mmol/L, or specific treatment of this abnormality),
- Reduced HDL cholesterol (<1.03 mmol/L in males, and <1.29 mmol/L in females, or specific treatment of this abnormality),
- Raised BP (systolic BP $\geq$ 130 or diastolic BP $\geq$ 85 mm Hg, or treatment of previously diagnosed hypertension), and
- Raised fasting plasma glucose ($\geq$5.6 mmol/L, or previously diagnosed type 2 diabetes).

---

thrombophilia, and the predisposition to atherosclerosis. Later, insulin resistance was hypothesized as the underlying factor and the term syndrome X was used to denote the many unknown aspects of the condition. This was followed by the recognition of central adiposity as an important factor and increasing evidence of insulin resistance.[11] Around the turn of the century, several efforts have been made toward the definition of the metabolic syndrome (**Box 1**) with the National Cholesterol Education Program/Adult Treatment Panel III (NCEP/ATP III) and the International Diabetes Federation (IDF) being the most widely used definition.[9,10,12,13] There was heated debate around the definition of metabolic syndrome, many reminiscences of the current debate on the new nomenclature for NAFLD. The term NAFLD does not attribute the disease to its underlying cause, is not in line with the reality that more than one cause of the chronic liver disease can and often coexist in the same patient, may trivialize the disease, and is considered to be stigmatizing by some patients.[14] Thus, a new term, metabolic dysfunction-associated fatty liver disease (MAFLD), was proposed in 2020. MAFLD is diagnosed based on the presence of hepatic steatosis in a person who is overweight or obese, has T2DM or has at least two metabolic risk abnormalities.[15] At the time of this review, the term MAFLD has been endorsed by several international and national organizations but has not been universally accepted.

TYPE 2 DIABETES AND INSULIN RESISTANCE

Studies have consistently demonstrated a close relationship between T2DM and NAFLD. Even before the development of diabetes, insulin resistance is almost ubiquitous in NAFLD.[16] In a systematic review and meta-analysis of 80 studies, the global prevalence of NAFLD among patients with T2DM is estimated at 55.5%.[17] On the flip side, NAFLD increases the risk of incident diabetes by twofold.[18] T2DM is also associated with the severity of NAFLD, with 37% having NASH and 15% to 20% having significant or advanced fibrosis.[17,19] In 3 years, 12% of patients with T2DM have a ≥30% relative increase in liver stiffness measurement by transient elastography suggestive of fibrosis progression.[20] In patients with NAFLD-related cirrhosis, the presence of T2DM increases the risk of hepatic decompensation and HCC by twofold.[21]

Despite the link between diabetes and NAFLD, it is difficult if not impossible to screen all 500 million people living with diabetes for NAFLD. Among patients with both T2DM and NAFLD, more than 90% of liver-related complications develop after the age of 50.[22] In contrast, the incidence of liver-related complications seems linear with the duration of diabetes.

Both hepatic lipid accumulation and inflammation are known to increase the risk of T2DM, and there is a complex interplay between the two. Putative mechanisms underlying the increased risk of T2DM in NAFLD include common dietary factors (eg, fructose and saturated fat), gut microbiota dysbiosis and increased gut permeability, adipose tissue dysfunction and changes in de novo ceramide synthesis, and increased hepatic glucose production.[23]

OVERWEIGHT AND OBESITY

The pooled prevalence of obesity is estimated at 51.3% among NAFLD.[24] Conversely, the prevalence of NAFLD in obese subjects ranges between 10% and over 90% and is particularly higher in morbid obesity cohorts.[25]

In a meta-analysis of 21 cohort studies involving 381,655 subjects, obesity was independently associated with a 3.5-fold increased risk of NAFLD development, compared with normal weight. Moreover, for every 1-unit rise in body mass index (BMI), there was a 1.2-fold increase in relative risk of NAFLD.[26] The independent impact of obesity on NAFLD may be further reiterated by studies on obese individuals without metabolic dysfunction. Coined metabolically healthy obesity (MHO), some obese individuals do not have any metabolic disturbances such as dyslipidemia, insulin resistance, or hypertension.[27] In a longitudinal study of 14,779 Korean overweight/ obese subjects deemed MHO and without NAFLD at baseline, even a modest weight increase of 1% to 5% translated into a 56% increased risk of incident NAFLD, whereas weight loss by the same amount would reduce the said risk by 17%.[28] Separately, NAFLD may be associated with the transition from metabolically healthy to metabolically unhealthy obesity.[29]

Obesity also impacts the severity of NAFLD, augmenting the risk of NASH, fibrosis, and cirrhosis. A meta-analysis of eight studies illustrated that overweight/obese patients with NAFLD had a higher NAFLD activity score and fibrosis stage, whereas non-obese patients with NAFLD had a 40% lower risk of having NASH.[30] Furthermore, obesity is associated with fibrosis progression with a 1.2-fold increased risk of severe liver disease events among patients with NAFLD.[31,32]

Obesity plays a major role in the pathogenesis of NAFLD. Obesity increases adipose tissue mass, driving a multitude of pathologic changes, including adipocyte dysfunction, increasing insulin resistance, and enhancing lipolysis, resulting in excess circulating free fatty acids and ensuing intrahepatic fat accumulation.[25] Lipotoxicity, mitochondrial dysfunction, activation of inflammatory pathways, and oxidative stress are implicated as part of the obesity-driven pathogenesis of NAFLD-NASH.[25] Obesity also impacts the liver via dysregulation of adipokines such as increased leptin and reduced adiponectin, which drives the liver to a more steatogenic, inflammatory, and fibrotic state.[33]

HYPERTENSION

Mounting evidence suggests a close relationship between hypertension and NAFLD, independent of other metabolic risk factors.[34,35] Prevalence of hypertension is higher in patients with NAFLD than in the general population; in a meta-analysis, the pooled odds ratio for prevalent hypertension was 1.24 in subjects with NAFLD compared with those without.[36]

Prospective longitudinal studies demonstrate that NAFLD was associated with incident hypertension, with odds ratios ranging from 1.58 to 3.1.[37–39] In addition, the risk magnitude of developing hypertension is suggested to parallel NAFLD severity. In a prospective 5-year cohort study on 22,090 Korean men without hypertension, incidence rate of hypertension increased according to the degree of NAFLD. Relative to subjects without NAFLD, adjusted hazard ratios for hypertension were higher in the mild (1.07) and moderate-to-severe (1.14) NAFLD groups.[40]

Separately, hypertension promotes the development of NAFLD, with prospective cohort studies reporting that hypertension predicted incident NAFLD, with the risk of NAFLD increasing progressively over blood pressure categories.[41–43] More importantly, in a meta-analysis of 411 biopsy-proven patients with NAFLD, there was a 1.94-fold increased odds of fibrosis progression in subjects with hypertension compared with those without.[4]

The bidirectional NAFLD-Hypertension relationship was further exemplified by findings that although presence of NAFLD predicted the onset of hypertension, the development of hypertension also predicted the onset of NAFLD.[44] Though causal mechanisms remain to be fully elucidated, several postulations have been proposed. Systematic inflammation upregulated pro-inflammatory cytokines and oxidative stress have been implicated in the activation of the sympathetic nervous system and renin-angiotensin-aldosterone system, which in turn mediate blood pressure/hypertension.[45–47] Similarly, the roles of insulin resistance, endothelial dysfunction, and increased vasoconstriction mediated by NAFLD have also been postulated.[34,35]

DYSLIPIDEMIA

Dyslipidemia in patients with NAFLD involves changes in serum cholesterol (hypercholesterolemia), triglycerides (hypertriglyceridemia), or both (combined dyslipidemia). The overall prevalence of combined dyslipidemia in patients with NAFLD or NASH was as common as 69% and 72%, respectively.[24] Such a high prevalence was confirmed in a landmark clinical trial, the REGENERATE study for obeticholic acid, in which 68% to 70% of the recruited NAFLD subjects suffered from combined dyslipidemia at baseline.[48] Although NAFLD dramatically increases the risk of dyslipidemia by 3 to 5 times, dyslipidemia is also a well-established risk factor of NAFLD with an adjusted hazard ratio of two to three.[49,50] Advanced fibrosis in NAFLD is associated with dyslipidemia, yet the effect size is generally smaller than that of T2DM.[51]

Different pathways are involved in dyslipidemia in patients with NAFLD, for example, inadequate uptake of circulating lipids, increased hepatic *de novo* lipogenesis, insufficient enhancement of fatty acid oxidation, and altered export of lipids as components of very-low-density lipoprotein cholesterol.[52] Insulin resistance is another important driver for the lipoprotein abnormalities in NAFLD, leading to dyslipidemia on top of hyperglycemia and activation of oxidative stress and inflammation.[49] Triglyceride-rich lipoproteins containing apolipoprotein C3 are important activators of inflammatory response leading to inflammasome activation and apoptotic cell death, and later stimulation of inflammation, tissue regeneration, and fibrogenesis in NASH.[51,53]

CLINICAL OUTCOMES
Liver-related events

Metabolic syndrome is a risk factor for liver-related events in patients with NAFLD (**Fig. 2**). In a meta-analysis of 18 studies, presence of T2DM in patients with NAFLD is associated with a 2.3-fold increased risk of developing liver-related events including cirrhosis, hepatic decompensation, and HCC.[32] Obesity is also associated with a 20% increase in the risk of developing liver-related events.[32] Moreover, the risk of disease progression increased with the number of metabolic risk components. Patients with coexisting hypertension and dyslipidemia had a 1.8-fold higher risk of progression, whereas patients who had all diabetes, obesity, dyslipidemia, and hypertension were at a 2.6-fold higher risk. Among the four metabolic risk factors, diabetes seemed to have the strongest association with HCC.[54] In contrast, a good control on the metabolic syndrome results in a reduced risk of HCC in patients with NAFLD. For example, an adequate glycemic control of hemoglobin A_{1c} <7% over time confers a 31% lower risk of HCC in patients with NAFLD.

Cardiovascular events

Presence of metabolic syndrome are associated with more cardiovascular events in patients with NAFLD.[55,56] Also, a higher fibrosis stage is also associated with a higher risk of cardiovascular events after considering other traditional risk factors and cardiovascular risk scores.[56] In contrast, among obese patients with NAFLD, patients who

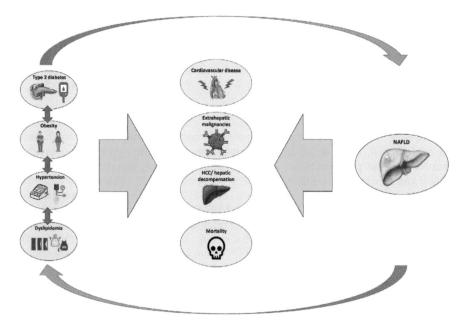

Fig. 2. Interaction between metabolic risk factors and NAFLD in clinical outcomes.

undergo bariatric surgery are associated with a lower risk of cardiovascular events than those who received nonsurgical management.[57] On the other hand, coexisting NAFLD is a risk factor for cardiovascular events in patients with metabolic syndrome. In a meta-analysis of 11 studies, coexisting NAFLD in patients with T2DM contributes to the development of cardiovascular events.[58]

Extrahepatic Malignancies

NAFLD has been linked with a higher risk of different extrahepatic malignancies including gastrointestinal cancers, lung cancer, breast cancer, and gynecologic or urinary system cancers independent of diabetes and obesity.[59] Most evidence of the association between NAFLD, metabolic syndrome, and extrahepatic malignancies comes from colorectal cancer. The presence of metabolic syndrome and NAFLD may synergistically increase the risk of colorectal cancer.[60]

Overall Mortality

Extrahepatic malignancies and cardiovascular diseases are the top killers in patients with NAFLD, whereas liver disease is the leading cause of death in patients with NAFLD-related cirrhosis.[61] NAFLD patients with metabolic syndrome have a higher mortality risk than those without metabolic syndrome; an increasing number of components of metabolic syndrome was also associated with higher mortality risk.[62] A good control of components of metabolic syndrome is beneficial. The increased mortality risk due to presence of hypertension in patients with NAFLD can be attenuated by good blood pressure control.[55] On the other hand, the use of a new definition of MAFLD may better identify patients with elevated mortality risk than the original definition of NAFLD.[63] In a US study, MAFLD was associated with an increased risk of all-cause mortality, whereas the association between NAFLD and increased mortality risk disappeared after adjusting for metabolic risk factors.

SCREENING

Although the prevalence of NAFLD is high in the general population, screening everyone for NAFLD is not recommended due to limited effective treatment options, and lack of knowledge related to long-term benefits and cost-effectiveness. Instead, international guidelines recommend focusing on the population who have a higher risk of NAFLD with advanced fibrosis including patients with T2DM, obesity, and metabolic syndrome, as liver fibrosis is the most important predictor of liver and non-liver outcomes (**Box 2**). Common serum fibrosis scores including fibrosis-4 index and NAFLD fibrosis score, as well as noninvasive assessments such as transient elastography, can be used to identify and exclude advanced fibrosis. Lifestyle modification remains important in preventing adverse clinical outcomes in patients with NAFLD. International guidelines generally recommend the assessment of dietary and physical activity habits at NAFLD screening.

To facilitate the systematic screening of NAFLD with advanced fibrosis at the primary care setting, the American Gastroenterological Association proposed a clinical care pathway with multidisciplinary experts (**Fig. 3**).[64] At-risk patients with T2DM, two or more metabolic risk factors, and an incidental finding of hepatic steatosis or elevated liver enzymes are identified and recommended to screen for alcohol use and receive blood tests for calculating serum fibrosis scores. Those with elevated liver enzymes should be evaluated for other chronic liver and biliary diseases. Those classified as low risk by serum fibrosis score are unlikely to have advanced fibrosis and can generally repeat the calculation after 2 to 3 years, whereas those classified as

---

Box 2
Current guidelines on case identification and screening for nonalcoholic fatty liver disease (NAFLD) or metabolic dysfunction-associated fatty liver disease (MAFLD)

American Association for the Study of Liver Diseases (AASLD) 2018[50]
- Routine screening for NAFLD in high-risk groups attending primary care, diabetes, or obesity clinics is not advised at this time because of uncertainties surrounding diagnostic tests and treatment options, along with lack of knowledge related to long-term benefits and cost-effectiveness of screening.
- There should be a high index of suspicion for NAFLD and nonalcoholic steatohepatitis (NASH) in patients with type 2 diabetes (T2DM). Clinical decision aids such as NAFLD fibrosis score or fibrosis-4 index (FIB-4) or vibration-controlled transient elastography (VCTE) can be used to identify those at low or high risk for advanced fibrosis (bridging fibrosis or cirrhosis).
- Systematic screening of family members for NAFLD is not recommended currently.

European Association for the Study of the Liver (EASL) 2016[72]
- Screening for NAFLD in the population at risk should be in the context of the available resources, considering the burden for the national health care systems, and the currently limited effective treatments.
- Patients with insulin resistance and/or metabolic risk factors (ie, obesity or metabolic syndrome [MetS]) should undergo diagnostic procedures for the diagnosis of NAFLD, which relies on the demonstration of excessive liver fat.
- In subjects with obesity or MetS, screening for NAFLD by liver enzymes and/or ultrasound should be part of a routine workup. In high-risk individuals (age >50 years, T2DM, MetS) case finding of advanced disease (ie, NASH with fibrosis) is advisable.
- Family screening is not generally advisable, with the exception of cases with defined inherited diseases (eg, lysosomal acid lipase deficiency).
- The assessment of dietary and physical activity habits is part of comprehensive NAFLD screening

Asian Pacific Association for the Study of the Liver (APASL) 2020[73]
- Screening for MAFLD by ultrasonography should be considered in at-risk populations such as patients with overweight/obesity, T2DM, and MetS.
- Patients with MAFLD should be assessed for other components of MetS and treated accordingly.
- Patients with MAFLD should receive advice and support for lifestyle interventions to reduce the risk of events from metabolic and cardiovascular disease, and to resolve fatty liver disease.

---

high risk should be referred to hepatologists. Those classified as intermediate risk by serum fibrosis score can perform liver stiffness measurement for confirmation. Those remaining at intermediate risk can be referred to hepatologists for further assessment.

TREATMENT IMPLICATIONS

Because of the close relationship between NAFLD and metabolic risk factors, it comes as no surprise that metabolic treatments can benefit both. Lifestyle intervention with a healthy diet and regular exercise is the cornerstone for the management of obesity-related diseases. Approximately 7% and 10% weight reduction are often quoted as the thresholds for NASH resolution and fibrosis improvement, respectively, though improvements in NAFLD can be seen with modest weight loss, especially if the patient has a lower baseline BMI.[65–67]

The current American guidelines support the use of vitamin E and pioglitazone in selected patients with NASH.[50] Pioglitazone, a peroxisome proliferator-activated receptor-gamma agonist, is an insulin sensitizer that reduced hepatic steatosis and inflammation in a few clinical trials. Nevertheless, its use is limited by the side effects

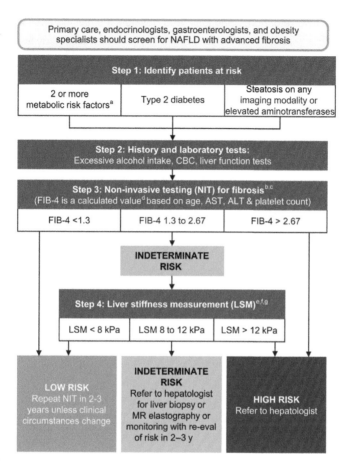

Fig. 3. The American Gastroenterological Association Clinical Care Pathway for NAFLD as an example of a multidisciplinary approach for patient assessment, depending on the local availability of various tests. HCC, hepatocellular carcinoma; NAFLD, non-alcoholic fatty liver disease. [a]Metabolic risk factors: central obesity, high triglycerides, low HDL cholesterol, hypertension, prediabetes, or insulin resistance. [b]For patients 65+, USE fib-4<2.0 as the lower cutoff. The higher cutoff does not change. [c]Other NITs derived from routine laboratories can be used instead of FIB-4. [d]Many online FIB-4 calculators are available such as https://www. mdcalc.com/fibrosis-4-fib-4-index-liver-fibrosis. [e]Ultrasound is acceptable if vibration-controlled transient elastography (VCTE, FibroScan) is unavailable. Consider referral to a hepatologist for patients with hepatic steatosis on ultrasound who are indeterminate or high-risk based on FIB-4. [f]LSM values are for VCTE (FibroScan). Other techniques such as bi-dimensional shear wave elastography or point shear wave elastography can also be used to measure LSM. Proprietary commercially available blood NITs may be considered for patients considered indeterminate or high risk based on FIB-4 or APRI, or where LSM is unavailable. [g]Eddowes and colleagues[38] used 8.2 and 12.1 kPa as cutoffs for LSM using VCTE. Validation of simple (rounded) cutoffs reported by Papatheodoridi and colleagues.[41] (*Adapted from* Kanwal F, Shubrook JH, Adams LA, Pfotenhauer K, Wai-Sun Wong V, et. al Clinical Care Pathway for the Risk Stratification and Management of Patients With Nonalcoholic Fatty Liver Disease. Gastroenterology. 2021 Nov;161(5):1657-1669. https://doi.org/10.1053/j. gastro.2021.07.049. Epub 2021 Sep 20. PMID: 34602251; PMCID: PMC8819923.)

of weight gain, fluid retention, bone loss, and possibly a small increase in the risk of bladder cancer.

Glucagon-like peptide-1 receptor agonists are new anti-diabetic drugs that decrease appetite, delay gastric emptying, and improve insulin sensitivity in various organs. This class of drugs has been shown to improve cardiovascular outcomes and overall survival. In a phase 2b study, subcutaneous semaglutide 0.4 mg daily for 72 weeks led to NASH resolution with no worsening of fibrosis in 59% of patients, compared with 17% in the placebo arm.[68] However, the drug failed to resolve NASH or improve fibrosis at 48 weeks in patients with compensated NASH-related cirrhosis.[69]

Sodium-glucose co-transporter-2 inhibitors lead to glycosuria and can improve glycemic control, blood pressure, cardiovascular and renal outcomes as well as survival. They also reduce liver enzymes and hepatic steatosis on imaging studies in patients with NAFLD, but data on histologic benefits are limited to small uncontrolled studies.[70]

Metformin, statins, aspirin, and angiotensin-converting enzyme inhibitors have not been shown to improve liver histology in NAFLD, but observational data suggest they may reduce the risk of cirrhotic complications and HCC.[22,71] Notwithstanding the caveats of observational studies, these metabolic drugs have various benefits for the cardiovascular system and kidneys. Mounting evidence also supports their safety in patients with chronic liver disease.

In patients with severe obesity, bariatric surgery is currently the most effective method for weight reduction. It can also lead to remission of diabetes and NASH resolution and liver fibrosis improvement. Recent data also suggest a benefit in reducing major liver-related events.[57]

SUMMARY

NAFLD is not a standalone liver disease but an integral part of the metabolic syndrome; two conditions are bidirectionally related. With an increasing prevalence worldwide, NAFLD is a major contributor to mortality, not only from liver-related complications but more often from cardiovascular events and extrahepatic malignancies, which are strongly associated with metabolic syndrome. NAFLD generally increases the risk of various metabolic risk factors, specifically T2DM and insulin resistance, overweight and obesity, hypertension, and dyslipidemia. The presence of these metabolic risk factors in return intensifies the risks of NAFLD. Poorly-controlled metabolic risk factors are linked to more severe NAFLD like NASH, advanced fibrosis, and cirrhosis, and hence worse clinical outcomes. All such interlinked relationships make NAFLD not simply a liver disease but a hepatic manifestation of systemic metabolic dysfunction. Targeted screening for NAFLD in patients with T2DM, obesity, and metabolic syndrome is recommended by international guidelines, whereas the long-term benefits and cost-effectiveness of screening are to be established. Multidisciplinary care pathways including lifestyle modifications, adequate control of metabolic factors, and hopefully the coming-soon pharmacologic treatments for NAFLD are crucial to improve the clinical outcomes of patients with NAFLD.

CLINICS CARE POINTS

- NAFLD is the most common chronic liver disease worldwide, which represents significant clinical burden.
- As an integral part of metabolic syndrome, NAFLD exibits a close bi-directional relationship with the various components of metabolic syndrome.

- A multidisciplinary approach including targetted screening and optimisation of metabolic factors are important to improve clinical outcomes in NAFLD care.

DISCLOSURE

T.C-F. Yip has served as an advisory committee member and a speaker for Gilead Sciences. G.L-H. Wong has served as an advisory committee member for Gilead Sciences and Janssen, and as a speaker for Abbott, Abbvie, Ascletis, Bristol-Myers Squibb, Echosens, Gilead Sciences, Janssen, and Roche. She has also received a research grant from Gilead Sciences. V.W-S. Wong has served as a consultant or advisory committee member for AbbVie, Boehringer Ingelheim, Echosens, Gilead Sciences, Intercept, Inventiva, Merck, Novo Nordisk, Pfizer, ProSciento, Sagimet Biosciences, and TARGET PharmaSolutions; and a speaker for Abbott, AbbVie, Echosens, Gilead Sciences, and Novo Nordisk. He has received a research grant from Gilead Sciences, and is a co-founder of Illuminatio Medical Technology Limited. G.B-B. Goh has served as an advisory board member for Gilead Science, Boehringer Ingelheim, and a speaker for Echosens and Novo Nordisk. W-K. Chan has served as a consultant for Abbvie, Boehringer Ingelheim and Novo Nordisk; and a speaker for Viatris and Hisky Medical.

REFERENCES

1. Wong VWS, Chan WK, Chitturi S, et al. Asia–Pacific Working Party on Non-alcoholic Fatty Liver Disease guidelines 2017—part 1: definition, risk factors and assessment. J Gastroenterol Hepatol 2018;33:70–85.
2. Kuchay MS, Martinez-Montoro JI, Choudhary NS, et al. Non-Alcoholic Fatty Liver Disease in Lean and Non-Obese Individuals: Current and Future Challenges. Biomedicines 2021;9:1346.
3. Le MH, Yeo YH, Li X, et al. 2019 Global NAFLD Prevalence: A Systematic Review and Meta-analysis. Clin Gastroenterol Hepatol 2021;20(12):2809–17, e28.
4. Singh S, Allen AM, Wang Z, et al. Fibrosis progression in nonalcoholic fatty liver vs nonalcoholic steatohepatitis: a systematic review and meta-analysis of paired-biopsy studies. Clin Gastroenterol Hepatol 2015;13:643–54, e1-9; [quiz: e39-40].
5. Dulai PS, Singh S, Patel J, et al. Increased risk of mortality by fibrosis stage in nonalcoholic fatty liver disease: Systematic review and meta-analysis. Hepatology 2017;65:1557–65.
6. Huang DQ, El-Serag HB, Loomba R. Global epidemiology of NAFLD-related HCC: trends, predictions, risk factors and prevention. Nat Rev Gastroenterol Hepatol 2021;18:223–38.
7. Wong RJ, Aguilar M, Cheung R, et al. Nonalcoholic steatohepatitis is the second leading etiology of liver disease among adults awaiting liver transplantation in the United States. Gastroenterology 2015;148:547–55.
8. Wong RJ, Cheung R, Ahmed A. Nonalcoholic steatohepatitis is the most rapidly growing indication for liver transplantation in patients with hepatocellular carcinoma in the U.S. Hepatology 2014;59:2188–95.
9. National Cholesterol Education Program. Expert Panel on Detection E, Treatment of High Blood Cholesterol in A. Third Report of the National Cholesterol Education Program (NCEP) Expert Panel on Detection, Evaluation, and Treatment of High Blood Cholesterol in Adults (Adult Treatment Panel III) final report. Circulation 2002;106:3143–421.

10. Alberti KG, Zimmet P, Shaw J, et al. The metabolic syndrome–a new worldwide definition. Lancet 2005;366:1059–62.
11. Sarafidis PA, Nilsson PM. The metabolic syndrome: a glance at its history. J Hypertens 2006;24:621–6.
12. Alberti KG, Zimmet PZ. Definition, diagnosis and classification of diabetes mellitus and its complications. Part 1: diagnosis and classification of diabetes mellitus provisional report of a WHO consultation. Diabet Med 1998;15:539–53.
13. Balkau B, Charles MA. Comment on the provisional report from the WHO consultation. European Group for the Study of Insulin Resistance (EGIR). Diabet Med 1999;16:442–3.
14. Chan WK, Wong VW. Meaning of non-overlapping patients between the MAFLD and NAFLD definitions. Liver Int 2022;42:271–3.
15. Eslam M, Newsome PN, Sarin SK, et al. A new definition for metabolic dysfunction-associated fatty liver disease: An international expert consensus statement. J Hepatol 2020;73:202–9.
16. Wong VW, Hui AY, Tsang SW, et al. Prevalence of undiagnosed diabetes and postchallenge hyperglycaemia in Chinese patients with non-alcoholic fatty liver disease. Aliment Pharmacol Ther 2006;24:1215–22.
17. Younossi ZM, Golabi P, de Avila L, et al. The global epidemiology of NAFLD and NASH in patients with type 2 diabetes: A systematic review and meta-analysis. J Hepatol 2019;71:793–801.
18. Mantovani A, Petracca G, Beatrice G, et al. Non-alcoholic fatty liver disease and risk of incident diabetes mellitus: an updated meta-analysis of 501 022 adult individuals. Gut 2021;70:962–9.
19. Kwok R, Choi KC, Wong GL, et al. Screening diabetic patients for non-alcoholic fatty liver disease with controlled attenuation parameter and liver stiffness measurements: a prospective cohort study. Gut 2016;65:1359–68.
20. Lee HW, Wong GL, Kwok R, et al. Serial Transient Elastography Examinations to Monitor Patients With Type 2 Diabetes: A Prospective Cohort Study. Hepatology 2020;72:1230–41.
21. Calzadilla-Bertot L, Vilar-Gomez E, Wong VW, et al. ABIDE: An Accurate Predictive Model of Liver Decompensation in Patients With Nonalcoholic Fatty Liver-Related Cirrhosis. Hepatology 2021;73:2238–50.
22. Zhang X, Wong GL, Yip TC, et al. Risk of liver-related events by age and diabetes duration in patients with diabetes and nonalcoholic fatty liver disease. Hepatology 2022;76(5):1409–22.
23. Targher G, Corey KE, Byrne CD, et al. The complex link between NAFLD and type 2 diabetes mellitus - mechanisms and treatments. Nat Rev Gastroenterol Hepatol 2021;18:599–612.
24. Younossi ZM, Koenig AB, Abdelatif D, et al. Global epidemiology of nonalcoholic fatty liver disease-Meta-analytic assessment of prevalence, incidence, and outcomes. Hepatology 2016;64:73–84.
25. Polyzos SA, Kountouras J, Mantzoros CS. Obesity and nonalcoholic fatty liver disease: From pathophysiology to therapeutics. Metabolism 2019;92:82–97.
26. Li L, Liu DW, Yan HY, et al. Obesity is an independent risk factor for non-alcoholic fatty liver disease: evidence from a meta-analysis of 21 cohort studies. Obes Rev 2016;17:510–9.
27. Smith GI, Mittendorfer B, Klein S. Metabolically healthy obesity: facts and fantasies. J Clin Invest 2019;129:3978–89.

28. Cho IY, Chang Y, Sung E, et al. Weight Change and the Development of Nonal-coholic Fatty Liver Disease in Metabolically Healthy Overweight Individuals. Clin Gastroenterol Hepatol 2022;20:e583–99.
29. Lonardo A, Mantovani A, Lugari S, et al. Epidemiology and pathophysiology of the association between NAFLD and metabolically healthy or metabolically un-healthy obesity. Ann Hepatol 2020;19:359–66.
30. Sookoian S, Pirola CJ. Systematic review with meta-analysis: the significance of histological disease severity in lean patients with nonalcoholic fatty liver disease. Aliment Pharmacol Ther 2018;47:16–25.
31. Fassio E, Alvarez E, Dominguez N, et al. Natural history of nonalcoholic steatohe-patitis: a longitudinal study of repeat liver biopsies. Hepatology 2004;40:820–6.
32. Jarvis H, Craig D, Barker R, et al. Metabolic risk factors and incident advanced liver disease in non-alcoholic fatty liver disease (NAFLD): A systematic review and meta-analysis of population-based observational studies. Plos Med 2020;17:e1003100.
33. Polyzos SA, Kountouras J, Mantzoros CS. Adipokines in nonalcoholic fatty liver disease. Metabolism 2016;65:1062–79.
34. Zhao YC, Zhao GJ, Chen Z, et al. Nonalcoholic Fatty Liver Disease: An Emerging Driver of Hypertension. Hypertension 2020;75:275–84.
35. Oikonomou D, Georgiopoulos G, Katsi V, et al. Non-alcoholic fatty liver disease and hypertension: coprevalent or correlated? Eur J Gastroenterol Hepatol 2018;30:979–85.
36. Wu S, Wu F, Ding Y, et al. Association of non-alcoholic fatty liver disease with ma-jor adverse cardiovascular events: A systematic review and meta-analysis. Sci Rep 2016;6:33386.
37. Stranges S, Trevisan M, Dorn JM, et al. Body fat distribution, liver enzymes, and risk of hypertension: evidence from the Western New York Study. Hypertension 2005;46:1186–93.
38. Bonnet F, Gastaldelli A, Pihan-Le Bars F, et al. Gamma-glutamyltransferase, fatty liver index and hepatic insulin resistance are associated with incident hyperten-sion in two longitudinal studies. J Hypertens 2017;35:493–500.
39. Lau K, Lorbeer R, Haring R, et al. The association between fatty liver disease and blood pressure in a population-based prospective longitudinal study. J Hypertens 2010;28:1829–35.
40. Ryoo JH, Suh YJ, Shin HC, et al. Clinical association between non-alcoholic fatty liver disease and the development of hypertension. J Gastroenterol Hepatol 2014;29:1926–31.
41. Zhang T, Zhang C, Zhang Y, et al. Metabolic syndrome and its components as predictors of nonalcoholic fatty liver disease in a northern urban Han Chinese population: a prospective cohort study. Atherosclerosis 2015;240:144–8.
42. Aneni EC, Oni ET, Martin SS, et al. Blood pressure is associated with the pres-ence and severity of nonalcoholic fatty liver disease across the spectrum of car-diometabolic risk. J Hypertens 2015;33:1207–14.
43. Sorrentino P, Terracciano L, D'Angelo S, et al. Predicting fibrosis worsening in obese patients with NASH through parenchymal fibronectin, HOMA-IR, and hy-pertension. Am J Gastroenterol 2010;105:336–44.
44. Ma J, Hwang SJ, Pedley A, et al. Bi-directional analysis between fatty liver and cardiovascular disease risk factors. J Hepatol 2017;66:390–7.
45. Carnagarin R, Matthews V, Zaldivia MTK, et al. The bidirectional interaction be-tween the sympathetic nervous system and immune mechanisms in the patho-genesis of hypertension. Br J Pharmacol 2019;176:1839–52.

46. Satou R, Penrose H, Navar LG. Inflammation as a Regulator of the Renin-Angiotensin System and Blood Pressure. Curr Hypertens Rep 2018;20:100.

47. Lee HJ, Lee CH, Kim S, et al. Association between vascular inflammation and non-alcoholic fatty liver disease: Analysis by (18)F-fluorodeoxyglucose positron emission tomography. Metabolism 2017;67:72–9.

48. Younossi ZM, Ratziu V, Loomba R, et al. Obeticholic acid for the treatment of non-alcoholic steatohepatitis: interim analysis from a multicentre, randomised, placebo-controlled phase 3 trial. Lancet 2019;394:2184–96.

49. Amor AJ, Perea V. Dyslipidemia in nonalcoholic fatty liver disease. Curr Opin Endocrinol Diabetes Obes 2019;26:103–8.

50. Chalasani N, Younossi Z, Lavine JE, et al. The diagnosis and management of nonalcoholic fatty liver disease: Practice guidance from the American Association for the Study of Liver Diseases. Hepatology 2018;67:328–57.

51. Powell EE, Wong VW, Rinella M. Non-alcoholic fatty liver disease. Lancet 2021; 397:2212–24.

52. Ipsen DH, Lykkesfeldt J, Tveden-Nyborg P. Molecular mechanisms of hepatic lipid accumulation in non-alcoholic fatty liver disease. Cell Mol Life Sci 2018; 75:3313–27.

53. Zewinger S, Reiser J, Jankowski V, et al. Apolipoprotein C3 induces inflammation and organ damage by alternative inflammasome activation. Nat Immunol 2020; 21:30–41.

54. Kanwal F, Kramer JR, Li L, et al. Effect of Metabolic Traits on the Risk of Cirrhosis and Hepatocellular Cancer in Nonalcoholic Fatty Liver Disease. Hepatology 2020;71:808–19.

55. Ng CH, Wong ZY, Chew NWS, et al. Hypertension is prevalent in non-alcoholic fatty liver disease and increases all-cause and cardiovascular mortality. Front Cardiovasc Med 2022;9:942753.

56. Pitisuttithum P, Chan WK, Goh GB, et al. Gamma-glutamyl transferase and cardiovascular risk in nonalcoholic fatty liver disease: The Gut and Obesity Asia initiative. World J Gastroenterol 2020;26:2416–26.

57. Aminian A, Al-Kurd A, Wilson R, et al. Association of Bariatric Surgery With Major Adverse Liver and Cardiovascular Outcomes in Patients With Biopsy-Proven Nonalcoholic Steatohepatitis. JAMA 2021;326:2031–42.

58. Zhou YY, Zhou XD, Wu SJ, et al. Synergistic increase in cardiovascular risk in diabetes mellitus with nonalcoholic fatty liver disease: a meta-analysis. Eur J Gastroenterol Hepatol 2018;30:631–6.

59. Mantovani A, Petracca G, Beatrice G, et al. Non-alcoholic fatty liver disease and increased risk of incident extrahepatic cancers: a meta-analysis of observational cohort studies. Gut 2022;71:778–88.

60. Chen ZF, Dong XL, Huang QK, et al. The combined effect of non-alcoholic fatty liver disease and metabolic syndrome on colorectal carcinoma mortality: a retrospective in Chinese females. World J Surg Oncol 2018;16:163.

61. Zhang X, Wong GL, Yip TC, et al. Angiotensin-converting enzyme inhibitors prevent liver-related events in nonalcoholic fatty liver disease. Hepatology 2022;76: 469–82.

62. Golabi P, Otgonsuren M, de Avila L, et al. Components of metabolic syndrome increase the risk of mortality in nonalcoholic fatty liver disease (NAFLD). Medicine (Baltimore) 2018;97:e0214.

63. Kim D, Konyn P, Sandhu KK, et al. Metabolic dysfunction-associated fatty liver disease is associated with increased all-cause mortality in the United States. J Hepatol 2021;75:1284–91.

64. Kanwal F, Shubrook JH, Adams LA, et al. Clinical Care Pathway for the Risk Stratification and Management of Patients With Nonalcoholic Fatty Liver Disease. Gastroenterology 2021;161:1657–69.
65. Vilar-Gomez E, Martinez-Perez Y, Calzadilla-Bertot L, et al. Weight Loss Through Lifestyle Modification Significantly Reduces Features of Nonalcoholic Steatohepatitis. Gastroenterology 2015;149:367–78, e5; quiz e14-5.
66. Wong VW, Chan RS, Wong GL, et al. Community-based lifestyle modification programme for non-alcoholic fatty liver disease: a randomized controlled trial. J Hepatol 2013;59:536–42.
67. Wong VW, Wong GL, Chan RS, et al. Beneficial effects of lifestyle intervention in non-obese patients with non-alcoholic fatty liver disease. J Hepatol 2018;69: 1349–56.
68. Newsome PN, Buchholtz K, Cusi K, et al. A Placebo-Controlled Trial of Subcutaneous Semaglutide in Nonalcoholic Steatohepatitis. N Engl J Med 2021;384: 1113–24.
69. Loomba R, Abdelmalek MF, Armstrong M, et al. Semaglutide 2.4 mg once weekly improved liver and metabolic parameters, and was well tolerated, in patients with non-alcoholic steatohepatitis-related cirrhosis: a randomised, placebo-controlled phase 2 trial. J Hepatol 2022;77(S1):S10.
70. Hsiang JC, Wong VW. SGLT2 Inhibitors in Liver Patients. Clin Gastroenterol Hepatol 2020;18:2168–2172 e2.
71. Lange NF, Radu P, Dufour JF. Prevention of NAFLD-associated HCC: Role of lifestyle and chemoprevention. J Hepatol 2021;75:1217–27.
72. European Association for the Study of the Liver (EASL), European Association for the Study of Diabetes (EASD), European Association for the Study of Obesity (EASO). EASL-EASD-EASO Clinical Practice Guidelines for the management of non-alcoholic fatty liver disease. J Hepatol 2016;64:1388–402.
73. Eslam M, Sarin SK, Wong VW, et al. The Asian Pacific Association for the Study of the Liver clinical practice guidelines for the diagnosis and management of metabolic associated fatty liver disease. Hepatol Int 2020;14:889–919.

Hepatic Manifestations of Systemic Diseases

Humberto C. Gonzalez, MD[a,b],*, Stuart C. Gordon, MD[a,b]

KEYWORDS

- Tuberculosis • Brucellosis • Histoplasmosis • Covid-19 • Cytomegalovirus (CMV)
- Epstein-Barr (EBV) • Sarcoidosis • Amyloidosis

KEY POINTS

- Several systemic infectious and infiltrative diseases can affect the liver.
- Hepatic manifestations of systemic infections are more common and severe among immune-compromised patients (including those who are human immunodeficiency virus positive or transplant recipients).
- Liver manifestations of systemic infiltrative diseases may vary from relatively benign to acute liver failure and death.
- Signs and symptoms may be non-specific—such as elevated aminotransferases—or absent; clinical suspicion and careful differentials may be necessary for diagnosis.

INFECTIONS

Tuberculosis

Worldwide, tuberculosis (TB)—caused by *Mycobacterium tuberculosis*—accounts for approximately 10 million infections and 1.5 million deaths each year (**Table 1**).[1] In the United States, poverty (which may result in inadequate health care access) and human immunodeficiency virus (HIV)/acquired immunodeficiency syndrome (AIDS) are major contributors to TB prevalence. Approximately 20% of infections present with extrapulmonary TB (EPTB); risk factors for EPTB include female sex, non-US place of birth, and HIV infection.[2] Notably, the risk of EPTB among HIV+ persons increases with a declining cluster of differentiation 4 (CD4) counts.[3]

Gastrointestinal/hepatic TB may present as part of active pulmonary disease or as a primary infection, arising as a consequence of reactivation of latent TB, by ingestion or biliary secretion of the bacilli, or by hematogenous or lymphatic spread from a distant site or direct extension from adjacent tissues.[4] Studies suggest that hepatic TB occurs in roughly 1% of all cases of active TB, but lack of familiarity with this disease likely contributes to underreporting.[5]

[a] Division of Gastroenterology and Hepatology, Henry Ford Health, 2799 West Grand Boulevard, Detroit, MI 48202, USA; [b] Wayne State University School of Medicine, 540 E Canfield St, Detroit, MI 48201, USA
* Corresponding author.
E-mail address: hgonzal1@hfhs.org

Med Clin N Am 107 (2023) 465–489
https://doi.org/10.1016/j.mcna.2023.01.008
0025-7125/23/© 2023 Elsevier Inc. All rights reserved.

Table 1
Systemic illnesses affecting the liver

Systemic Illnesses Affecting the Liver			
Viral	**Bacterial**	**Spirochetal**	**Helminthic**
Adenovirus	Actinomycosis	*Leptospirosis**	Ascariasis
Chikungunya	*Brucellosis**	Lyme disease	Capillariasis
*COVID-19**	Campylobacter	Syphilis	Fascioliasis
Dengue	Cat scratch disease	**Rickettsial**	Opisthorchiasis
Ebola	Chlamydia	Ehrlichiosis	Schistosomiasis
Hepatitis A B C E	Leprosy	Q fever	**Protozoal**
Herpesviruses (HSV, EBV, CMV*, VZV)*	Listeriosis	Rocky mountain Spotted fever	Leishmaniasis
Lassa fever	*Tuberculosis**		Toxoplasmosis
Malaria	MAC	**Fungal**	Trypanosomiasis
Parvovirus B19	Melioidosis	Actinomycosis	**Malignant**
Rubella	Neisseria	Blastomycosis	Infiltrative HCC
Yellow fever	Nocardiosis	Candidiasis	Lymphoma
Infiltrative	Psittacosis	Coccidioidomycosis	Metastatic breast cancer
*Amyloidosis**	Salmonella	*Histoplasmosis**	Metastatic small cell
*Sarcoidosis**	Tularemia	Mucormycosis	lung cancer

Conditions marked with an (*) are covered in this review.

Hepatic TB can be variously categorized, based on presentation: (1) disseminated/ miliary TB, also known as micronodular TB; (2) local/granulomatous TB, also called granulomatous hepatitis; (3) isolated macronodular TB, also known as tuberculoma; and (4) hepatobiliary TB.[6] Miliary TB is the most common form, representing roughly 79% of cases, and results from the hematogenous spread of the infection. It usually involves the spleen and occurs with hepatosplenomegaly. Miliary TB may be mistaken for sarcoidosis, fungal abscess, or pneumocystis jirovecii.[4] Granulomatous TB presents with hepatomegaly, diffuse hepatic infiltration without recognizable pulmonary involvement, and elevated alkaline phosphatase (ALP).[7,8] The differential diagnosis of granulomatous TB is broad and includes brucellosis, listeriosis, Q fever, syphilis, and toxoplasmosis, among others.[8] Macronodular TB results after multiple hepatic granulomas have undergone caseation and liquefaction, which coalesce and form a larger tumor or tubercular abscess[7]; it may be mistaken for pyogenic abscess, metastatic disease, or other liver tumors.[9] Hepatobiliary TB comprises isolated hepatic, biliary, or hepatobiliary involvement, including tuberculous pseudotumor, tuberculous cholangitis, and tuberculous liver abscess.[10]

Biochemical and clinical manifestations of hepatic TB are generally nonspecific. In laboratory tests, hepatic TB presents with elevated ALP and gamma-glutamyl transferase; reversed albumin/globulin ratios, mild hyperbilirubinemia, and mild-to-moderate elevations of aspartate aminotransferase and alanine aminotransferase may also be observed.[11] Symptoms include fever (67%), respiratory symptoms (66%), abdominal pain (60%), and weight loss (57%). The most common signs include hepatomegaly (80%), splenomegaly (30%), ascites (23%), and jaundice (20%). Miliary TB is associated with more respiratory symptoms, whereas local TB presents more frequently with diffuse abdominal pain.[4,5]

Uncommon hepatic manifestations of TB include acute liver failure, which is a rare but universally fatal complication of systemic TB.[12,13] Liver failure has also been described during antituberculosis treatment; transplantation in these cases is frequently unsuccessful.[14] Portal hypertension can be caused by tuberculous lymph-adenopathy, splenic vein occlusion, or direct involvement of the liver and abdominal vasculature (including the portal vein); it may lead to the development of esophageal varices and variceal hemorrhage.[15,16] Multiple cases of obstructive jaundice resulting from tuberculous lymphadenitis have also been reported, as well as biliary stricture of the common bile duct, pancreatic head enlargement, or retroperitoneal abscess.[17] Painless jaundice and weight loss are cardinal symptoms. The condition may mimic cholangiocarcinoma or pancreatic cancer on imagining; endoscopic cholangiography with cytology may be required for diagnosis.[18]

Radiologically, miliary TB presents with tiny hypodense lesions on computed tomography (CT). Minimal peripheral enhancement is seen with intravenous contrast. However, lesions are frequently too small to be observed and hepatosplenomegaly may be the only finding. In more advanced cases, calcified lesions may be seen. Isolated TB is characterized by hepatomegaly and a single or multiple low attenuation lesions with central enhancement and a peripheral rim, or with calcifications in chronic cases.[19]

A diagnosis of hepatic TB should be suspected if hepatic granulomas are present when TB is diagnosed.[20] In TB endemic regions, hepatic granulomas warrant a course of anti-TB therapy.[21] In nonendemic regions, liver biopsy is generally necessary for diagnosis. Histology usually reveals necrotizing granulomas with central caseation, but this finding is not specific to TB; additional pathological characteristics that may assist the diagnosis include giant epithelioid and giant Langhans cells (**Fig. 1**). Biopsies should be sent for acid-fast bacilli (AFB) and mycobacterial culture, but the

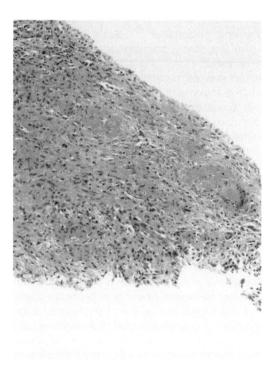

Fig. 1. Liver biopsy in a patient with hepatic tuberculosis. H&E stain. Multiple caseating (tuberculoid) granulomas. (*Courtesy of* Ejas Palathingal Bava MD, Sanam Husain MD and Brian K. Theisen MD. Department of Pathology Henry Ford Hospital.)

accuracy of both is limited; both sensitivity and specificity of AFB are low, and despite better sensitivity, the specificity of culture is limited. Polymerase chain reaction (PCR), with a sensitivity of ~86%, is recommended. Moreover, new testing modalities show promise. The Xpert MTB/RIF test, designed to identify pulmonary and meningeal TB, shows high sensitivity and specificity, shortens diagnosis time, and detects rifampicin resistance.[5] Although the accuracy of Xpert MTB/RIF has not been specifically assessed for hepatic TB, a Cochrane database analysis showed a sensitivity of greater than 80% for urine, bone, and other tissue, as well as a specificity of greater than 98% for cerebrospinal fluid, urine, and peritoneal fluid.[22,23]

A recent metanalysis determined that infant bacille Calmette-Guerin (BCG) vaccination was only protective against TB (including EPTB) in young children, but ineffective in adolescents and adults.[24] Standard treatment of hepatic TB is isoniazid, rifampicin, pyrazinamide, and ethambutol for 2 months, followed by isoniazid and rifampicin for 4 months.[25] However, drug-induced liver injury (DILI) is more likely to occur in patients with advanced liver disease and is a common reason for treatment interruptions. Routine biochemical monitoring is recommended.[25] If DILI occurs, streptomycin, levofloxacin, cycloserine, and ethambutol are alternative therapeutic options. Among HIV+ persons, immune reconstitution syndrome is a significant concern, particularly for those with low baseline and rapidly increasing CD4 counts.[26] Prednisone can be used for prevention or treatment.[27]

Brucellosis

Brucellosis—a zoonotic infection caused in humans by brucella species *Brucella melitensis*, *B abortus*, and *B suis*[28]—is most commonly acquired by the ingestion of unpasteurized milk from infected animals or by exposure (aerosolization) of laboratory specimens by processing personnel.[29,30] Human-to-human transmission is very rare, but may occur via pregnancy, breastfeeding, blood transfusion, bone marrow transplant, or sexual activity.[31]

Brucellosis can present in acute, subacute, or chronic forms; although it is rarely fatal, it frequently evolves into granulomatous disease, which may be debilitating.[29] Although it can affect any organ, brucellosis most commonly infects the reticuloendothelial system; as the largest reticuloendothelial organ, the liver is universally involved.[32] The most frequent symptom is tender hepatomegaly, but splenomegaly, undulant fever, weakness, lymphadenopathy, testicular swelling, and arthralgias are also common.[28,33] Biochemical profiles show mild-to-moderate elevation of aminotransferases in 25% of patients, inversely correlated with age.[34] Chronic hepatosplenic suppurative brucellosis (or brucelloma), characterized radiographically by a hypodense lesion with central calcification, is a rare and late complication most common in Mediterranean countries where *B melitensis* is prevalent.[35] These abscesses result from the bacteria's capacity to cause caseous necrosis. Symptoms tend to be insidious and prolonged.[36]

Diagnosis of brucellosis may be done via blood culture; yield depends on disease phase, prior antibiotic use, and methodology (lower for Ruiz-Castaneda and higher for centrifugation). Bone marrow culture, which provides higher sensitivity and shorter culture times, is superior when there has been prior antibiotic use. In facilities that have no access to culture, Rose Bengal can be used for screening, with positive confirmation by serum agglutination test, which is based on antibody reactivity against smooth lipopolysaccharide.[29] Limitations include low antibodies titers in early phases of infection, the persistence of antibodies after recovery from infection (affecting diagnostic value), and cross reactivity with gram-negative bacteria. Nucleic acid amplification tests can help diagnose brucellosis in a few hours; however, a positive test can also indicate low inoculum, DNA of dead bacteria, and a convalescent state.[30] Liver biopsy usually shows mild lobular or portal inflammation with lymphocytes; non-caseating granulomas are also common (**Fig. 2**).[37]

Owing to the ability of brucella to persist in macrophages, which may result in therapeutic failure and recurrence, 6 weeks of combined antibiotic treatment with doxycycline/gentamycin/streptomycin or doxycycline/rifampin is recommended. For deep abscesses (brucelloma), drainage or surgery plus antibiotic therapy are recommended.[38]

Leptospirosis

Leptospirosis is a zoonotic infection with broad geographic distribution, but is most commonly found in tropical regions. It infects 1 million individuals annually and is responsible for 60,000 deaths.[39] Pathogenic leptospira are excreted into the soil or water by infected animals (chronic carriers) from the renal tubules. They infect humans when the leptospira enters the body through skin abrasions, the oral cavity, and conjunctiva.[40]

Leptospirosis typically presents as a biphasic illness: anicteric (also known as acute or septicemic phase) and fulminant (icterohemorrhagic form). The acute phase, which usually lasts for roughly a week, is characterized by a febrile illness of sudden onset, but up to 70% of cases are subclinical. Additional symptoms in this phase include fever, myalgia, headache, nausea, vomiting, jaundice, conjunctival suffusion, and muscle tenderness (particularly the back and calves); these last two symptoms are classic physical findings. Fever resolution coincides with antibody formation and spirochete excretion in the urine. Recurrence of fever (3 to 4 days after remission) marks the initiation of the biphasic illness. Headache, retro-orbital pain, and photophobia resemble dengue. Mild rhabdomyolysis is common. Aseptic meningitis is seen in up to 25% of

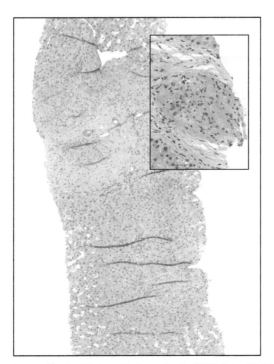

Fig. 2. Liver biopsy in a patient with hepatic brucellosis. H&E stain. Multiple, small, poorly formed granulomata without necrosis are seen in portal tracts and hepatic lobules. (*Courtesy of* Brian K. Theisen MD. Department of Pathology Henry Ford Hospital.)

cases. Weil's disease is the most severe form of the second phase of this illness, and it is characterized by jaundice, renal failure (non-oliguric), and bleeding. Bilirubin elevates to the 30 - 40 mg/dL range, likely resulting from cholestasis of sepsis. Indications associated with mortality include pulmonary involvement, hemodynamic instability, acute renal failure, hyperkalemia, and thrombocytopenia. The fatality rate is 5% to 15%.[41]

Diagnostic testing should be based on the stage of the disease: blood in the first week (leptospiremia), and urine in the second week (leptospiruria). Detection of pathogenic lepstospira species from sterile sites, positive PCR, detection by histology, immunostaining, or histochemistry, a microscopic agglutination test (MAT) titer of $\geq$1:400 or a fourfold MAT titer increase of acute or convalescent plasma is diagnostic of leptospirosis.[42] The BioFire Global Fever Panel, a multiplex nucleic acid amplification test, has been used to detect common agents of acute febrile illnesses and has a reported sensitivity of 94% and specificity of 99% for leptospirosis.[43]

The classic treatments for leptospirosis include penicillin and doxycycline; however, few randomized trials have been conducted; they have also yielded mixed results when assessing mortality, duration of fever, kidney dysfunction, and hospital stay.[39,44] Experts recommend doxycycline in early leptospirosis. Antibiotic use remains controversial in late and severe diseases but no study has found adverse effects. Corticosteroids are suggested in severe leptospirosis with pulmonary involvement.[44] Chemoprophylaxis with doxycycline has been suggested, but a Cochrane metanalysis found its efficacy questionable.[45,46]

Histoplasmosis

Histoplasmosis is caused by *Histoplasma capsulatum*, an organism present in bat guano, bird droppings, and soil contaminated with such material. Humans are infected by inhaling spores during cave exploration or via occupational exposure (eg, renovation or demolition of buildings, cleaning chicken coops, or pest waste removal).[47] Globally, 500,000 infections occur each year; 20% of these present as the disseminated form, which has a 30% to 50% mortality rate.[48] Histoplasmosis is endemic in Latin America, the Caribbean, parts of North America (in the Mississippi and Ohio River basins), Southeast Asia, and eastern Africa.[48,49]

After inhalation, histoplasma spores reach the alveoli and convert to a yeast form; in the lung, the organism is phagocytosed by macrophages and spreads via the lymphatic system to organs rich in reticuloendothelial cells before cellular immunity develops. Manifestations range from asymptomatic/self-limited disease to presentation with pulmonary involvement (acute, subacute, chronic cavitary, and nodules), mediastinal (adenitis, granuloma, and fibrosis), and progressive disseminated infections. Severity is generally dependent on host immune status; in immune-competent individuals, the infection is generally eliminated by cytokines, which can result in the formation of granulomas, but in immunosuppressed patients, the risk of more serious presentations increases.[47,48] This risk varies by patient age, degree of immunosuppression, and the size of the inoculum.[47,50]

Liver involvement occurs in 90% of disseminated histoplasmosis cases.[48] Symptoms are non-specific; fever, fatigue, nausea, vomiting, weight loss, elevated liver biochemistries, lymphadenopathy, splenomegaly, and hepatomegaly.[47,51] Primary liver histoplasmosis (without lung involvement) is quite rare and presentation varies, ranging from isolated liver lesions,[52] portal hypertension,[48] idiopathic granulomatous liver disease,[53] and hemophagocytic lymphohistocytosis syndrome.[54] Laboratory results vary according to the disease process, spanning from abnormal aminotransferases to jaundice with cholestasis.[55]

The gold standard for diagnosis of histoplasmosis is culture from a clinical specimen; a limitation of this approach is that growth can take up to 8 weeks, although 2 to 4 weeks is average. Gomori methenamine silver or periodic Acid-Schiff stains can be used to help identify budding yeast in histopathological specimens (**Fig. 3**).[56] Serological antibody tests (immunodiffusion, complement fixation, and enzyme immunoassay) are useful in the subacute and chronic forms of the disease, but accuracy suffers in immunocompromised patients.[47] Antigen tests are rapid, noninvasive, and accurate; they are generally used in urine and serum, but can also be used for cerebrospinal fluid and bronchial alveolar lavage specimens.[47,57] Response to treatment can also be monitored by antigen clearance.[58] Liver histology is characterized by lymphocytolytic inflammation and sinusoidal Kupffer cell hyperplasia. The fungal organisms are seen in the portal and sinusoidal macrophages. Discrete granulomas may be observed in the portal and lobular regions.[55]

Prompt initiation of antifungal therapy is critical for improving survival, especially in immunocompromised patients. The preferred treatment of the disseminated disease is liposomal amphotericin B for 1 to 2 weeks, followed by a minimum 12-month course of itraconazole.[48]

Coronavirus Disease-2019

Although coronavirus disease-2019 (COVID-19) is primarily a respiratory illness that may be complicated by pneumonia and acute respiratory distress syndrome, gastrointestinal symptoms—such as diarrhea, nausea, vomiting, and abdominal pain—are common and often precede respiratory symptoms.[59] Likewise, extra-pulmonary manifestations are

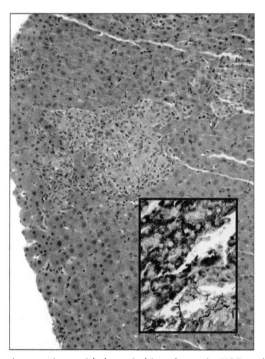

Fig. 3. Liver biopsy in a patient with hepatic histoplasmosis. H&E and GMS stain. Non-caseating granulomas in sinusoidal spaces with intracellular budding years forms are highlighted by GMS stain (*inset*). (*Courtesy* Sanam Husain and Brian Theisen MD Department of Pathology Henry Ford Hospital.)

well described and involve the cardiovascular, hematological, renal, gastrointestinal, hepatobiliary, endocrine, ophthalmological, and dermatological systems.[60,61] Risk factors for increased morbidity and mortality in COVID-19 infection include advancing age, obesity, diabetes, heart disease, malignancy, and chronic liver disease.[62,63] In patients with cirrhosis, increased 30-day mortality has been reported, particularly among those with more severe Model of End-stage Liver Disease and Child-Pugh classifications.[64,65] Nonalcoholic fatty liver disease (NAFLD) has been associated with worse COVID progression, a six-fold risk of severe disease, and longer viral shedding.[66,67]

Abnormal liver biochemistries are reported in 15% to 65% of COVID-19-infected patients.[68] Generally, values are mildly elevated at 1 to 2 times the upper limit of normal, with AST higher than ALT. Hyperbilirubinemia, hypoalbuminemia, and synthetic dysfunction are rare except in cases of severe disease.[68]

COVID has been associated with acute-on-chronic liver failure or acute decompensation in up to 20% of patients with cirrhosis.[69] Although specific evidence of severe acute respiratory syndrome coronavirus 2 (SARS-CoV2) hepatotropism is lacking, the liver is a potential target given its expression of ACE-2, which is 20-fold higher in cholangiocytes versus hepatocytes. Angiotensin converting enzyme 2 (ACE-2) is also expressed in the hepatic sinusoids and Kupffer cells.[60] Liver injury may be a result of multiple mechanisms; direct viral injury due to viral replication, DILI, hypoxia, shock, and ischemia.[70] Histologically, the liver shows steatosis, mild lymphocytic hepatitis, aggregate of Kupffer cells, and hepatocellular regenerative changes (**Fig. 4**).[71] Autopsy liver histopathology has shown steatosis (55%), congestion (35%) and vascular thrombosis (30%), fibrosis (20%), Kupffer cell hyperplasia (14%), portal inflammation (13%), and lobular inflammation (13%).[72]

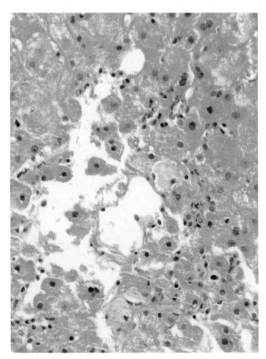

Fig. 4. Liver biopsy in a patient with COVID-19. H&E stain. Mild lobular inflammation with hepatocellular dropout and rare macrophages. (*Courtesy of* Ejas Palathingal Bava MD, Sanam Husain MD and Brian K. Theisen MD. Department of Pathology Henry Ford Hospital.)

Cases of COVID-associated cholangiopathy have been reported among a few patients 3 to 4 months after recovery from severe COVID. Possible causes include ischemic injury related to microvascular coagulopathy, hypotension secondary to sepsis, and/or viral injury of the biliary epithelium, given its high ACE-2 levels.[73] The syndrome is characterized by elevated ALP, hyperbilirubinemia, variable elevation of aminotransferases, and bile duct injury on imaging. Beading of the intrahepatic bile duct resembles sclerosing cholangitis. On biopsy, acute and/or chronic large duct obstruction without clear bile duct loss is observed. There is no specific treatment of this syndrome and few patients have been referred for a liver transplant.

Corticosteroids, convalescent plasma, neutralizing antibodies, tocilizumab, and remdesivir have been used to treat COVID-19, but there are no specific medications to treat the liver-associated manifestations.[74] Primary prevention via vaccination remains the first line of defense. Multiple vaccines have been developed worldwide; as of November 2022, 12.8 billion doses have been administered.[75] mRNA vaccines are one of the most common and have been widely used. These have shown a high degree of efficacy in preventing symptomatic illness, severe disease, hospitalization, and mortality.[76,77] Vaccines for COVID-19 have associated local and systemic side effects, presenting in 13% to 33% of patients. These are described as moderate in frequency, mild in severity, and short-lived.[78] However, there are recent descriptions of a very rare side effect of the BNT162b2 mRNA vaccine — an autoimmune-like hepatitis that is CD8 T-cell predominant. This condition responds to corticosteroids and immunosuppressants.[79]

Cytomegalovirus

Cytomegalovirus (CMV) is a double-stranded DNA virus that belongs to the herpesvirus family (HHV-5). Infection is associated with a wide range of clinical presentations, from asymptomatic to mononucleosis, congenital CMV, and severe disease. Host immune status impacts the risk of severe manifestations, particularly among transplant recipients and HIV-infected individuals.[80] CMV seroprevalence is roughly 85% in population-based studies, but rises to greater than 90% in HIV patients.[81,82] Prevalence is inversely related to the socioeconomic development of a country, being more prevalent in the Global South and Asia, and less common in Europe and the United States.[81,83,84] In the United States, seroprevalence increases with age, from 36% among children 6 to 11 years old to 91% among those greater than 90 years.[85] Ethnicity also plays a role, with rates 20% to 30% higher in non-white compared populations.[84]

CMV infection generally occurs during childhood or early adulthood. Transmission occurs due to exposure to bodily fluids, or through blood transfusions and organ transplantation. Primary CMV infection is generally asymptomatic but can also present as mononucleosis, with fever and lymphadenopathy. After a self-limited course, CMV remains in a latent form in fibroblasts, epithelial, endothelial, and muscle cells where it replicates and travels via monocytes and circulating endothelial cells to distant areas of the body.[80] Secondary infection presents later in life, reflecting reactivation or reinfection with a new strain.[86]

Primary infection leads to CMV-specific IgM and later IgG antibody formation.[87] Intermittent reactivation in immunocompetent individuals leads to immunologic memory activation which offers effective viral replication control.[88] However, in HIV-positive individuals and transplant recipients (solid or hematopoietic stem cell), CMV-specific CD4+ and CD8+ T cells are lost, allowing unchecked viral replication and clinical disease.[89]

Diagnosis of CMV is established with PCR testing, or by a fourfold rise in paired CMV-IgM and CMV-IgG specimens drawn 2 weeks apart. Symptomatic CMV in the immunocompetent host usually presents with a mononucleosis like-syndrome characterized by fever, atypical lymphocytes, lymphadenopathy, and negative heterophile antibody testing. In comparison to the Epstein–Barr virus, CMV-mononucleosis has less lymphadenopathy, splenomegaly, and tonsillar exudates.[90] Most patients (90%) will have abnormal liver biochemistries, usually greater than 3 times ULN, and up to a third have hepatomegaly.[91] Granulomatous hepatitis with a sinusoidal fibrin ring of lymphocytes and eosinophilic infiltrates has been described in association with CMV.[92] Rare cases of liver failure requiring transplantation have been reported.[93] Non-malignant non-cirrhotic portal venous system thrombosis (PVT) has been linked to CMV infection; it should be suspected in patients with recent mononucleosis-like symptoms and new onset PVT. Notably, more than half of CMV-associated PVTs have been related to the prothrombin G20210A gene variant, suggesting a synergistic effect.[94]

In solid organ transplantation, donor and recipient CMV serostatus determine infection risk. Primary infection occurs when a CMV-seropositive (D+) allograft is transplanted to a CMV-seronegative recipient (R-).[95] In this setting the recipient has no preexisting immunity, and with the addition of immunosuppression, is unable to control the infection. This D+/R- CMV mismatch constitutes the highest risk scenario for CMV infection.[80] Secondary infection occurs in CMV-seropositive recipients (R+), due to reactivation (CMV negative donor) or superinfection (positive donor), usually in the setting of intense immunosuppression (eg, use of anti-thymocyte-immunoglobulin).[95] In this setting, CMV can present with a subclinical course or with a symptomatic disease which can be further subdivided into CMV syndrome and tissue-invasive disease. In the subclinical presentation, the CMV virus is detected in the bloodstream without any signs or symptoms of the disease. CMV syndrome generally occurs with fever, malaise, and myelosuppression. The tissue-invasive disease generally involves the gastrointestinal tract and the transplanted allograft.[80] Indirect effects of CMV in solid organ transplant recipients include predisposition to other opportunistic infections and acute and chronic allograft injury.[95,96]

In bone marrow transplant recipients, allogenic stimulation and immunosuppression to prevent rejection and graft-versus-host disease increase the risk of CMV disease. Allogenic-hematopoietic cell transplant recipients (HSCT) are at higher risk of CMV compared with autologous HSCT.[97] In contrast to solid organ transplantation, CMV-positive serostatus in recipients confers the highest risk of disease, approaching an incidence of 70% with seronegative donors (D-/R+; reversed mismatch).[98]

Diagnosis of CMV hepatitis requires a liver biopsy to identify viral inclusions and antigens by immunohistochemistry.[99] PCR in sera is commonly used to assist in the diagnosis and allows monitoring of disease activity. Antigenemia tests and cultures have limitations and are not generally used.[100] Liver biopsy findings depend on host immune status. In immunocompromised patients, the direct viral cytopathic effect allows more extensive necrosis and the classic mononuclear inflammatory infiltrate is less prominent than in immunocompetent patients. Microabscesses are common in liver transplant recipients with CMV hepatitis, whereas giant cell granulomas are seen in immunocompetent individuals (**Fig. 5**).[100]

Treatment is generally not necessary in immunocompetent persons with asymptomatic illness or mononucleosis like-syndrome, as the disease is self-limited; if the illness is protracted, antiviral therapies may be used. Among solid organ transplant recipients, at least 3 months of prophylaxis and CMV monitoring with preemptive therapy when positive are standard. The preferred treatment regimens are valganciclovir or ganciclovir, which have similar efficacy. Foscarnet and cidofovir are reserved for UL97 (enzyme required for the activation of ganclyclovir) resistant cases given its nephrotoxic effects.[100] In CMV-positive HSCT recipients, letermovir is indicated for prophylaxis and treatment; this drug exerts its antiviral effect by interfering with the pUL56 gene and disrupts the viral terminase complex.[101] Maribavir, a CMV enzyme

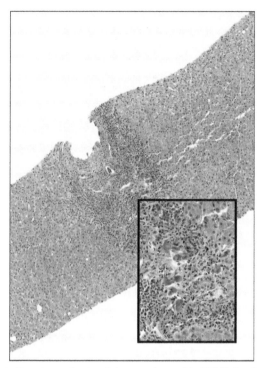

Fig. 5. Liver biopsy in liver transplant recipient patient with CMV infection. H&E stain. Intranuclear owls eye inclusions and intracytoplasmic eosinophilic inclusions (*inset*). (*Courtesy of* Brian K. Theisen MD and Sanam Husain Department of Pathology Henry Ford Hospital.)

pUL97 kinase inhibitor, is now approved for the treatment of post-transplant infection/disease that is refractory to ganciclovir, valganciclovir, cidofovir or foscarnet.[102]

Epstein–Barr Virus

Epstein-Barr virus (EBV) is a linear double-stranded DNA virus that belongs to the herpes virus (HHV4) family. Infection is nearly universal, with the prevalence of more than 90% of the adult population worldwide. EBV is generally acquired during childhood or adolescence by exposure to infected oral secretions. The virus replicates in oropharyngeal cells and is shed into the saliva.[103,104] EBV can also be transmitted through blood transfusions or transplantation of bone marrow or solid organs.[105] Infection involves interaction with the host B cells, replication, viral genome changes, and establishment of latency.[103,104] Presentation varies, ranging from minimal to no symptoms, to mononucleosis syndrome, chronic active EBV, and lymphoproliferative cancers.

Primary EBV infection in infants and children is usually asymptomatic; however, adolescents and adults generally present with infectious mononucleosis. EBV is responsible for 90% of all mononucleosis cases, over half of which is characterized by fever, lymphadenopathy, and pharyngitis.[104,106] Roughly 10% to 20% of patients also present with splenomegaly, hepatomegaly, palatal petechiae, periorbital and eyelid edema, as well as rash, generally after exposure to penicillin derivatives.[104,105] Rare complications include aplastic anemia, thrombocytopenia, myocarditis, genital ulcerations, Guillain-Barre syndrome, encephalitis, and meningitis.[104] Splenic rupture is a rare (0.1% to 0.2%) complication of acute mononucleosis that occurs as a consequence of splenomegaly and disrupted splenic architecture. Because it is usually seen in young athletes involved in contact sports, patients are recommended to refrain from physical activity for 3 weeks after diagnosis.[106]

Classic findings in infectious mononucleosis include lymphocytosis, atypical lymphocytes, and heterophile antibodies. In 75% of cases, there are signs of hepatocellular injury, with elevated ALT; this may be subclinical and generally normalizes in 2 to 3 weeks. Less frequently, a mixed or cholestatic pattern can present. Cholestasis is thought to be secondary to bile duct inflammation and canalicular transport dysfunction,[107] and usually presents with elevated bilirubin (avg 12 mg/dL) and ALP (avg 750 iu/L).[108] Acute liver failure due to EBV accounts for less than 1% of US cases reported by the Acute Liver Failure Study Group.[109]

EBV is known to be a trigger of classic autoimmune hepatitis (AIH, type 1 and 2), 3 to 5 months after infection. Chronic active EBV can also mimic AIH triggered by EBV. Differentiation is critical as AIH responds favorably to immunosuppression, whereas chronic active EBV does not. EBV-induced AIH generally presents with declining EBV-IgM titers at the time of positive autoimmune markers, absence of the virus and EBV-encoded RNA in peripheral mononuclear cells, and classic liver histology for AIH.[110] EBV has also been linked to granulomatous hepatitis,[111] vanishing bile duct syndrome,[112] and viral-precipitated ACLF.[113]

In rare instances, EBV-infected patients develop chronic active EBV disease. This lymphoproliferative disorder presents in otherwise healthy individuals with acute EBV, in whom mononucleosis-like symptoms persist and progress (>6 months). It is characterized by elevated levels of the virus in blood, high levels of viral RNA in protein or tissues, and histologic evidence of end-organ damage. The most common symptoms are fever, lymphadenopathy, and thrombocytopenia; less common are hepatomegaly, anemia, bone marrow hypoplasia, rash, hypersensitivity to mosquito bites, oral ulcers, uveitis, hemophagocytic syndrome, coronary artery aneurysms, liver failure, lymphoma, and interstitial pneumonia. This illness has mainly been described among patients in whom the virus is detected within T cells or NK cells, versus B cells; Asian and Native American patients appear to be at higher risk than other groups. Currently, the only effective treatment is HSCT, as patients otherwise experience progressive immunodeficiency and die from infections or lymphoproliferative disease.[104,114]

Nasopharyngeal carcinoma, gastric carcinoma, Hodgkin's lymphoma, Burkitt's lymphoma, diffuse large B Cell lymphoma, and extranodal NK/T-cell lymphoma have been associated with EBV virus. However, only a small fraction of the EBV-infected population develops such cancers, given that multiple factors (environmental, genetics, co-infections, etc.) influence the risk.[103]

Post-transplant lymphoproliferative disorder (PTLD) is a group of lymphoid conditions—ranging from indolent polyclonal proliferation to aggressive lymphomas—that complicate solid organ and bone marrow transplants.[110] Incidence varies by transplanted organ, from 1% of liver and 2% to 5% of a kidney transplant, to 20% of intestine transplants. EBV-driven B cell proliferation in the setting of chronic T-cell immunosuppression is the likely mechanism, although 30% of PTLD cases are EBV-negative.[115] Extranodal disease is the most common presentation, with symptoms related to the site involved. A biopsy is the diagnostic gold standard.[110] In contrast to other solid organ transplants, PTLD after a liver transplant tends to present with liver involvement.[110,116] Lymphomas in this setting tend to be high-grade and aggressive.[117] Treatment involves reduction of immunosuppression, as well as rituximab alone or in combination with cytotoxic chemotherapy for CD20+ PTLD.[118]

On histopathology, EBV hepatitis presents with diffuse single file or "string of beads" lymphocytic infiltrate in the portal tracts, which tend to be expanded (**Fig. 6**). Less

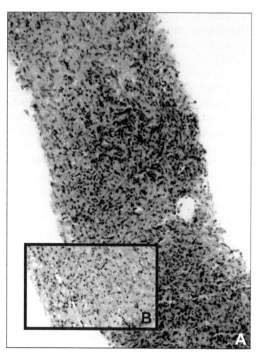

Fig. 6. Liver biopsy in a patient with EBV. H&E. Diffuse sinusoidal dense lymphocytic infiltrate (A) with positive EBV (EBER) stain (*inset* B). (*Courtesy of* Ejas Palathingal Bava MD, Sanam Husain MD and Brian K. Theisen MD. Department of Pathology Henry Ford Hospital.)

commonly, fibrin ring granulomas, endotheliolitis, bile duct damage, and erythrophagocytosis are observed. PCR and in situ hybridization staining of EBV-encoded RNA can assist in the diagnosis.[119]

The majority of EBV infections require only supportive care and no specific treatment as they resolve spontaneously. In EBV-hepatitis, anti-viral medications such as ganciclovir and valganciclovir—with or without corticosteroids—have been used successfully.[110,120] For chronic active EBV hepatitis, the antivirals IVIG and IFN have shown response.[114] In PTLD, reduction of immunosuppression and administration of rituximab, with cytotoxic chemotherapy in selected cases, is recommended.[118] In EBV-related acute liver failure, a transplant may be the only course of action.[109]

INFILTRATIVE DISEASES
Sarcoidosis

Sarcoidosis is a multisystemic inflammatory disease characterized by the formation of non-caseating granulomas. It primarily affects the lungs, and 50% of cases also present with extrapulmonary involvement,[121] most commonly the lymph nodes, liver, skin, eyes, or a combination of these sites.[122] Although the exact pathogenesis of sarcoidosis remains unknown, a combination of environmental, genetic, and immunologic factors are believed to be responsible. As a result, prevalence varies widely in different regions and ethnic groups. In parts of Asia (Japan, South Korea, and Taiwan) prevalence ranges from 1 to 5 cases per 100,000, whereas in countries like Sweden and Canada, prevalence is 30 to 100 times higher (140 to 160 cases per 100,000). In the United States, the prevalence is highest among African

Americans. Peak incidence is in middle-aged adults, with a slight predominance among women.[123] The clinical course is also highly variable, ranging from spontaneous resolution to chronic fibrosis and/or irreversible organ failure, and management remains challenging.[122]

Hepatic sarcoidosis is common, as documented in 50% to 70% of cases in an autopsy series. It is more frequently associated with lung parenchymal involvement versus hilar lymphadenopathy.[124] Isolated hepatic sarcoidosis is rare (<5% of cases). Liver-related symptoms usually encompass fatigue, pruritus, abdominal pain (from Glisson's capsule distention, 15%), hepatosplenomegaly (50% to 70%), and fever (3% to 28%); additional symptoms include nausea, vomiting, and arthralgia, but jaundice is rare.[124–126] However, the majority of cases remain asymptomatic, with only 11% to 30% of patients having a clinically significant disease.[124,127]

Hepatic sarcoidosis can be complicated by portal hypertension, with gastrointestinal hemorrhage from varices as the presenting symptom. Although portal hypertension in this setting may be secondary to cirrhosis, it more commonly occurs as a consequence of presinusoidal hypertension from portal granulomas and fibrosis.[128] Granulomatous phlebitis of the hepatic and portal veins have also been described as contributors to portal hypertension.[129] Budd-Chiari syndrome has been noted to be a very rare complication of hepatic sarcoidosis; it is presumed that external compression of the hepatic veins or its involvement by sarcoid granulomas results in narrowing of the lumen, leading to stasis and thrombotic occlusion.[130,131] Only ~6% of patients with hepatic sarcoidosis develop cirrhosis,[132] which is thought to be secondary to fibrosis from granulomatous inflammation or vascular injury.[124]

The diagnosis of hepatic sarcoidosis is challenging, generally requiring a combination of laboratory, clinical, and histological tests.[133] Cholestatic liver diseases, primary biliary cholangitis, primary sclerosing cholangitis, DILI, and lymphoma must be excluded.[134]

Sarcoidosis results in the elevation of ALP and/or gamma-glutamyl transpeptidase (cholestatic pattern), roughly 3 times the upper limit of normal (ULN). Aminotransferases may also be elevated, usually less than two times the ULN.[127] Degree of elevation correlates with histopathological changes, granulomatous inflammation, and severity of fibrosis.[135] Other biochemical abnormalities may include hypercalcemia, which may be observed in 10% to 20% of cases. High levels of ACE have low sensitivity, but in conjunction with other pulmonary tests can assist in differentiating sarcoidosis from antimitochondrial antibody-negative primary biliary cholangitis.[133,136] Hepatosplenomegaly, hepatic heterogeneity, and lymphadenopathy are commonly noted on imaging (ultrasound, CT, or MRI). Small (0.5 to 1.5 cm) hypodense focal hepatic lesions with or without calcifications may be observed and confused with metastatic disease; T2-weighted MRI sequences can help differentiate both entities.[137,138]

On biopsy, the typical finding is a non-caseating granuloma composed of mononuclear cells, usually macrophages that are sometimes multinucleated, and giant cells. The rim has lymphocytes and fibroblasts. Ziehl-Neelsen, Grocott, and GMS stains are negative. Additional findings include an inflammatory infiltrate in the portal and lobular regions, granulomas of different ages, areas of focal necrosis, ductopenia, and intrahepatic cholestasis (**Fig. 7**).[124,127,139]

The majority of patients with hepatic sarcoidosis are asymptomatic and generally do not require specific treatment.[121] Spontaneous improvement of biochemical abnormalities have been documented, making the necessity and timing of therapy unclear. Treatment indications are often guided by extra-hepatic manifestations.[124] In subjects with symptomatic liver disease, at risk of severe complications or cholestasis, pharmacological therapy should be offered.[121] However, there are currently

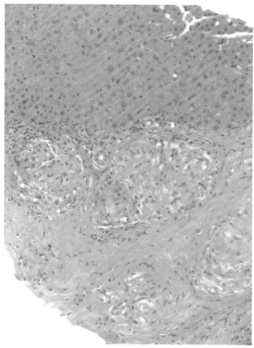

Fig. 7. Liver biopsy in a patient with sarcoidosis. Multiple, non-caseating granulomata with epithelioid histiocytes and subtle lymphoid cuff. (*Courtesy of* Sanam Husain MD and Brian K. Theisen MD. Department of Pathology Henry Ford Hospital.)

no guidelines or standardized treatments. Corticosteroids have long been the backbone of therapy; the rate of response, either complete or partial, ranges from 60% to 83%. The impact of corticosteroids on disease progression is not clearly understood. A small case series of biochemical responders to corticosteroids showed that 60% of patients had histological improvement and 40% progressed to cirrhosis.[140] In chronic cholestasis with portal hypertension, corticosteroids improve symptoms and hepatomegaly but do not prevent the progression of the disease. Corticosteroids are generally administered for 4 to 6 weeks at 20 to 40 mg a day, followed by a 5 to 10 mg taper for 4 to 8 weeks. Tapering or discontinuation can lead to recrudescence of the disease.[121]

Ursodeoxycholic acid (UDCA) is generally prescribed for cholestasis or bile duct injury associated with hepatic sarcoidosis. A retrospective study comparing UCDA, prednisolone, or no treatment in symptomatic hepatic sarcoidosis showed that UCDA resulted in greater improvement in pruritus, fatigue, and liver biochemistries.[141] The usual UDCA dose is 10 to 15 mg/kg/d. For individuals who are steroids-dependent, non-responders, or intolerant, azathioprine (50 to 150 mg/d) and methotrexate (10 to 15 mg/wk) have been used.[121,142] Other options include cyclosporine, cyclophosphamide, thalidomide, pentoxifylline, and infliximab.[121] Anti-TNF agents may be useful in necrotizing sarcoidosis.[143] Liver transplantation may be required in advanced hepatic sarcoidosis, with similar 1-, 3-, 5-, and 10- year post-transplant survival to cholestatic liver disease.[144] However, sarcoidosis can recur in the transplanted liver allograft. This is generally managed with corticosteroids.[121]

Amyloidosis

Amyloidosis is a group of disorders secondary to misfolding of extracellular proteins, with subsequent deposition in tissues, causing organ dysfunction. The aberrant precursor protein defines the specific amyloid type. Diagnosis requires histopathological confirmation using Congo red dye to show green birefringence under cross-polarized light.[145] Amyloidosis can occur as a systemic disease, where amyloidogenic protein is produced by an organ (bone marrow, liver, etc.) and deposited in a distant site, or as a localized process where abnormal amyloid is both produced and deposited in the same organ.[146] At least 36 different pathogenic amyloid proteins have been described, 17 of which are known to cause systemic disease.[147] Amyloidosis can be a hereditary or acquired disorder, and can manifest with the following syndromes: systemic amyloid light chain (AL); systemic amyloid A (AA); hereditary transthyretin amyloid (ATTR); beta2-microglobulin (B2M); and senile amyloidosis.

Systemic AL amyloidosis is the most common type seen in the developed world. It is usually seen in patients with hematologic disorders, including 15% observed in patients with multiple myeloma. Manifestations relate to the affected organ: proteinuria with kidney infiltration, gastrointestinal dysfunction when there is autonomic systemic affection, and restrictive cardiomyopathy in cardiac involvement.[145] In systemic AL amyloidosis, the liver is a common site of amyloid deposition, and the key manifestations include hepatomegaly (80%) and ALP in the 500 mg/dL range (86%). The infiltration with amyloid enlarges the liver and gives it an elastic rubbery appearance.[145,148] Portal hypertension has been described as a rare consequence of sinusoidal infiltration by amyloid.[149] Indicators of poor prognosis include heart failure, platelets greater than 500*10^9/L, and elevated bilirubin.[148] Liver biopsy-associated bleeding has been reported; spontaneous liver rupture is an exceedingly rare occurrence.[148] Treatment is targeted to eliminate the amyloidogenic light chain production by plasma cells. Initial therapy is with bortezomib-based treatment regimens, which generally induce rapid and effective responses.[146,150]

Systemic AA amyloidosis is associated with neoplastic, infectious, or inflammatory disorders. The pathogenic fibrils are derived from the acute phase reactants in the serum. Rheumatoid arthritis accounts for almost half of AA amyloidosis cases. Crohn's disease, lupus, primary biliary cholangitis, and ankylosing spondylitis have also been linked. Proteinuric kidney disease is the universal manifestation.[145] In systemic AA amyloidosis, the liver is involved in roughly 20% of cases, with ALP elevated to 1.5 times the ULN and hepatomegaly in less than 10% of cases.[151] Liver involvement is regarded as a feature of advanced disease. Treatment is directed toward controlling the inflammatory etiology.[145]

Hereditary systemic amyloidosis is a rare autosomal dominant disorder with variable penetrance, resulting from a single amino acid substitution in the TTR gene. Over 100 pathogenic mutations have now been described, the most common being TTR V30M. This aberrant protein is produced by the liver, resulting in sensory and autonomic neuropathy, as well as cardiomyopathy that progresses to wasting, malnutrition, and death within 3 to 15 years of diagnosis.[145,152] Carpal tunnel syndrome, usually bilateral, precedes the diagnosis by 5 to 10 years in 30% to 50% of patients.[146] Historically, the only disease-modifying therapeutic strategy was liver transplantation, as the liver is the main source of unstable protein production. The 5-year survival rate is excellent—nearly 100% for those with a V30 mutation and 59% for non-TTR V30. Worse survival is noted in late-onset and long duration of the disease, cardiomyopathy, and malnutrition. Sepsis and cardiac complications are the main causes of death after a liver transplant. Liver/kidney or liver/heart transplantation has been attempted

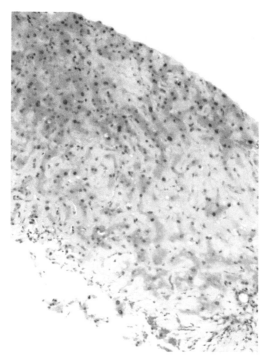

Fig. 8. Liver biopsy in a patient with amyloidosis. H&E stain. Sinusoidal amorphous pink deposits are consistent with amyloidosis. (*Courtesy of* Ejas Palathingal Bava MD, Sanam Husain MD and Brian K. Theisen MD. Department of Pathology Henry Ford Hospital.)

in small series and constitutes a reasonable alternative (in experienced centers) for those patients with advanced kidney disease or heart failure.[153] Early hepatic artery thrombosis is a known complication.[154,155] Domino or sequential transplantation with a TTR liver is an option for selected patients with end-stage liver disease; however, neuropathy can present as early as within 6 years.[154,156] In randomized clinical trials that included V30 and non-V30 mutation patients, diflunisal (TTR stabilizer), patisiran (TTR small interfering RNA), and inotersen (TTR antisense oligonucleide) reduced peripheral neuropathy as compared with placebo,[157–159] constituting reasonable treatment options.

Liver histology in amyloidosis includes portal fibrosis and inflammation, fatty infiltration, passive congestion, and iron deposition. Bile duct injury, interface hepatitis, and atrophy of the hepatic cords due to amyloid infiltration of the sinusoids have been described. Deposition of AA amyloid in the liver is generally seen in the blood vessels, whereas in non-AA amyloid, deposits appear in a mixed pattern, blood vessels, sinusoids, and portal stroma (**Fig. 8**).[160]

CLINICS CARE POINTS

- Disseminated or miliary tuberculosis is the most common presentation of hepatic tuberculosis and generally presents with fever, hepatomegaly and respiratory symptoms
- Hepatomegaly is a common feature of tuberculosis, brucellosis, histoplasmosis, cytomegalovirus, Epstein Barr infection, sarcoidosis and amyloidosis

- The combination of immunosuppressed state, cholestatic liver panel and fever should alert for uncommon illnesses that affect the liver
- Liver histology can assist in clarifying infiltrative, infectious and malignant processes involving the liver, as symptoms related to these illnesses tend to be non-specific

DISCLOSURE

The authors have nothing to disclose.

REFERENCES

1. WHO. Global tuberculosis report 2020. Geneva (Switzerland): World Health Organization; 2020.
2. Peto HM, Pratt RH, Harrington TA, et al. Epidemiology of extrapulmonary tuberculosis in the United States, 1993-2006. Clin Infect Dis 2009;49:1350–7.
3. Jones BE, Young SM, Antoniskis D, et al. Relationship of the manifestations of tuberculosis to CD4 cell counts in patients with human immunodeficiency virus infection. Am Rev Respir Dis 1993;148:1292–7.
4. Eraksoy H. Gastrointestinal and abdominal tuberculosis. Gastroenterol Clin North Am 2021;50:341–60.
5. Hickey AJ, Gounder L, Moosa MY, et al. A systematic review of hepatic tuberculosis with considerations in human immunodeficiency virus co-infection. BMC Infect Dis 2015;15:209.
6. Gordon S, Gonzalez H. Hepatic manifestations of systemic disease. In: Schiff E, Maddrey W, Reddy K, editors. Schiff's diseases of the liver. 12th edition. Hoboken, NJ: Wiley-Blackwell; 2017. p. 218.
7. Sonika U, Kar P. Tuberculosis and liver disease: management issues. Trop Gastroenterol 2012;33:102–6.
8. Choudhury A, Shukla J, Mahajan G, et al. Hepatic tuberculosis: myriad of hues. Germs 2021;11:310–3.
9. Kwan CK, Ernst JD. HIV and tuberculosis: a deadly human syndemic. Clin Microbiol Rev 2011;24:351–76.
10. Alvarez SZ. Hepatobiliary tuberculosis. J Gastroenterol Hepatol 1998;13:833–9.
11. Chien RN, Lin PY, Liaw YF. Hepatic tuberculosis: comparison of miliary and local form. Infection 1995;23:5–8.
12. Toptas T, Ilhan B, Bilgin H, et al. Miliary tuberculosis induced acute liver failure. Case Rep Infect Dis 2015;2015:759341.
13. Hussain W, Mutimer D, Harrison R, et al. Fulminant hepatic failure caused by tuberculosis. Gut 1995;36:792–4.
14. Bartoletti M, Martelli G, Tedeschi S, et al. Liver transplantation is associated with good clinical outcome in patients with active tuberculosis and acute liver failure due to anti-tubercular treatment. Transpl Infect Dis 2017;19:e12658.
15. Jazet IM, Perk L, De Roos A, et al. Obstructive jaundice and hematemesis: two cases with unusual presentations of intra-abdominal tuberculosis. Eur J Intern Med 2004;15:259–61.
16. Mojtahedzadeh M, Otoukesh S, Shahsafi MR, et al. Case report: portal hypertension secondary to isolated liver tuberculosis. Am J Trop Med Hyg 2012;87:162–4.
17. Ocak Serin S, Isiklar A, Cakit H, et al. A case of tuberculosis presented by obstructive jaundice tuberculosis-related mechanical icterus. J Infect Dev Ctries 2020;14:1221–4.

18. Inal M, Aksungur E, Akgül E, et al. Biliary tuberculosis mimicking cholangiocarcinoma: treatment with metallic biliary endoprothesis. Am J Gastroenterol 2000; 95:1069–71.

19. Ladumor H, Al-Mohannadi S, Ameerudeen FS, et al. TB or not TB: a comprehensive review of imaging manifestations of abdominal tuberculosis and its mimics. Clin Imaging 2021;76:130–43.

20. Diaz ML, Herrera T, Lopez-Vidal Y, et al. Polymerase chain reaction for the detection of Mycobacterium tuberculosis DNA in tissue and assessment of its utility in the diagnosis of hepatic granulomas. J Lab Clin Med 1996;127:359–63.

21. Puri A. Hepatic tuberculosis. Indian J Tubercul 1994;41:131.

22. Kohli M, Schiller I, Dendukuri N, et al. Xpert(®) MTB/RIF assay for extrapulmonary tuberculosis and rifampicin resistance. Cochrane Database Syst Rev 2018;(8):CD012768.

23. Kohli M, Schiller I, Dendukuri N, et al. Xpert MTB/RIF Ultra and Xpert MTB/RIF assays for extrapulmonary tuberculosis and rifampicin resistance in adults. Cochrane Database Syst Rev 2021;(1):CD012768.

24. Martinez L, Cords O, Liu Q, et al. Infant BCG vaccination and risk of pulmonary and extrapulmonary tuberculosis throughout the life course: a systematic review and individual participant data meta-analysis. Lancet Glob Health 2022;10: e1307–16.

25. Sharma SK, Ryan H, Khaparde S, et al. Index-TB guidelines: guidelines on extrapulmonary tuberculosis for India. Indian J Med Res 2017;145:448–63.

26. Xue M, Xie R, Pang Y, et al. Prevalence and risk factors of paradoxical tuberculosis associated immune reconstitution inflammatory syndrome among HIV-infected patients in Beijing, China. BMC Infect Dis 2020;20:554.

27. Meintjes G, Stek C, Blumenthal L, et al. Prednisone for the prevention of paradoxical tuberculosis-associated IRIS. N Engl J Med 2018;379:1915–25.

28. Liu CM, Suo B, Zhang Y. Analysis of clinical manifestations of acute and chronic brucellosis in patients admitted to a public general hospital in Northern China. Int J Gen Med 2021;14:8311–6.

29. Franco MP, Mulder M, Gilman RH, et al. Human brucellosis. Lancet Infect Dis 2007;7:775–86.

30. Di Bonaventura G, Angeletti S, Ianni A, et al. Microbiological laboratory diagnosis of human brucellosis: an overview. Pathogens 2021;10:1623.

31. Tuon FF, Gondolfo RB, Cerchiari N. Human-to-human transmission of Brucella - a systematic review. Trop Med Int Health 2017;22:539–46.

32. Akritidis N, Tzivras M, Delladetsima I, et al. The liver in brucellosis. Clin Gastroenterol Hepatol 2007;5:1109–12.

33. Ozturk-Engin D, Erdem H, Gencer S, et al. Liver involvement in patients with brucellosis: results of the Marmara study. Eur J Clin Microbiol Infect Dis 2014; 33:1253–62.

34. Gür A, Geyik MF, Dikici B, et al. Complications of brucellosis in different age groups: a study of 283 cases in southeastern Anatolia of Turkey. Yonsei Med J 2003;44:33–44.

35. Heller T, Bélard S, Wallrauch C, et al. Patterns of hepatosplenic brucella abscesses on cross-sectional imaging: a review of clinical and imaging features. Am J Trop Med Hyg 2015;93:761–6.

36. Ariza J, Pigrau C, Cañas C, et al. Current understanding and management of chronic hepatosplenic suppurative brucellosis. Clin Infect Dis 2001;32:1024–33.

37. Young EJ, Hasanjani Roushan MR, Shafae S, et al. Liver histology of acute brucellosis caused by Brucella melitensis. Hum Pathol 2014;45:2023–8.

38. Bosilkovski M, Keramat F, Arapović J. The current therapeutical strategies in human brucellosis. Infection 2021;49:823–32.
39. Guzmán Pérez M, Blanch Sancho JJ, Segura Luque JC, et al. Current evidence on the antimicrobial treatment and chemoprophylaxis of human leptospirosis: a meta-analysis. Pathogens 2021;10:1125.
40. De Brito T, Silva A, Abreu PAE. Pathology and pathogenesis of human leptospirosis: a commented review. Rev Inst Med Trop Sao Paulo 2018;60:e23.
41. Bharti AR, Nally JE, Ricaldi JN, et al. Leptospirosis: a zoonotic disease of global importance. Lancet Infect Dis 2003;3:757–71.
42. Koizumi N. Laboratory diagnosis of leptospirosis. Methods Mol Biol 2020;2134:277–87.
43. Manabe YC, Betz J, Jackson O, et al. Clinical evaluation of the BioFire Global Fever Panel for the identification of malaria, leptospirosis, chikungunya, and dengue from whole blood: a prospective, multicentre, cross-sectional diagnostic accuracy study. Lancet Infect Dis 2022;22:1356–64.
44. Faucher JF, Hoen B, Estavoyer JM. The management of leptospirosis. Expert Opin Pharmacother 2004;5:819–27.
45. Takafuji ET, Kirkpatrick JW, Miller RN, et al. An efficacy trial of doxycycline chemoprophylaxis against leptospirosis. N Engl J Med 1984;310:497–500.
46. Brett-Major DM, Lipnick RJ. Antibiotic prophylaxis for leptospirosis. Cochrane Database Syst Rev 2009;(3):CD007342.
47. Araúz AB, Papineni P. Histoplasmosis. Infect Dis Clin North Am 2021;35:471–91.
48. Sayeed M, Benzamin M, Nahar L, et al. Hepatic histoplasmosis: an update. J Clin Transl Hepatol 2022;10:726–9.
49. Thompson GR 3rd, Le T, Chindamporn A, et al. Global guideline for the diagnosis and management of the endemic mycoses: an initiative of the European Confederation of Medical Mycology in cooperation with the International Society for Human and Animal Mycology. Lancet Infect Dis 2021;21:e364–74.
50. Donnelly JP, Chen SC, Kauffman CA, et al. Revision and update of the consensus definitions of invasive fungal disease from the European Organization for Research and Treatment of Cancer and the Mycoses Study Group Education and Research Consortium. Clin Infect Dis 2020;71:1367–76.
51. Assi MA, Sandid MS, Baddour LM, et al. Systemic histoplasmosis: a 15-year retrospective institutional review of 111 patients. Medicine (Baltimore) 2007;86:162–9.
52. Martin RC 2nd, Edwards MJ, McMasters KM. Histoplasmosis as an isolated liver lesion: review and surgical therapy. Am Surg 2001;67:430–1.
53. Rihana NA, Kandula M, Velez A, et al. Histoplasmosis presenting as granulomatous hepatitis: case report and review of the literature. Case Rep Med 2014;2014:879535.
54. Columbus-Morales I, Maahs L, Husain S, et al. A case of hemophagocytic lymphohistiocytosis secondary to disseminated histoplasmosis. Case Reports Hepatol 2020;2020:6901514.
55. Lamps LW, Molina CP, West AB, et al. The pathologic spectrum of gastrointestinal and hepatic histoplasmosis. Am J Clin Pathol 2000;113:64–72.
56. Azar MM, Hage CA. Clinical perspectives in the diagnosis and management of histoplasmosis. Clin Chest Med 2017;38:403–15.
57. Scheel CM, Gómez BL. Diagnostic methods for histoplasmosis: focus on endemic countries with variable infrastructure levels. Curr Trop Med Rep 2014;1:129–37.

58. Hage CA, Kirsch EJ, Stump TE, et al. Histoplasma antigen clearance during treatment of histoplasmosis in patients with AIDS determined by a quantitative antigen enzyme immunoassay. Clin Vaccine Immunol 2011;18:661–6.
59. Wang D, Hu B, Hu C, et al. Clinical characteristics of 138 hospitalized patients with 2019 novel coronavirus-infected pneumonia in Wuhan, China. JAMA 2020; 323:1061–9.
60. Spearman CW, Aghemo A, Valenti L, et al. COVID-19 and the liver: a 2021 update. Liver Int 2021;41:1988–98.
61. Gupta A, Madhavan MV, Sehgal K, et al. Extrapulmonary manifestations of COVID-19. Nat Med 2020;26:1017–32.
62. Williamson EJ, Walker AJ, Bhaskaran K, et al. Factors associated with COVID-19-related death using OpenSAFELY. Nature 2020;584:430–6.
63. Hashemi N, Viveiros K, Redd WD, et al. Impact of chronic liver disease on outcomes of hospitalized patients with COVID-19: a multicentre United States experience. Liver Int 2020;40:2515–21.
64. Iavarone M, D'Ambrosio R, Soria A, et al. High rates of 30-day mortality in patients with cirrhosis and COVID-19. J Hepatol 2020;73:1063–71.
65. Mohammed A, Paranji N, Chen PH, et al. COVID-19 in chronic liver disease and liver transplantation: a clinical review. J Clin Gastroenterol 2021;55:187–94.
66. Targher G, Mantovani A, Byrne CD, et al. Risk of severe illness from COVID-19 in patients with metabolic dysfunction-associated fatty liver disease and increased fibrosis scores. Gut 2020;69:1545–7.
67. Ji D, Qin E, Xu J, et al. Non-alcoholic fatty liver diseases in patients with COVID-19: a retrospective study. J Hepatol 2020;73:451–3.
68. Marjot T, Webb GJ, Barritt ASt, et al. COVID-19 and liver disease: mechanistic and clinical perspectives. Nat Rev Gastroenterol Hepatol 2021;18:348–64.
69. Sarin SK, Choudhury A, Lau GK, et al. Pre-existing liver disease is associated with poor outcome in patients with SARS CoV2 infection; The APCOLIS Study (APASL COVID-19 Liver Injury Spectrum Study). Hepatol Int 2020;14:690–700.
70. Amin M. COVID-19 and the liver: overview. Eur J Gastroenterol Hepatol 2021;33: 309–11.
71. Fassan M, Mescoli C, Sbaraglia M, et al. Liver histopathology in COVID-19 patients: a mono-institutional series of liver biopsies and autopsy specimens. Pathol Res Pract 2021;221:153451.
72. Díaz LA, Idalsoaga F, Cannistra M, et al. High prevalence of hepatic steatosis and vascular thrombosis in COVID-19: a systematic review and meta-analysis of autopsy data. World J Gastroenterol 2020;26:7693–706.
73. Faruqui S, Okoli FC, Olsen SK, et al. Cholangiopathy after severe COVID-19: clinical features and prognostic implications. Am J Gastroenterol 2021;116: 1414–25.
74. Welte T, Ambrose LJ, Sibbring GC, et al. Current evidence for COVID-19 therapies: a systematic literature review. Eur Respir Rev 2021;30:200384.
75. World Health Organization. WHO coronavirus (COVID-19) dashboard. 2022, 2022. Available at: https://covid19.who.int/. Accessed December 12, 2022.
76. Baden LR, El Sahly HM, Essink B, et al. Efficacy and safety of the mRNA-1273 SARS-CoV-2 vaccine. N Engl J Med 2021;384:403–16.
77. Dagan N, Barda N, Kepten E, et al. BNT162b2 mRNA Covid-19 vaccine in a nationwide mass vaccination setting. N Engl J Med 2021;384:1412–23.
78. Menni C, Klaser K, May A, et al. Vaccine side-effects and SARS-CoV-2 infection after vaccination in users of the COVID symptom study app in the UK: a prospective observational study. Lancet Infect Dis 2021;21:939–49.

79. Boettler T, Csernalabics B, Salié H, et al. SARS-CoV-2 vaccination can elicit a CD8 T-cell dominant hepatitis. J Hepatol 2022;77:653–9.
80. Dioverti MV, Razonable RR. Cytomegalovirus. Microbiol Spectr 2016;4(4).
81. Zuhair M, Smit GSA, Wallis G, et al. Estimation of the worldwide seroprevalence of cytomegalovirus: a systematic review and meta-analysis. Rev Med Virol 2019; 29:e2034.
82. Hoehl S, Berger A, Ciesek S, et al. Thirty years of CMV seroprevalence-a longitudinal analysis in a German university hospital. Eur J Clin Microbiol Infect Dis 2020;39:1095–102.
83. Ho M. Epidemiology of cytomegalovirus infections. Rev Infect Dis 1990; 12(Suppl 7):S701–10.
84. Cannon MJ, Schmid DS, Hyde TB. Review of cytomegalovirus seroprevalence and demographic characteristics associated with infection. Rev Med Virol 2010;20:202–13.
85. Staras SA, Dollard SC, Radford KW, et al. Seroprevalence of cytomegalovirus infection in the United States, 1988-1994. Clin Infect Dis 2006;43:1143–51.
86. Ross SA, Arora N, Novak Z, et al. Cytomegalovirus reinfections in healthy seroimmune women. J Infect Dis 2010;201:386–9.
87. Vauloup-Fellous C, Berth M, Heskia F, et al. Re-evaluation of the VIDAS(®) cytomegalovirus (CMV) IgG avidity assay: determination of new cut-off values based on the study of kinetics of CMV-IgG maturation. J Clin Virol 2013;56:118–23.
88. Dunn HS, Haney DJ, Ghanekar SA, et al. Dynamics of CD4 and CD8 T cell responses to cytomegalovirus in healthy human donors. J Infect Dis 2002;186: 15–22.
89. Watkins RR, Lemonovich TL, Razonable RR. Immune response to CMV in solid organ transplant recipients: current concepts and future directions. Expert Rev Clin Immunol 2012;8:383–93.
90. Klemola E, Von Essen R, Henle G, et al. Infectious-mononucleosis-like disease with negative heterophil agglutination test. clinical features in relation to Epstein-Barr virus and cytomegalovirus antibodies. J Infect Dis 1970;121:608–14.
91. Cohen JI, Corey GR. Cytomegalovirus infection in the normal host. Medicine (Baltimore) 1985;64:100–14.
92. Tjwa M, De Hertogh G, Neuville B, et al. Hepatic fibrin-ring granulomas in granulomatous hepatitis: report of four cases and review of the literature. Acta Clin Belg 2001;56:341–8.
93. Yu YD, Park GC, Park PJ, et al. Cytomegalovirus infection-associated fulminant hepatitis in an immunocompetent adult requiring emergency living-donor liver transplantation: report of a case. Surg Today 2013;43:424–8.
94. De Broucker C, Plessier A, Ollivier-Hourmand I, et al. Multicenter study on recent portal venous system thrombosis associated with cytomegalovirus disease. J Hepatol 2022;76:115–22.
95. Razonable RR, Humar A. Cytomegalovirus in solid organ transplantation. Am J Transplant 2013;13(Suppl 4):93–106.
96. Beam E, Razonable RR. Cytomegalovirus in solid organ transplantation: epidemiology, prevention, and treatment. Curr Infect Dis Rep 2012;14:633–41.
97. George B, Pati N, Gilroy N, et al. Pre-transplant cytomegalovirus (CMV) serostatus remains the most important determinant of CMV reactivation after allogeneic hematopoietic stem cell transplantation in the era of surveillance and preemptive therapy. Transpl Infect Dis 2010;12:322–9.
98. Hebart H, Jahn G, Sinzger C, et al. CMV infection in bone marrow and solid organ transplant patients in the era of antiviral prophylaxis. Herpes 2000;7:13–7.

99. Humar A, Mazzulli T, Moussa G, et al. Clinical utility of cytomegalovirus (CMV) serology testing in high-risk CMV D+/R- transplant recipients. Am J Transplant 2005;5:1065–70.

100. Da Cunha T, Wu GY. Cytomegalovirus hepatitis in immunocompetent and immunocompromised hosts. J Clin Transl Hepatol 2021;9:106–15.

101. Imlay HN, Kaul DR. Letermovir and Maribavir for the treatment and prevention of cytomegalovirus infection in solid organ and stem cell transplant recipients. Clin Infect Dis 2021;73:156–60.

102. Kang C. Maribavir: first approval. Drugs 2022;82:335–40.

103. Wong Y, Meehan MT, Burrows SR, et al. Estimating the global burden of Epstein-Barr virus-related cancers. J Cancer Res Clin Oncol 2022;148:31–46.

104. Cohen JI. Epstein-Barr virus infection. N Engl J Med 2000;343:481–92.

105. Dunmire SK, Hogquist KA, Balfour HH. Infectious mononucleosis. Curr Top Microbiol Immunol 2015;390:211–40.

106. Fugl A, Andersen CL. Epstein-Barr virus and its association with disease - a review of relevance to general practice. BMC Fam Pract 2019;20:62.

107. Noor A, Panwala A, Forouhar F, et al. Hepatitis caused by herpes viruses: a review. J Dig Dis 2018;19:446–55.

108. Shaukat A, Tsai HT, Rutherford R, et al. Epstein-Barr virus induced hepatitis: an important cause of cholestasis. Hepatol Res 2005;33:24–6.

109. Mellinger JL, Rossaro L, Naugler WE, et al. Epstein-Barr virus (EBV) related acute liver failure: a case series from the US Acute Liver Failure Study Group. Dig Dis Sci 2014;59:1630–7.

110. Bunchorntavakul C, Reddy KR. Epstein-Barr Virus and cytomegalovirus infections of the liver. Gastroenterol Clin North Am 2020;49:331–46.

111. Biest S, Schubert TT. Chronic Epstein-Barr virus infection: a cause of granulomatous hepatitis? J Clin Gastroenterol 1989;11:343–6.

112. Kikuchi K, Miyakawa H, Abe K, et al. Vanishing bile duct syndrome associated with chronic EBV infection. Dig Dis Sci 2000;45:160–5.

113. Gupta E, Ballani N, Kumar M, et al. Role of non-hepatotropic viruses in acute sporadic viral hepatitis and acute-on-chronic liver failure in adults. Indian J Gastroenterol 2015;34:448–52.

114. Cohen JI, Jaffe ES, Dale JK, et al. Characterization and treatment of chronic active Epstein-Barr virus disease: a 28-year experience in the United States. Blood 2011;117:5835–49.

115. Al-Mansour Z, Nelson BP, Evens AM. Post-transplant lymphoproliferative disease (PTLD): risk factors, diagnosis, and current treatment strategies. Curr Hematol Malig Rep 2013;8:173–83.

116. Bunchorntavakul C, Reddy KR. Hepatic manifestations of lymphoproliferative disorders. Clin Liver Dis 2019;23:293–308.

117. Parker A, Bowles K, Bradley JA, et al. Management of post-transplant lymphoproliferative disorder in adult solid organ transplant recipients - BCSH and BTS guidelines. Br J Haematol 2010;149:693–705.

118. Allen UD, Preiksaitis JK. Post-transplant lymphoproliferative disorders, Epstein-Barr virus infection, and disease in solid organ transplantation: guidelines from the American Society of Transplantation Infectious Diseases Community of Practice. Clin Transplant 2019;33:e13652.

119. Schechter S, Lamps L. Epstein-Barr Virus Hepatitis: a review of clinicopathologic features and differential diagnosis. Arch Pathol Lab Med 2018;142:1191–5.

120. Adams LA, Deboer B, Jeffrey G, et al. Ganciclovir and the treatment of Epstein-Barr virus hepatitis. J Gastroenterol Hepatol 2006;21:1758–60.
121. Kumar M, Herrera JL. Sarcoidosis and the liver. Clin Liver Dis 2019;23:331–43.
122. Drent M, Crouser ED, Grunewald J. Challenges of sarcoidosis and its management. N Engl J Med 2021;385:1018–32.
123. Arkema EV, Cozier YC. Sarcoidosis epidemiology: recent estimates of incidence, prevalence and risk factors. Curr Opin Pulm Med 2020;26:527–34.
124. Rossi G, Ziol M, Roulot D, et al. Hepatic sarcoidosis: current concepts and treatments. Semin Respir Crit Care Med 2020;41:652–8.
125. Dulai PS, Rothstein RI. Disseminated sarcoidosis presenting as granulomatous gastritis: a clinical review of the gastrointestinal and hepatic manifestations of sarcoidosis. J Clin Gastroenterol 2012;46:367–74.
126. Nolan JP, Klatskin G. The fever of sarcoidosis. Ann Intern Med 1964;61:455–61.
127. Ungprasert P, Crowson CS, Simonetto DA, et al. Clinical characteristics and outcome of hepatic sarcoidosis: a population-based study 1976-2013. Am J Gastroenterol 2017;112:1556–63.
128. Valla D, Pessegueiro-Miranda H, Degott C, et al. Hepatic sarcoidosis with portal hypertension. a report of seven cases with a review of the literature. Q J Med 1987;63:531–44.
129. Moreno-Merlo F, Wanless IR, Shimamatsu K, et al. The role of granulomatous phlebitis and thrombosis in the pathogenesis of cirrhosis and portal hypertension in sarcoidosis. Hepatology 1997;26:554–60.
130. Russi EW, Bansky G, Pfaltz M, et al. Budd-Chiari syndrome in sarcoidosis. Am J Gastroenterol 1986;81:71–5.
131. Ennaifer R, Bacha D, Romdhane H, et al. Budd-Chiari syndrome: an unusual presentation of multisystemic sarcoidosis. Clin Pract 2015;5:768.
132. Syed U, Alkhawam H, Bakhit M, et al. Hepatic sarcoidosis: pathogenesis, clinical context, and treatment options. Scand J Gastroenterol 2016;51:1025–30.
133. Ryland KL. Hepatic sarcoidosis: incidence, monitoring, and treatment. Clinical Liver Disease 2020;16:208–11.
134. Zakim D, Boyer T. Hepatology: a textbook of liver diseases. Philadelphia: WB Saunders; 1996. p. 1472.
135. Cremers J, Drent M, Driessen A, et al. Liver-test abnormalities in sarcoidosis. Eur J Gastroenterol Hepatol 2012;24:17–24.
136. Modaresi Esfeh J, Culver D, Plesec T, et al. Clinical presentation and protocol for management of hepatic sarcoidosis. Expet Rev Gastroenterol Hepatol 2015;9:349–58.
137. Warshauer DM, Dumbleton SA, Molina PL, et al. Abdominal CT findings in sarcoidosis: radiologic and clinical correlation. Radiology 1994;192:93–8.
138. Fetzer DT, Rees MA, Dasyam AK, et al. Hepatic sarcoidosis in patients presenting with liver dysfunction: imaging appearance, pathological correlation and disease evolution. Eur Radiol 2016;26:3129–37.
139. Maddrey WC, Johns CJ, Boitnott JK, et al. Sarcoidosis and chronic hepatic disease: a clinical and pathologic study of 20 patients. Medicine (Baltimore) 1970;49:375–95.
140. Kennedy PT, Zakaria N, Modawi SB, et al. Natural history of hepatic sarcoidosis and its response to treatment. Eur J Gastroenterol Hepatol 2006;18:721–6.
141. Bakker GJ, Haan YC, Maillette de Buy Wenniger LJ, et al. Sarcoidosis of the liver: to treat or not to treat? Neth J Med 2012;70:349–56.
142. Ayyala US, Padilla ML. Diagnosis and treatment of hepatic sarcoidosis. Curr Treat Options Gastroenterol 2006;9:475–83.

143. Sebode M, Weidemann S, Wehmeyer M, et al. Anti-TNF-α for necrotizing sarcoid granulomatosis of the liver. Hepatology 2017;65:1410–2.

144. Bilal M, Satapathy SK, Ismail MK, et al. Long-term outcomes of liver transplantation for hepatic sarcoidosis: a single center experience. J Clin Exp Hepatol 2016;6:94–9.

145. Syed U, Ching Companioni RA, Alkhawam H, et al. Amyloidosis of the gastrointestinal tract and the liver: clinical context, diagnosis and management. Eur J Gastroenterol Hepatol 2016;28:1109–21.

146. Muchtar E, Dispenzieri A, Magen H, et al. Systemic amyloidosis from A (AA) to T (ATTR): a review. J Intern Med 2021;289:268–92.

147. Benson MD, Buxbaum JN, Eisenberg DS, et al. Amyloid nomenclature 2018: recommendations by the International Society of Amyloidosis (ISA) nomenclature committee. Amyloid 2018;25:215–9.

148. Park MA, Mueller PS, Kyle RA, et al. Primary (AL) hepatic amyloidosis: clinical features and natural history in 98 patients. Medicine 2003;82:291–8.

149. Bion E, Brenard R, Pariente EA, et al. Sinusoidal portal hypertension in hepatic amyloidosis. Gut 1991;32:227–30.

150. Oliva L, Orfanelli U, Resnati M, et al. The amyloidogenic light chain is a stressor that sensitizes plasma cells to proteasome inhibitor toxicity. Blood 2017;129:2132–42.

151. Lachmann HJ, Goodman HJ, Gilbertson JA, et al. Natural history and outcome in systemic AA amyloidosis. N Engl J Med 2007;356:2361–71.

152. Gertz MA. Hereditary ATTR amyloidosis: burden of illness and diagnostic challenges. Am J Manag Care 2017;23:S107–12.

153. Sickels A, Shah KB, Ruch B, et al. Combined heart-liver and domino liver transplantation in familial amyloidosis. Am Surg 2022;88:2267–73.

154. Carvalho A, Rocha A, Lobato L. Liver transplantation in transthyretin amyloidosis: issues and challenges. Liver Transplant 2015;21:282–92.

155. Bispo M, Marcelino P, Freire A, et al. High incidence of thrombotic complications early after liver transplantation for familial amyloidotic polyneuropathy. Transpl Int 2009;22:165–71.

156. Lladó L, Baliellas C, Casasnovas C, et al. Risk of transmission of systemic transthyretin amyloidosis after domino liver transplantation. Liver Transplant 2010;16:1386–92.

157. Berk JL, Suhr OB, Obici L, et al. Repurposing diflunisal for familial amyloid polyneuropathy: a randomized clinical trial. JAMA 2013;310:2658–67.

158. Adams D, Gonzalez-Duarte A, O'Riordan WD, et al. Patisiran, an RNAi therapeutic, for hereditary transthyretin amyloidosis. N Engl J Med 2018;379:11–21.

159. Benson MD, Waddington-Cruz M, Berk JL, et al. Inotersen treatment for patients with hereditary transthyretin amyloidosis. N Engl J Med 2018;379:22–31.

160. Sarsik B, Sen S, Kirdok FS, et al. Hepatic amyloidosis: morphologic spectrum of histopathological changes in AA and nonAA amyloidosis. Pathol Res Pract 2012;208:713–8.

Liver Cirrhosis and Portal Hypertension

How to Deal with Esophageal Varices?

Dinesh Jothimani, FRCP[a], Mohamed Rela, FRCS[a],
Patrick S. Kamath, MD[b],*

KEYWORDS

- Cirrhosis • Portal hypertension • Hepatic decompensation • Transient elastography
- Esophageal varices • Nonselective beta blocker • Vasoactive drugs • Band ligation

KEY POINTS

- Clinically significant portal hypertension is a presymptomatic stage in patients with liver cirrhosis associated with significantly reduced survival.
- Esophagogastroduodenoscopy is necessary for the identification of esophageal and gastric varices at risk for bleeding.
- Patients with varices ≥ 5 mm diameter are recommended nonselective beta blocker therapy to prevent index variceal bleed.
- Acute variceal bleeding is a major life-threatening complication of portal hypertension that requires endoscopic band ligation.
- Early TIPS should be considered in those with refractory bleed or in endoscopic treatment failure.

INTRODUCTION

Variceal hemorrhage, ascites, and hepatic encephalopathy are complications of portal hypertension and define hepatic decompensation in patients with cirrhosis.[1] Portal pressure is a product of volume of portal blood flow and resistance to blood flow. In cirrhosis, the initiating event leading to portal hypertension is increased resistance to portal blood flow largely due to distortion of hepatic architecture by nodular regeneration of the liver and is perpetuated by an increase in splanchnic blood flow. As a means of decreasing pressure in the portal system, portosystemic collaterals develop but are insufficient to normalize portal pressure. The venous collaterals at the

[a] Institute of Liver Disease and Transplantation, Dr Rela Institute and Medical Centre, 7, CLC Works Road, Chrompet, Chennai, India-600044; [b] Division of Gastroenterology and Hepatology, Mayo Clinic College of Medicine and Science, 200 First Street Southwest, Rochester, MN 55906, USA
* Corresponding author.
E-mail address: kamath.patrick@mayo.edu

Med Clin N Am 107 (2023) 491–504
https://doi.org/10.1016/j.mcna.2023.01.002
0025-7125/23/© 2023 Elsevier Inc. All rights reserved.

gastroesophageal junction, termed gastroesophageal varices, are the usual cause of gastrointestinal bleeding in most of the patients with portal hypertension.

The risk of developing small esophageal varices is approximately 7% per year, and increase in size of varices from small to large occurs at the rate of 10% to 15% per year, but may be higher with hepatic decompensation. With progression of liver disease, the risk of variceal bleed increases from 5% to 25% and to 50% in patients with Child A, Child B, and Child C cirrhosis, respectively.[2] Variceal bleeding is a major complication in patients with cirrhosis with an annual incidence of 10% to 15% depending on the size of varices, red wale signs on endoscopy, and degree of hepatic dysfunction.[3] Despite advances in endoscopic and pharmacologic therapy, mortality associated with variceal bleed is approximately 20% at 6 weeks and may increase to 30% in patients with Child C cirrhosis.[4,5] Gastric varices develop in 20% of patients with portal hypertension and hemorrhage accounts for about 10% to 15% of all bleeding episodes in patients with cirrhosis.[6] Bleeding from ectopic varices including rectal varices is uncommon.

In this review, the authors discuss recent updates on portal hypertension and management of esophageal varices.

Pathogenesis of Portal Hypertension

The understanding of portal hypertension continues to evolve. Two major pathogenic changes occur in patients with cirrhosis leading to portal hypertension: increase in resistance to portal blood flow and increase in portal flow. The increased resistance may be structural related to hepatic fibrosis and distortion of the normal hepatic architecture or may be related to vasoactive factors. Cirrhosis is characterized by structural changes that occur in the hepatic sinusoids: chronic and progressive hepatocyte injury and cell death along with sinusoidal endothelial damage causes loss of its fenestrations where these cells acquire 'capillarisation' phenotype leading to increased secretion of vasoactive factors.[7] Release of one such factor, endothelin-1 (ET-1) activates dormant hepatic stellate cells into myofibroblast phenotype upon which there is accelerated collagen deposition in the extracellular matrix resulting in fibrogenesis.[8] This process of increased hepatic fibrosis occurs over years before culminating in portal hypertension. In addition to fibrosis, two unique pathogenic changes occur in patients progressing to cirrhosis; areas of parenchymal extinction, and significant vascular remodeling, causing sinusoidal collapse and architectural distortion.[9] Proliferation of hepatocytes in these areas of extinction leads to the formation of regenerative nodules. Combination of structural distortion compounded by increased intrahepatic vascular resistance due to an increase in vasoconstrictors such as ET-1, and a reduction in the intrahepatic circulation of vasodilators such as nitric oxide (NO) results in increased resistance to portal blood flow. In addition, portal hypertension is propagated by splanchnic arteriolar vasodilatation contributing to the increased blood flow across the portal venous system. The combination of increased flow and increased resistance to flow results in portal hypertension.

Recent evidences point toward existence of a prothrombotic state in patients with cirrhosis that may contribute to disease progression in patients with liver cirrhosis. Presence of intimal fibrosis attributed to healed hepatic vein (HV) or portal vein (PV) thrombosis have been described in livers explanted during transplantation. HV thrombosis tends to be patchy and confined to veins between 0.1 and 3 mm in diameter. PV lesions occur more uniformly across the liver. HV lesions are associated with confluent fibrosis (focal parenchymal extinction), whereas PV lesions are associated with regional variation in the size of cirrhotic nodules and a history of bleeding varices. These observations suggest that thrombosis of medium and large PVs and HVs is a frequent occurrence in cirrhosis and these events are important in causing progression of cirrhosis.[10] More recent studies have described the role of gut bacteria in the pathogenesis of cirrhosis. There has been a growing interest in bacterial dysbiosis and altered intestinal permeability in cirrhosis which may also contribute to portal hypertension by the release endotoxins and other pro-inflammatory cytokines.[11]

Acute decompensation manifests as variceal hemorrhage, ascites, or hepatic encephalopathy, whereas acute-on-chronic liver failure (ACLF) exhibits with the presence of one or more organ failures, usually precipitated by sepsis. These manifestations of cirrhosis can be life-threatening with rapid increase in portal pressure, which may be contributed by altered gut microbes, increased intestinal translocation of bacteria and bacterial products. This process triggers the release of pro-inflammatory cytokine, which leads to severe systemic inflammatory response triggering propagation and rapid progression of portal hypertension.[12,13] Unlike the systemic circulation, the portal circulation is a smaller and relatively a closed compartment. Therefore, the gastrointestinal vascular system goes through several adaptive mechanisms to accommodate and overcome the increase in portal pressure over years. Splenomegaly opening of new and embryonic vessels that occur as a compensatory mechanism unfortunately is ineffective in normalizing portal pressure.

Diagnosis of Portal Hypertension

Portal pressure measurement using the hepatic venous pressure gradient (HVPG) is the most precise method for assessing the severity of portal hypertension. It is measured by wedging an occlusion balloon catheter into the right HV. With the balloon inflated and occluding a hepatic venule, the pressure recorded is the wedged HV pressure (WHVP). The pressure recorded in the right HV on deflation of the balloon is the free HV pressure (FHVP). The difference between WHVP and FHVP is the HVPG, which represents hepatic sinusoidal pressure;[14] that is, HVPG represents hepatic sinusoidal pressure and is normally less than 5 mm Hg. An HVPG $\geq$5 mm Hg is diagnostic of portal hypertension. However, varices or ascites do not develop till the HVPG is $\geq$ 10 mm Hg,[15] and thus, clinically significant portal hypertension (CSPH) is defined as HVPG $\geq$ 10 mm Hg.

In a prospective study by Ripoll and colleagues, where HVPG measurement was carried out on 213 patients with compensated cirrhosis, an HVPG level less than 10 mm Hg was associated over 90% chance of remaining stable in contrary to those with HVPG $\geq$10 mm Hg[16] confirming that CSPH occurs only when HVPG is $\geq$ 10 mm Hg. Variceal bleeding defining severe portal hypertension occurs with HVPG $\geq$12 mmHg.[17] Interestingly, HVPG measurements correlate best with portal pressure in patients with cirrhosis secondary to alcohol or viral related hepatitis rather than cirrhosis from other disease etiologies.[18]

The onset of CSPH determines the key prognostic milestone in the natural history of patients with cirrhosis; it is presymptomatic and predicts the development of varices. Ascites is the most common event that defines "decompensation" which reduces the median survival from 10 to 2 years. Importantly, CSPH is associated with a sixfold increased risk of Hepatocellular carcinoma (HCC).[19] Although HVPG is accurate in diagnosing the severity of portal hypertension, it is impractical to implement on all cirrhotic patients outside clinical trials. Being an invasive procedure HVPG measurement requires a higher level of expertise, and limited by its lack of wider availability due to cost factor. Hence, noninvasive methods of evaluation of portal hypertension are increasingly developed, tested, and used in day-to-day clinical practice.

Liver stiffness measurement (LSM) came in to use as a noninvasive alternative tool for fibrosis assessment in patients with chronic viral hepatitis. Utility of LSM by transient elastography (TE) in comparison to HVPG has been evaluated in several studies. A meta-analysis of 11 studies with 1399 patients showed a correlation coefficient of 0.783 for TE against overall HVPG and 0.552 to 0.858 for CSPH.[20] An LSM-TE greater than 20 to 25 kPa or splenic stiffness (SS) greater than 40 to 45 kPa indicate a high likelihood of CSPH. Interestingly, SS has a better correlation with portal hypertension than LSM.[21] Although CSPH can be identified noninvasively by a TE or the presence of portosystemic collaterals on imaging, it cannot be ruled out with confidence by these parameters alone.

As cirrhosis is technically a histopathological diagnosis, and with an increasing use of TE as a noninvasive alternative for biopsy to assess degree of hepatic fibrosis in patients with chronic liver disease, the term compensated advanced chronic liver disease (cACLD) may be used in place of compensated "cirrhosis." TE less than 10 kPa excludes cACLD, whereas 10 to 15 is suggestive and greater than 15 kPa highly suggestive of cACLD. In patients with cACLD, the presence of TE less than 15 kPa with platelet count greater than 150/mm³ rules out CSPH with a sensitivity and a negative predictive value of greater than 90%. Patients without CSPH do not require screening endoscopy for esophageal varices, whereas patients with TE 15 to 20 kPa with platelet less than 110/mm³ or TE 20 to 25 kPa with platelet count less than 150/mm³ possess 60% chance of CSPH. TE $\geq$ 25 kPa is highly suggestive of CSPH with a positive predictive value greater than 90%, particularly in patients with cirrhosis due to viral, alcohol, and nonobese non-alcohol related steatohepatitis (**Fig. 1**). These patients are likely to have endoscopic features of portal hypertension and risk of hepatic decompensation.[22] Therefore, these patients must be screened for varices. Spleen stiffness measurement less than 40 kPa rules out CSPH. Thus, noninvasive tests using platelet counts, liver stiffness, and spleen stiffness may be quite beneficial in selecting patients for surveillance endoscopy for varices.[23]

Portal phase CT has been studied to assess esophageal varices in 104 patients who underwent endoscopic variceal surveillance. CT showed a good correlation (kappa = 0.88) with endoscopy for esophageal varices with a receiver operating curve (ROC) between 0.77 and 0.91.[24] Despite noninvasive alternatives, esophagogastroduodenoscopy (EGD) remains the "gold standard in the diagnosis and management of esophageal varices.

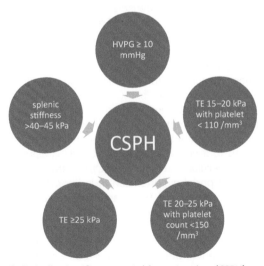

Fig. 1. Illustration of clinically significant portal hypertension (CSPH).

Diagnosis and Surveillance for Varices

Endoscopic examination of the upper gastrointestinal tract is necessary for identification of esophageal and gastric varices at risk of bleeding. EGD provides information on the size of esophageal varices (< 5mm-small; >5 mm-large), the presence of red wale signs indicating the risk of bleeding; gastric varices; changes of gastric antral vascular ectasia and portal hypertensive gastropathy. If no varices are found at the initial endoscopy, repeat surveillance endoscopy may be carried out in 2 to 3 years, earlier if patient has hepatic decompensation. If small varices are seen, follow-up surveillance endoscopy is carried out in 1 year.[25]

Prevention of First Variceal Bleed: Primary Prophylaxis

Effective reduction of portal pressure delays the onset of hepatic decompensation and development of varices. Reversal of the etiologic factor of cirrhosis, for example, in patients with alcohol-related liver disease and chronic hepatitis B or C infections ameliorates portal hypertension. Improvement in liver function and resolution of complications of portal hypertension is termed "recompensation of cirrhosis." The Baveno VII consensus recommends using the term "recompensation" for those patients who fulfill all three of the following criteria: (1) reversal of the etiology of cirrhosis (viral elimination for hepatitis C, sustained viral suppression for hepatitis B, sustained alcohol abstinence for alcohol-induced cirrhosis); (2) resolution of ascites, encephalopathy, and absence of recurrent variceal hemorrhage for 1 year in the absence of any treatment; and (3) normalization of liver biochemistry.[26] In a recent study of 283 chronic hepatitis B patients with decompensated cirrhosis on entecavir for 120 weeks, 56.2% patients achieved recompensation.[27] Thus, every effort should be attempted to allow patients with cirrhosis to "recompensate" so as to reduce risk of variceal bleeding.

Nonselective beta blocker

Patients with varices $\geq$ 5 mm diameter are recommended nonselective beta blocker (NSBB) therapy to prevent index variceal bleed. NSBB has no role in preventing development of varices in patients with normal index endoscopy.

Basic understanding of adrenergic receptors may help selecting drugs in the management of portal hypertension. Adrenergic or sympathetic receptors possess two major receptor categories: α and β, with a subcategory of $\alpha 1$ and $\alpha 2$ and $\beta 1$, $\beta 2$, and the more recently described $\beta 3$ receptor. The α_1-adrenoceptors are the predominant α-receptors located on vascular smooth muscle. α-agonists constrict both arteries and veins; arterial vasoconstriction increases systemic vascular resistance, whereas venous constriction increases venous pressure. Among β-adrenoreceptors, $\beta 1$ activation causes positive chronotropic and inotropic effects on the heart, increasing cardiac output, whereas $\beta 2$ receptor activation causes splanchnic vasodilation with an increase in portal blood flow.

Propranolol, a nonselective β-adrenergic blocker, has been used in the treatment of portal hypertension for over four decades. Blockade of $\beta 1$ receptors result in negative chrono- and inotropic effects in the heart, thereby reducing cardiac output. Through its $\beta 2$-antagonistic effects, propranolol inhibits smooth muscle relaxation in the splanchnic vessels allowing unopposed α-adrenergic effects that lead to splanchnic vasoconstriction and consequently lowering portal blood flow and reduction in portal pressure.[28–30]

Primary prophylaxis refers to the use of propranolol in the prevention of index variceal bleed. Propranolol reduces the risk of variceal bleed by 10% and the absolute risk of first variceal bleed to 9% over 2 years in placebo-controlled trials. In a large randomized double-blinded controlled trial, propranolol showed a reduction in the incidence of variceal bleed (4% vs 22%, $P < .01$) over a period of 16 months and was cost-effective.[31,32] NSBB is indicated for prevention of bleeding in patients with large esophageal varices and in patients with small esophageal varices with red wale signs or Child-Pugh class B or C severity.

Several randomized controlled studies have compared propranolol with primary endoscopic band ligation (EBL) in preventing the index variceal bleed. In a study of cirrhotic patients with large esophageal varices, 39 received EBL and 36 received propranolol. With a median follow-up over 4.5 years, variceal bleed occurred in 12% vs 25% in the EBL and propranolol group, respectively, with no statistical difference ($P = .17$); however, esophageal variceal bleed was less in the primary EBL group (5.1% vs 25%, $P = .027$).[33,34] A meta-analysis of 16 studies showed EBL was associated with a significant reduction in the index variceal bleed. However, on an average, three sessions of EBL were required for eradication of varices and 33 sessions were the number required for prevention of one index bleed. Moreover, there was no difference in mortality. In contrary, NSBB (propranolol 40 mg twice a day) is cost-effective, widely available with easy to use and monitor for adverse events, and associated with reduction in all-cause mortality,[35] NSBB is thus the preferred modality for primary prophylaxis.

Carvedilol is increasing used in the management of portal hypertension. In addition to β-adrenergic blockade, carvedilol reduces intrahepatic vascular resistance by anti-alpha 1 adrenergic effect and has shown higher efficacy than propranolol. A recent meta-analysis of four randomized controlled trial (RCT) comparing 181 patients treated with carvedilol with 171 controls showed a significant reduction in the risk of hepatic decompensation sub-distribution hazard ratio (SHR 0.506, $P = .017$), reduced ascites formation (SHR 0.491, $P = .042$), and more importantly, carvedilol use was associated with reduced mortality (SHR 0.417, $P = .025$).[36] The dose of carvedilol was 6.25 mg a day and may increased to 12.5 mg per day if tolerated. Patients with CSPH may be started on NSBB for the prevention of decompensation in patients with compensated cirrhosis, but this is yet uncertain.

A large multicenter randomized study comparing carvedilol ($n = 77$) to EBL ($n = 75$) was conducted by Tripathi and colleagues. There was a lower rate of index variceal bleed in the carvedilol arm (10% vs 23%, hazard ratio 0.41; 95%CI 0.19–0.96; $P = .04$) over a period of 20 months without a difference in mortality ($P = .71$).[37] Interestingly, these findings were not observed in another large randomized controlled study involving 209 cirrhotic patients. The risk of variceal bleeding observed was similar in both carvedilol and EBL arms, 8.5% and 6.9%, respectively.[38]

Careful monitoring of heart rate should be carried out in patients on NSBB therapy. An heart rate of 50 to 55 beats per minute indictes adequate betablockade. NSBB should be avoided in patients with second- and third-degree heart blocks, peripheral vascular disease, uncontrolled diabetes, bronchial asthma, and in patients with peripheral vascular disease. NSBB should not be initiated in patients with systolic blood pressure less than 90 mm Hg and in patients with uncontrolled ascites or worsening renal function. Patients with contraindications for NSBB should be considered for EBL.

Statins

Statins are well-established drug in the management of dyslipidemia and coronary artery disease. In addition to the lipid-lowering effect, statins have shown to reduce oxidative stress and exert anti-inflammatory activity on vascular endothelium, thereby improving endothelial function by enhancing NO production. Similar effects have been observed in experimental studies in the liver, thereby decreasing intrahepatic vascular resistance and reducing portal pressure.[39] Simvastatin given for a month reduced HVPG by 8.3% in an RCT.[40] Simvastatin when used in combination with propranolol was found to reduce variceal bleeding (27.3 vs 4.7%, $P = .036$) compared with NSBB alone. However, this effect was not observed in patients who received in addition to carvedilol.[41] Moreover, a multicenter placebo-controlled trial showed addition of simvastatin to NSBB or EBL did not reduce rebleeding rates.[42] Thus, the exact role of statins in the treatment of patients with portal hypertension awaits further studies.

Risk of bleeding from esophageal varices occurs with HVPG $\geq$12 mm Hg. Reduction in HVPG to less than 12 mmHg or by greater than 20% from baseline is associated with reduced risk of variceal bleeding. NSBB is started preferably as a single dose of nadolol 20 to 40 mg or long-acting propranolol 60 to 80 mg in the evening or with carvedilol 3.125 mg every 12 hours. The medication dose is titrated up every 5 days to the maximum tolerated dose or reduction in the resting heart rate by 25% or to 50 to 55 beats per minute. Fatigue, cold extremities, depression, and erectile dysfunction are potential side-effects warranting discontinuation of treatment. In patients who are intolerant to NSBB or have contraindications to NSBB, endoscopic variceal ligation may be initiated. Varices are ligated in the lower one-third of the esophagus in a spiral fashion to avoid the risk of esophageal strictures. Complications of EBL include banding ulcers which may rarely be associated with life-threatening bleeds, aspiration pneumonia, and esophageal strictures. EBL is continued at 3 to 4 weekly intervals till complete obliteration. Follow-up sessions may be at 6 monthly intervals initially and then annually.

The decision to select either NSBB or EBL for primary prophylaxis is made after discussion with the patient and taking into consideration patient preferences. Given the low cost, ease of use, equivalent efficacy, and absence of life-threatening complications, NSBB is preferred over EBL. There is no role for a combination of NSBB and EBL for primary prophylaxis against variceal hemorrhage.

Control of Variceal Bleed

Acute variceal bleed (AVB) is a life-threatening emergency following rupture of varices leading to torrential blood loss and the second most common cause of hepatic decompensation after ascites in patients with cirrhosis. Severity and mortality of variceal varies with the severity of underlying liver disease as determined by Child-Pugh, MELD score, and HVPG. Variceal bleed may be aggravated by underlying sepsis and concomitantly variceal bleed may precipitate infection due to bacterial translocation.[43]

Varices bleed when there is an increase is variceal wall tension which is directly proportional to variceal diameter and transmural pressure gradient and inversely proportional to variceal wall thickness. Management should be geared toward volume resuscitation, preventing infection, and control of bleeding using a combination of pharmacologic and endoscopic therapy. Patients should be admitted via the emergency department and treated in the intensive care unit if there is active bleeding. Adequate resuscitation with packed red blood cell transfusion is mandatory to maintain hemoglobin greater than 7 G/dL and to maintain tissue perfusion. Caution should be excised regarding the risk of over transfusion which can aggravate bleeding. Villeneuve and colleagues studied restrictive (transfuse to maintain hemoglobin > 7 G/dL) versus liberal (transfuse to maintain hemoglobin > 9 G/dL) transfusions in 921 cirrhotic patients with variceal bleed and found increased rebleeding rates (10% vs 16%, $P = .01$) and importantly higher mortality in patients with liberal transfusion (5% vs 9%, $P = .02$).[44]

Vasoactive drug such as intravenous (IV) terlipressin should be commenced at the suspicious of AVB. Terlipressin controls bleeding within 48 hours of commencement

(OR 2.94, P = .0008) and reduced mortality related to the bleed (Odds ratio 0.31, P = 0.0008).[45] The dose of terlipressin is 2 mg IV followed by 1 mg every sixth hourly for 3 to 5 days is recommended.[1] Recent studies support the use of terlipressin continuous infusion better tolerated at relatively lower doses with similar efficacy than bolus doses. However, this was in the setting of hepatorenal syndrome and not bleed variceal bleed.[46]

Terlipressin may cause bradycardia and arrhythmias; therefore, cardiac monitoring is necessary for patients on terlipressin. In the absence of terlipressin, intravenous octreotide may be used as an intravenous bolus of 50 µg followed by an infusion of 25 to 50 µg/h. A large (n = 324) double-blind randomized controlled trial showed similar efficacy profile for control of bleeding between terlipressin and octreotide (92.6% vs 95.6%), but length of hospital stay was less with terlipressin (108.4 vs 126.3 hours, P < .001) for terlipressin and octreotide arms, respectively.[47,48]

AVB increases the risk of gut bacterial translocation, and sepsis increases the risk of rebleeding. Therefore, prophylactic antibiotics are recommended in all patients with cirrhosis and gastrointestinal bleeding, not specifically in variceal bleeding alone. Ceftriaxone (1 g/24 h) is the first choice in patients with decompensated cirrhosis, especially in those on quinolone prophylaxis, or when there is a high prevalence of quinolone-resistant bacterial infections. Oral quinolones (norfloxacin 400 mg twice a day; ciprofloxacin 50 mg twice a day) are used in other patients. In patients with ascites, a diagnostic paracentesis for spontaneous bacterial peritonitis should be performed, if possible, before administration of prophylactic antibiotics.

EGD remains the cornerstone in the management of AVB. Studies on timing of endoscopy in variceal bleed showed conflicting results.[49,50] Experts recommend that therapeutic endoscopic procedure should be performed by an experienced endoscopist within 12 hours of admission, following resuscitation, and infusion of the selected vasoactive agent for at least 30 minutes; combination of both pharmacotherapy and endoscopic therapy has been shown to achieve better hemostasis.[51] EBL is the preferred modality of therapy in patients with AVB, with the first band being placed on the site of the bleeding varix[52] (**Fig. 2**).

Failure to control bleed is defined as ongoing blood loss requiring transfusions and in the presence of tachycardia and hypotension. In up to 20% of cirrhotic particularly in Child-Pugh C patients, bleeding can be torrential leading to poor endoscopic visualization. Mortality in these patients may be up to 50%. Model for End stage liver disease (MELD) score predicts mortality in these patients.[53] Treatment involves optimizing terlipressin dosage and a repeat endoscopy-guided therapeutic intervention. A self-expanding endoscopically retrievable endoscopic stent may be used to control bleeding as a bridge to TIPS. Recent evidence recommends early TIPS as the treatment of choice in patients with ongoing active bleed.

Early Transjugular intrahepatic portosystemic shunt (TIPS)

Previously, TIPS was recommended in patients with refractory variceal bleed following failure of endoscopic intervention. Interestingly, studies have shown early TIPS (within 72 hours) to improve survival in patients with high risk of treatment failure, particularly in patients with Child B with active bleed and Child C cirrhosis.[54] A recent multicenter, observational study on preemptive TIPS in 671 patients with AVB with above high-risk features of treatment failure showed reduced rebleeding rates in the high risk groups (92% vs 74%, P = .017) in comparison to drug and endoscopic management. Preemptive TIPS was associated with lower 1 year mortality (22% vs 47%, P = .002) in patients with Child C cirrhosis. The presence of ACLF or hepatic encephalopathy or jaundice is not absolute contraindications for TIPS in the presence of active bleed,

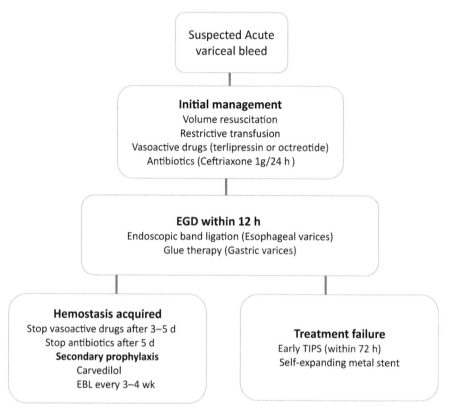

Fig. 2. Algorithmic approach to acute esophageal variceal bleed.

especially in patients who are candidates for liver transplantation Progressive-worsening liver failure as evidenced by lactate greater than 12, Child-Pugh score greater than 14, or MELD greater than 24 are contraindications for TIPS and if performed, back up liver transplantation should be available.[55] Unfortunately, the use of TIPS is limited by the lack of wider availability and limited availability of liver transplantation experts. Rebleeding in the first 5 days can be effectively managed by endoscopic measures followed by TIPS.

Secondary Prophylaxis

Recurrence of variceal bleed is associated with a 1-year mortality of 40%. Hence, following the control of variceal bleed, patients should be treated with a combination of NSBB and EBL with the intention of complete eradication. All patients with variceal bleeding should also be evaluated for liver transplantation. NSBB reduce the rate of rebleeding from 60% in untreated controls to approximately 40% and all-cause mortality. The combination of EBL and NSBB is more effective than EBL alone in decreasing the risk of rebleeding, but without a survival advantage. Thus, the combination of an NSBB and EBL is the recommended therapy for secondary prophylaxis of esophageal variceal bleeding. EBL is carried out every 3 to 4 weeks until variceal obliteration is achieved. If patients have a variceal bleed despite a combination of NSBB and EBL therapy then TIPS is recommended.[56]

Future Research

Although the management of portal hypertension, varices, and related bleeding has improved remarkably over the last couple of decades, several questions remain unanswered. With recent advances in the understanding of pathogenesis, in particular bacterial dysbiosis, endotoxin release, and the presence of systemic inflammatory response, there may be more treatment options.

Identification of patients at risk of variceal rupture remains less clear. It is probably appropriate time to seek the help of artificial intelligence (AI) and machine learning (ML). The application of AI and ML is changing the approach to several diseases. The role of these novel software tools have been studied in the diagnosis of portal hypertension. The role of portal phase CT was recently studied using deep learning. Auto-ML HVPG (aHVPG) was measured and validated using radiomics in 372 patients and identified linear correlation with conventional HVPG readings. aHVPG correlated well with HVPG greater than 10 (area under the curve [AUC] 0.833), HVPG greater than 12 mmHg (AUC 0.774), HVPG greater than 16 mmHg (AUC 0.81), and HVPG greater than 20 (AUC 0.81).[57]

Identifying patients at risk of esophageal variceal bleed is challenging. This was recently studied using ML. In this study, 163 of 828 patients with cACLD and high-risk esophageal varices developed variceal bleed, where ML was able to predict future variceal bleed 98.7%, 93.7%, and 85.7% in the derivation, internal validation, and external validation cohorts, respectively. Interestingly, the combination of endoscopy and ML produced a better prediction for 3-year risk of variceal bleeding rates (64%–85%).[58] In another ML model, the outcome of variceal bleeding was evaluated using various clinical and biochemical parameters. The model predicted 1- and 12-month survival with an ROC 0.91.[59]

All these studies are retrospective in a smaller number of patients. A large metacentric, prospective study required to evaluate the utility of ML in patients with portal Hypertension.

SUMMARY

Understanding the pathogenesis of portal hypertension is continuing to evolve. The risk of portal hypertension and liver disease progression obtained through HVPG can be corroborated clinically using noninvasive tools. More validated studies are required to ascertain the exact role of these tools in the diagnosis and monitoring of patients with portal hypertension.

NSBB, in particular carvedilol, is the treatment of choice for patients with CSPH. Endoscopic screening is mandatory to identify patients with higher risk of variceal bleed. All patients with suspected variceal hemorrhage should be treated with vasoactive drugs. EBL remains the therapeutic modality of choice in patients with acute variceal hemorrhage. Early TIPS is recommended for those with failure to control bleed. The cause of liver disease should be identified, and every attempt should be made to treat the underlying disease to stabilize or to recompensate patients with cirrhosis.

CLINICS CARE POINTS

- Transient elastography and platelet count guides cirrhotic patients for screening EGD.
- Non-selective betablocker is the most effective therapy in reducing portal pressure and variceal bleed.

- Antibiotic prophylaxis is mandatory in the management of acute variceal bleed.
- Placement of TIPS within 72 hours improves survival in patients with high risk variceal bleed.
- Combination of EBL and NSBB reduces variceal rebleed.

ACKNOWLEDGEMENT

Not applicable.

FUNDING

None.

REFERENCES

1. Garcia-Tsao G, Abraldes JG, Berzigotti A, et al. Portal hypertensive bleeding in cirrhosis: risk stratification, diagnosis, and management: 2016 practice guidance by the American Association for the study of liver diseases. Hepatology 2017; 65(1):310–35 [Erratum appears in Hepatology 2017;66(1):304].
2. D'Amico G, Pagliaro L, Bosch J. The treatment of portal hypertension: a meta-analytic review. Hepatology 1995;22(1):332–54.
3. Merli M, Nicolini G, Angeloni S, et al. Incidence and natural history of small esophageal varices in cirrhotic patients. J Hepatol 2003;38(3):266–72.
4. Amitrano L, Guardascione MA, Manguso F, et al. The effectiveness of current acute variceal bleed treatments in unselected cirrhotic patients: refining short-term prognosis and risk factors. Am J Gastroenterol 2012;107(12):1872–8.
5. Fortune BE, Garcia-Tsao G, Ciarleglio M, et al, Vapreotide Study Group. Child-Turcotte-Pugh Class is Best at Stratifying Risk in Variceal Hemorrhage: Analysis of a US Multicenter Prospective Study. J Clin Gastroenterol 2017;51(5):446–53.
6. Sarin SK, Lahoti D, Saxena SP, et al. Prevalence, classification and natural history of gastric varices: a long-term follow-up study in 568 portal hypertension patients. Hepatology 1992;16(6):1343–9.
7. Gracia-Sancho J, Caparrós E, Fernández-Iglesias A, et al. Role of liver sinusoidal endothelial cells in liver diseases. Nat Rev Gastroenterol Hepatol 2021;18(6): 411–31.
8. Tsuchida T, Friedman SL. Mechanisms of hepatic stellate cell activation. Nat Rev Gastroenterol Hepatol 2017;14(7):397–411.
9. Wanless IR, Wong F, Blendis LM, et al. Hepatic and portal vein thrombosis in cirrhosis: possible role in development of parenchymal extinction and portal hypertension. Hepatology 1995;21(5):1238–47. PMID: 7737629.
10. Tripodi A. Hemostasis abnormalities in cirrhosis. Curr Opin Hematol 2015;22(5): 406–12.
11. Baffy G. Potential mechanisms linking gut microbiota and portal hypertension. Liver Int 2019;39(4):598–609.
12. Trebicka J, Macnaughtan J, Schnabl B, et al. The microbiota in cirrhosis and its role in hepatic decompensation. J Hepatol 2021;75(Suppl 1):S67–81.
13. Arab JP, Martin-Mateos RM, Shah VH. Gut-liver axis, cirrhosis and portal hypertension: the chicken and the egg. Hepatol Int 2018;12(Suppl 1):24–33.
14. Bosch J, Abraldes JG, Berzigotti A, et al. The clinical use of HVPG measurements in chronic liver disease. Nat Rev Gastroenterol Hepatol 2009;6(10):573–82.

15. Berzigotti A, Rossi V, Tiani C, et al. Prognostic value of a single HVPG measurement and Doppler-ultrasound evaluation in patients with cirrhosis and portal hypertension. J Gastroenterol 2011;46(5):687–95.

16. Ripoll C, Groszmann R, Garcia-Tsao G, et al, Portal Hypertension Collaborative Group. Hepatic venous pressure gradient predicts clinical decompensation in patients with compensated cirrhosis. Gastroenterology 2007;133(2):481–8.

17. de Franchis R. Updating consensus in portal hypertension: report of the Baveno III Consensus Workshop on definitions, methodology and therapeutic strategies in portal hypertension. J Hepatol 2000;33(5):846–52.

18. Hutchinson SJ, Bird SM, Goldberg DJ. Influence of alcohol on the progression of hepatitis C virus infection: a meta-analysis. Clin Gastroenterol Hepatol 2005; 3(11):1150–9.

19. Ripoll C, Groszmann RJ, Garcia-Tsao G, et al, Portal Hypertension Collaborative Group. Hepatic venous pressure gradient predicts development of hepatocellular carcinoma independently of severity of cirrhosis. J Hepatol 2009;50(5):923–8.

20. You MW, Kim KW, Pyo J, et al. A Meta-analysis for the Diagnostic Performance of Transient Elastography for Clinically Significant Portal Hypertension. Ultrasound Med Biol 2017;43(1):59–68.

21. Reiberger T. The Value of Liver and Spleen Stiffness for Evaluation of Portal Hypertension in Compensated Cirrhosis. Hepatol Commun 2022;6(5):950–64.

22. de Franchis R, VI Faculty B. Expanding consensus in portal hypertension: Report of the Baveno VI Consensus Workshop: Stratifying risk and individualizing care for portal hypertension. J Hepatol 2015;63(3):743–52.

23. Vuille-Lessard É, Rodrigues SG, Berzigotti A. Noninvasive Detection of Clinically Significant Portal Hypertension in Compensated Advanced Chronic Liver Disease. Clin Liver Dis 2021;25(2):253–89.

24. Jothimani D, Danielraj S, Nallathambi B, et al. Optimal diagnostic tool for surveillance of oesophageal varices during COVID-19 pandemic. Clin Radiol 2021; 76(7):550.e1–7.

25. Tripathi D, Stanley AJ, Hayes PC, et al. Clinical Services and Standards Committee of the British Society of Gastroenterology. U.K. guidelines on the management of variceal haemorrhage in cirrhotic patients. Gut 2015;64(11):1680–704.

26. de Franchis R, Bosch J, Garcia-Tsao G, et al, Baveno VII Faculty. Baveno VII - Renewing consensus in portal hypertension. J Hepatol 2022;76(4):959–74. Erratum in: J Hepatol. 2022 Apr 14.

27. Wang Q, Zhao H, Deng Y, et al. Validation of Baveno VII criteria for recompensation in entecavir-treated patients with hepatitis B-related decompensated cirrhosis. J Hepatol 2022;77(6):1564–72.

28. Lebrec D, Poynard T, Hillon P, et al. Propranolol for prevention of recurrent gastrointestinal bleeding in patients with cirrhosis: a controlled study. N Engl J Med 1981;305(23):1371–4.

29. Pascal JP, Cales P. Propranolol in the prevention of first upper gastrointestinal tract hemorrhage in patients with cirrhosis of the liver and esophageal varices. N Engl J Med 1987;317(14):856–61. Erratum in: N Engl J Med 1988 Apr 14;318(15):994.

30. Garcia-Tsao G, Bosch J. Management of varices and variceal hemorrhage in cirrhosis. N Engl J Med 2010;362(9):823–32. Erratum in: N Engl J Med. 2011 Feb 3;364(5):490. Dosage error in article text.

31. Conn HO, Grace ND, Bosch J, et al. Propranolol in the prevention of the first hemorrhage from esophagogastric varices: A multicenter, randomized clinical trial.

The Boston-New Haven-Barcelona Portal Hypertension Study Group. Hepatology 1991;13(5):902–12. PMID: 2029994.

32. Teran JC, Imperiale TF, Mullen KD, et al. Primary prophylaxis of variceal bleeding in cirrhosis: a cost-effectiveness analysis. Gastroenterology 1997;112(2):473–82.

33. Pérez-Ayuso RM, Valderrama S, Espinoza M, et al. Endoscopic band ligation versus propranolol for the primary prophylaxis of variceal bleeding in cirrhotic patients with high risk esophageal varices. Ann Hepatol 2010;9(1):15–22. PMID: 20308718.

34. Rockey DC. Pharmacologic therapy for gastrointestinal bleeding due to portal hypertension and esophageal varices. Curr Gastroenterol Rep 2006;8(1):7–13.

35. Burroughs AK, Tsochatzis EA, Triantos C. Primary prevention of variceal haemorrhage: a pharmacological approach. J Hepatol 2010;52(6):946–8.

36. Villanueva C, Torres F, Sarin SK, et al. Carvedilol-IPD-MA-group and the Baveno Cooperation: an EASL Consortium. Carvedilol reduces the risk of decompensation and mortality in patients with compensated cirrhosis in a competing-risk meta-analysis. J Hepatol 2022;77(4):1014–25.

37. Tripathi D, Ferguson JW, Kochar N, et al. Randomized controlled trial of carvedilol versus variceal band ligation for the prevention of the first variceal bleed. Hepatology 2009;50(3):825–33.

38. Shah HA, Azam Z, Rauf J, et al. Carvedilol vs. esophageal variceal band ligation in the primary prophylaxis of variceal hemorrhage: a multicentre randomized controlled trial. J Hepatol 2014;60(4):757–64.

39. Zafra C, Abraldes JG, Turnes J, et al. Simvastatin enhances hepatic nitric oxide production and decreases the hepatic vascular tone in patients with cirrhosis. Gastroenterology 2004;126(3):749–55.

40. Abraldes JG, Albillos A, Bañares R, et al. Simvastatin lowers portal pressure in patients with cirrhosis and portal hypertension: a randomized controlled trial. Gastroenterology 2009;136(5):1651–8.

41. Vijayaraghavan R, Jindal A, Arora V, et al. Hemodynamic Effects of Adding Simvastatin to Carvedilol for Primary Prophylaxis of Variceal Bleeding: A Randomized Controlled Trial. Am J Gastroenterol 2020;115(5):729–37.

42. Abraldes JG, Villanueva C, Aracil C, et al, BLEPS Study Group. Addition of Simvastatin to Standard Therapy for the Prevention of Variceal Rebleeding Does Not Reduce Rebleeding but Increases Survival in Patients With Cirrhosis. Gastroenterology 2016;150(5):1160–70, e3.

43. Thalheimer U, Triantos CK, Samonakis DN, et al. Infection, coagulation, and variceal bleeding in cirrhosis. Gut 2005;54(4):556–63.

44. Villanueva C, Colomo A, Bosch A, et al. Transfusion strategies for acute upper gastrointestinal bleeding. N Engl J Med 2013;368(1):11–21. Erratum in: N Engl J Med. 2013;368(24):2341.

45. Zhou X, Tripathi D, Song T, et al. Terlipressin for the treatment of acute variceal bleeding: A systematic review and meta-analysis of randomized controlled trials. Medicine (Baltimore) 2018;97(48):e13437.

46. Cavallin M, Piano S, Romano A, et al. Terlipressin given by continuous intravenous infusion versus intravenous boluses in the treatment of hepatorenal syndrome: A randomized controlled study. Hepatology 2016;63(3):983–92.

47. Abid S, Jafri W, Hamid S, et al. Terlipressin vs. octreotide in bleeding esophageal varices as an adjuvant therapy with endoscopic band ligation: a randomized double-blind placebo-controlled trial. Am J Gastroenterol 2009;104(3):617–23.

48. Seo YS, Park SY, Kim MY, et al. Lack of difference among terlipressin, somato-statin, and octreotide in the control of acute gastroesophageal variceal hemor-rhage. Hepatology 2014;60(3):954–63.

49. Yan X, Leng Z, Xu Q, et al. The influences of timing of urgent endoscopy in pa-tients with acute variceal bleeding: a cohort study. BMC Gastroenterol 2022; 22(1):506.

50. Thabut D, Bernard-Chabert B. Management of acute bleeding from portal hyper-tension. Best Pract Res Clin Gastroenterol 2007;21(1):19–29.

51. Bañares R, Albillos A, Rincón D, et al. Endoscopic treatment versus endoscopic plus pharmacologic treatment for acute variceal bleeding: a meta-analysis. Hep-atology 2002;35(3):609–15.

52. Garcia-Tsao G, Sanyal AJ, Grace ND, et al. Practice Guidelines Committee of American Association for Study of Liver Diseases; Practice Parameters Commit-tee of American College of Gastroenterology. Prevention and management of gastroesophageal varices and variceal hemorrhage in cirrhosis. Am J Gastroen-terol 2007;102(9):2086–102. Erratum in: Am J Gastroenterol. 2007 Dec;102(12): 2868.

53. Kumar S, Asrani SK, Kamath PS. Epidemiology, diagnosis and early patient man-agement of esophagogastric hemorrhage. Gastroenterol Clin North Am 2014; 43(4):765–82.

54. García-Pagán JC, Caca K, Bureau C, et al. Early TIPS (Transjugular Intrahepatic Portosystemic Shunt) Cooperative Study Group. Early use of TIPS in patients with cirrhosis and variceal bleeding. N Engl J Med 2010;362(25):2370–9.

55. Hernández-Gea V, Procopet B, Giráldez Á, et al. International Variceal Bleeding Observational Study Group and Baveno Cooperation. Preemptive-TIPS Improves Outcome in High-Risk Variceal Bleeding: An Observational Study. Hepatology 2019;69(1):282–93.

56. Jakab SS, Garcia-Tsao G. Evaluation and Management of Esophageal and Gastric Varices in Patients with Cirrhosis. Clin Liver Dis 2020;24(3):335–50.

57. Yu Q, Huang Y, Li X, et al. An imaging-based artificial intelligence model for non-invasive grading of hepatic venous pressure gradient in cirrhotic portal hyperten-sion. Cell Rep Med 2022;3(3):100563.

58. Agarwal S, Sharma S, Kumar M, et al. Development of a machine learning model to predict bleed in esophageal varices in compensated advanced chronic liver disease: A proof of concept. J Gastroenterol Hepatol 2021;36(10):2935–42.

59. Wang Y, Hong Y, Wang Y, et al. Automated Multimodal Machine Learning for Esophageal Variceal Bleeding Prediction Based on Endoscopy and Structured Data. J Digit Imaging 2022. https://doi.org/10.1007/s10278-022-00724-6.

Cirrhosis and Portal Hypertension
How Do We Deal with Ascites and Its Consequences

Marta Tonon, MD, PhD, Salvatore Piano, MD, PhD*

KEYWORDS

- Ascites • Complications of cirrhosis • Portal hypertension
- Large-volume paracentesis • Human albumin • Refractory ascites • TIPS

KEY POINTS

- Ascites is the most common complication of cirrhosis and is associated with high risk of mortality.
- Portal hypertension, systemic inflammation, and splanchnic arterial vasodilation are the main drivers of the development of ascites.
- The treatment of ascites aims to control ascites and prevent further decompensation and acute on chronic liver failure and should be stratified according to the grade of ascites and presence of complications.

INTRODUCTION

The development of complications of cirrhosis (ie, ascites, gastrointestinal bleeding, and hepatic encephalopathy) marks a fundamental turning point in the course of liver disease. In fact, the transition from compensated to decompensated cirrhosis involves a rapid worsening of the patient's prognosis, which reaches a 5-year mortality of 30% to 50%.[1,2] Ascites is the most common cause of decompensation in patients with cirrhosis, with a rate of development of about 5% to 10% per year.[3] Its occurrence is associated with a very high mortality rate.[4] Herein, the authors reviewed the pathophysiological mechanisms and therapeutic options for ascites in patients with cirrhosis.

Unit of Internal Medicine and Hepatology, Department of Medicine, University of Padova, Padova, Italy
* Corresponding author. Department of Medicine, University of Padova, Via Giustiniani 2, 35128, Padova, Italy
E-mail address: salvatorepiano@gmail.com

Med Clin N Am 107 (2023) 505–516
https://doi.org/10.1016/j.mcna.2022.12.004
0025-7125/23/© 2022 Elsevier Inc. All rights reserved.

DEFINITIONS

Ascites is defined as an abnormal buildup of fluid in the abdomen. It is important to point out that ascites due to liver cirrhosis represents about 80% of all abdominal effusions. In all other cases, it is associated with different possible causes, such as malignancies, congestive heart failure, nephrotic syndrome, and tuberculosis.[5]

The International Club of Ascites (ICA) classified ascites according to two different criteria, that is, its quantity and responsivity to medical treatment (**Table 1**).

Considering ascites according to its quantity, there are three different possible grades: Grade 1 ascites is detectable only by ultrasound examination and Grade 2 ascites is characterized by moderate symmetric distention of abdomen, whereas Grade 3 ascites is defined as large or gross ascites with marked abdominal distention.[5]

Considering responsivity to medical treatment, ascites is classically considered either responsive or refractory, that is, ascites that cannot be mobilized or the early recurrence of which (ie, after large-volume paracentesis [LVP]) cannot be satisfactorily prevented by medical therapy.[3,6] The refractoriness of ascites may be secondary to the inability to resolve despite maximal diuretic therapy (ie, spironolactone 400 mg/d and furosemide 160 mg/d and a salt-restricted diet for at least 1 week). In this case, it can be classified as a diuretic-resistant ascites. In other patients, ascites cannot be managed with an appropriate dosage of diuretics due to the development of complications, such as hepatic encephalopathy, renal impairment, hyponatremia, hypokalemia or hyperkalemia, or invalidating muscle cramps. This is defined as diuretic-intractable ascites and is the most common type of refractory ascites.[7]

However, a third category has been defined by ICA, that is, recurrent ascites, which is defined as an ascites that recurs (and needs to be managed with LVPs) at least on three occasions within a 12-month period despite dietary sodium restriction and adequate diuretic dosage.[6] Refractory ascites is associated with a very poor prognosis, with a median survival of about 6 months.[8] Patients with refractory ascites had significantly lower 36-month transplant-free survival than patients with responsive or recurrent ascites.[9] Therefore, recurrent ascites is remarkably different than refractory ascites. The occurrence of complications of ascites (refractory ascites, refractory hydrothorax, spontaneous bacterial peritonitis [SBP], and hepatorenal syndrome-acute kidney injury [HRS-AKI]) defines complicated ascites. SBP is defined as an infection of ascites without surgically treatable source. It is defined by a polymorphonuclear cells (PMN) count greater than 250 cells/μL.[7] HRS-AKI is defined as AKI in patients with ascites which does not resolve after 2 days of volume expansion with albumin (1 g/kg/d) and without signs of parenchymal kidney damage (no proteinuria, no hematuria, no use of nephrotoxic drugs, and no shock).[7]

PATHOPHYSIOLOGY

Portal hypertension is the main driver of the development of ascites in cirrhosis and is caused by an increased intrahepatic vascular resistance due to the disruption of liver architecture, fibrosis, and endothelial dysfunction. Portal hypertension leads to the production of endogenous vasodilating substances in the splanchnic circulation, such as nitric oxide (NO), endocannabinoids, and carbon monoxide causing a splanchnic arterial vasodilation.[10] The reduction in systemic vascular resistance causes the activation of neurohumoral pathways (renin-angiotensin-aldosterone system [RAAS], sympathetic nervous system, and non-osmotic secretion of vasopressin) that increase sodium and water retention, increase cardiac output, and cause vasoconstriction to maintain systemic blood pressure within normal ranges. However, as the disease progresses, the worsening of portal hypertension and splanchnic

Table 1
Definitions and existing classifications of ascites and its complications

According to the amount of fluid in the abdominal cavity	*Grade 1*: Mild ascites which is only detectable by ultrasound examination *Grade 2*: Moderate symmetric distension of abdomen *Grade 3*: Large or gross ascites with marked abdominal distension
According to the presence of complications	*Uncomplicated*: ascites that is not refractory, not infected (ie, SBP) nor associated with renal failure (ie, HRS) *Complicated*: ascites that is complicated by any of the above
According to the response to medical treatment	*Responsive*: ascites that is well controlled with diuretic treatment and sodium restriction *Recurrent*: ascites that recurs at least on 3 occasions within a 12-month period despite dietary sodium restriction and adequate diuretic dosage *Refractory*: ascites that cannot be mobilized or the early recurrence of which (ie, after LVP) cannot be satisfactorily prevented by medical therapy
Criteria for refractoriness	*Diuretic-resistant*: ascites that is refractory because of a lack of response to sodium restriction and diuretic treatment *Diuretic-intractable*: ascites that is refractory because of the development of diuretic-induced complications[a] that preclude the use of an effective diuretic dosage

[a] Diuretic-induced complications: Diuretic-induced hepatic encephalopathy, diuretic-induced renal impairment (increase of serum creatinine by >100% to a value > 2 mg/dL (177 mmol/L), diuretic-induced hyponatremia (a decrease of serum sodium by > 10 mmol/L to a serum sodium of <125 mmol/L), diuretic-induced hypo- or hyperkalemia, and invalidating muscle cramps.

vasodilation cannot be compensated by a further increase in cardiac output. The result is a further increase in sodium and water retention that are responsible for the development of ascites. Moreover, in most advanced stages, the maximal activation of endogenous vasoconstrictors system may cause renal vasoconstriction and hypoperfusion, causing HRS-AKI. A recently discovered mechanism contributing to the development of ascites and circulatory dysfunction is systemic inflammation, which is caused by a pathologic bacterial translocation from the gut to the systemic circulation and is favored by a cirrhosis associated immune dysfunction.[11,12] The maximal manifestation of bacterial translocation is SBP. Systemic inflammation contributes to the worsening of splanchnic arterial vasodilation and is also responsible for a reduction in cardiac contractility.[13] The occurrence of bacterial infections can precipitate the occurrence of overt ascites.[14] The pathophysiology of ascites has been schematically summarized in **Fig. 1**.

CLINICAL IMPLICATIONS

Patients with ascites have a poor prognosis[1,2] and about one-half of them will develop further decompensating events within a median of 11 months.[15] The most common further decompensating events are refractory ascites, hepatic encephalopathy, SBP, and HRS-AKI, with a 1-year incidence of 24%, 19%, 10%, and 8%, respectively.[15] The rate of further decompensation is higher for Grade 3 ascites than for

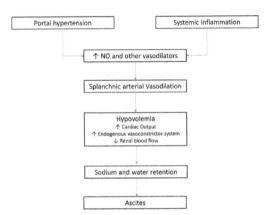

Fig. 1. Pathophysiology of ascites in cirrhosis.

Grade 2 ascites. Moreover, ascites is a risk factor for the occurrence of AKI and acute on chronic liver failure (ACLF).[16]

Prevention of Ascites

The prevention of occurrence of ascites can be obtained by treating the etiology of the disease or by the use of nonselective beta-blockers (NSBBs) in patients with clinically significant portal hypertension. Indeed, alcohol abstinence, hepatitis B virus (HBV) suppression, and hepatitis C virus (HCV) cure can almost abolish the risk of development of ascites in patients with compensated cirrhosis. Finally, in patients with compensated cirrhosis and clinically significant portal hypertension (hepatic venous pressure gradient [HVPG] >10 mm Hg) treatment with NSBBs proved to prevent decompensation, mainly reducing the occurrence of ascites.[17]

Therapeutic Options

All patients with ascites should be assessed for potential liver transplant indication/ eligibility and etiologic cure as well as screening endoscopy for esophageal varices.[18] Specific therapeutics options for ascites should be stratified according to the presence of complications (refractory ascites, SBP, and HRS-AKI) and the grade of ascites[7] (**Fig. 2**).

Treatment of Ascites

For patients with Grade 1 ascites, medical treatment is not recommended because there are no data on the actual benefit.[7] A recent study showed that patients with Grade 1 ascites had a similar 5-year mortality rate than patients with Grade 2 or 3 ascites, but the incidence of overt ascites was similar to those without ascites.[9] It is therefore suggested to monitor them closely because they are at higher risk of developing decompensation and ACLF.

For patients with Grade 2 ascites, the cornerstones of treatment are sodium restriction and diuretics (**Table 2**). As far as sodium restriction is concerned, it should be moderate (80–120 mmol/d). In fact, many studies demonstrate that an extreme salt restriction could favor hyponatremia and renal failure and worsen the precarious nutritional status of these patients due to a reduced calories intake and impaired food palatability.[7,19,20] Diuretic treatment should be started with the purpose of losing no more than 0.5 kg/d in those without edema and 1 kg/d in those with edema.

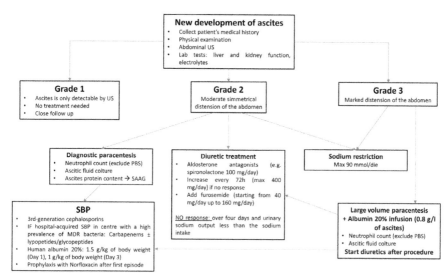

Fig. 2. Schematic approach to the treatment of ascites.

Antimineralocorticoid drugs (spironolactone, canrenone or K-canrenoate) are the drugs of choice as they counteract the consequence of RAAS activation. Antiminera-locorticoids can be aided by loop diuretics such as furosemide, which has been demonstrated to be more effective in mobilizing ascites than antimineralocorticoids alone in recurrent ascites.[21] The starting dose is 100 mg qd for antimineralocorticoids (increased stepwise up to 400 mg) and 20 to 25 mg bid for furosemide (increased step-wise up to 160 mg/d).

The treatment of choice for Grade 3 ascites is represented by LVPs. When the vol-ume of ascites drained is over 5L per paracentesis, plasma volume expansion is rec-ommended to avoid post-paracentesis circulatory dysfunction (PPCD).[22] PPCD can

Table 2	
Management of uncomplicated ascites	
Aldosterone antagonists	Starting dose: 100 mg/d Increase dose every 72 h if no response Maximum dosage: 400 mg/d
Furosemide	Starting dose: 20–25 mg BID (if no response with aldosterone antagonists alone) Maximum dosage: 160 mg/d
Sodium restriction	Maximum 90 mmol/L per day
Large-volume paracentesis	If needed

SBP prophylaxis with norfloxacin	Protein concentration in ascitic fluid <1.5 g/dL,
	    Child-Pugh ≥9
	Bilirubin ≥3 mg/dL or serum creatinine ≥1.2 mg/dL
	    or serum sodium ≤130 mmol/L)

Long-term albumin treatment
    (still under investigation)
	40 g twice a week for the first 2 wk followed by 40 gr per
	    week (only in patients with grade 2–3 ascites and at
	    least 200 mg of antialdosteronic drugs and furosemide)

No response: Mean weight loss of <0.8 kg over 4 days and urinary sodium output less than the sodium intake.

be prevented with 20% albumin solution (8 g/L removed) and is more effective than other plasma expanders.[23] A meta-analysis showed that albumin is superior to any other plasma expander not only in preventing PPCD but also its clinical consequences as well as mortality.[24] After a large-volume paracentesis, all patients should receive diuretics, when tolerated, to prevent early recurrence of ascites.[7]

It is important to state that both in patients with new onset Grade 2 or 3 ascites or other complications (encephalopathy, AKI, ACLF), or hospital admission, a paracentesis should be rapidly performed to rule out SBP.[7] A delay in performing paracentesis greater than 12 hours from admission is associated with higher mortality in patients with SBP.[25] When neutrophil count in ascitic fluid is higher than 250/mm^3, SBP is confirmed and an appropriate antibiotic treatment should be started, after performing ascitic fluid culture.[7]

For patients with refractory ascites, the first-line treatment is represented by periodic LVPs (Table 3). The performance of those, however, has no favorable impact on prognosis in these patients.[7] The placement of transjugular intrahepatic portosystemic shunt (TIPS) creates an artificial shunt between portal and hepatic vein, decreasing portal pressure and improving the control of ascites, therefore, should be considered in patients with refractory ascites.[26] In patients with recurrent/refractory ascites has been associated with an improvement of transplant free survival.[27] The main complication of TIPS, however, is the development of hepatic encephalopathy, which can be prevented by the use of rifaximin.[28] TIPS placement can be therefore considered in selected patients with recurrent ascites; however, the selection of patients' candidates for TIPS should be done by centers with relevant expertise and polytetrafluoroethylene-covered stents of 8 mm should be preferred.[7] Absolute

Table 3
Management of complicated ascites

Complication	Therapeutic Options
Refractory ascites	Large-volume paracentesis + albumin TIPS Liver transplantation
Recurrent ascites	Diuretic treatment Large-volume paracentesis + albumin if needed Consider TIPS Consider liver transplantation

SBP	Antibiotic treatment:
	  Third-generation cephalosporins or amoxicillin/clavulanic acid
	  Carbapenems ± lipopeptides/glycopeptides in hospital-acquired
	    episodes in centers with high prevalence of MDR bacteria
	Albumin:
	  1.5 g/kg of body weight on Day 1
	  1 g/kg of body weight on Day 3
	Prophylaxis with norfloxacin after first episode

HRS	Vasoconstrictors:
	  Terlipressin I.V. boluses starting from 1 mg/4–6 h to 2 mg/4–6 h OR
	    Continuous IV infusion starting from 2–3 mg/24 h to 12 mg/24 h
	  Midodrine/Octreotide Starting from 7.5 mg/8 h to 12.5 mg/8 h
	  Starting from 100 lg/8 h to 200 lg/8 h
	  Norepinephrine Continuous IV infusion starting from 0.5 mg/h to
	    3 mg/h
	Albumin:
	  20–40 g/d

contraindications to TIPS are recurrent hepatic encephalopathy (HE), hepatocellular carcinoma (HCC), intrahepatic masses, and heart failure. Relative contraindications to TIPS are model for end stage liver disease (MELD) $\geq$ 18, bilirubin greater than 3 mg/dL, advanced age (>70 year old), chronic kidney disease, and sarcopenia.

The use of automated low-flow ascites pump (alfapump) showed to be effective in reducing the need for LVP but was associated with a high rate of AKI and infections.[29]

The long-term administration of human albumin solution has been recently investigated in patients with ascites. Albumin aims to counteract the reduction of effective circulating volume and exerts anti-inflammatory activity due to its non-oncotic properties.[30] In the ANSWER trial, patients with ascites received human albumin (40 g twice a week for the initial 2 weeks and 40 g once a week thereafter) or standard of care for 18 months. Patients receiving albumin had a lower incidence of refractory ascites, SBP, renal failure, and liver-related hospitalizations and death than patients receiving standard of care.[31] A similar nonrandomized study showed that the use of human albumin (20 g twice a week) lead to a significantly lower 24-month mortality in patients with refractory ascites.[32] In the MACHT study, patients in waiting list for liver transplantation were randomized to receive either midodrine plus albumin (40 g every 15 days) or placebo.[33] The incidence of complications of cirrhosis was similar between the two groups. The discrepancy among those studies is likely related to the different population and duration of treatment. A new study is ongoing. Remarkably, no case of circulatory overload has been described with the long-term albumin administration, in contrast with findings in patients with acute decompensation of cirrhosis in whom albumin administration to reach 3 g/L was associated with no benefit and more serious adverse events.[34] The aim of this discussion is not to highlight the strengths or weaknesses of the various studies, but this is sufficient to consider the use of albumin in the treatment of ascites still not recommended in clinical practice guidelines (CPGs).

Other proposed treatment for ascites such as vaptans or splanchnic vasoconstrictors did not show enough encouraging results to justify their use in clinical practice do far.[7]

Treatment of Refractory Hydrothorax

Hepatic hydrothorax is defined by the accumulation of transudate fluids in the pleural cavity in a patient with cirrhosis without cardiopulmonary diseases. It is due to the aspiration of ascitic fluid from abdominal cavity to the thorax through a diaphragmatic defect because of the negative intrathoracic pressure. A diagnostic thoracentesis is needed in patients with hepatic hydrothorax to confirm the diagnosis and rule out spontaneous bacterial empyema.[7] Management of hepatic hydrothorax is similar to ascites and includes diuretics and thoracentesis to relief dyspnea.[7] Repeated thoracentesis can cause complications such as pneumothorax or bleeding. Evaluation of liver transplantation (LT) and/or TIPS placement is mandatory for these patients.[7] In those patients with contraindications to TIPS and LT, the placement of a permanent indwelling pleural catheter can be considered for palliative care.

Treatment of Spontaneous Bacterial Peritonitis

SBP is the most common infections in patients with cirrhosis.[35] Treatment of SBP involves both antibiotic treatment and plasma volume expansion with albumin. Antibiotic treatment should be adapted according to the local epidemiology, risk factors for multi drug resistant (MDR) bacteria, and presence of sepsis/septic shock.[36] Third-generation cephalosporins are appropriate for community acquired infections, whereas broad spectrum antibiotics (eg, carbapenems $\pm$ glycopeptides/lipopeptides) are needed for nosocomial ones.[37] Albumin expansion at the dose of 1.5 gr/kg of body weight on day 1 and 1 gr/kg of body weight on day 3 showed to reduce the incidence of AKI and improved survival in patients with SBP.[38] The effects were more evident in those with serum creatinine (SCr) greater than 1 mg/dL and bilirubin greater than 4 mg/dL.

There are three conditions in which antibiotic prophylaxis is indicated to prevent SBP, namely secondary prophylaxis, patients with variceal bleeding and those with protein count in ascites fluid below 1.5 g/dL and serum creatinine greater than 1.2 mg/dL or serum sodium less than 130 mmol/L or Child-Pugh score greater than B9 with bilirubin greater than 3 mg/dL.[7] Norfloxacin 400 mg/d can be used for the prophylaxis, but in patients with bleeding ceftriaxone was more effective.[39]

Treatment of Hepatorenal Syndrome-Acute Kidney Injury

HRS-AKI is the most severe form of AKI in cirrhosis, associated with a very high mortality rate. The management of HRS-AKI should follow the recommendations of the ICA.[40] Although the current differential diagnosis is far from being accurate, new urinary biomarkers, such as neutrophil gelatinase-associated lipocalin, could be of help in refining the differential diagnosis.[41,42] In patients with HRS-AKI, the treatment of choice is with terlipressin plus albumin.[43,44] Terlipressin is more effective than midodrine and octreotide,[45] whereas noradrenaline showed a similar efficacy in some trials[46] and inferiority in others.[47] Terlipressin has relevant potential side effects (arrhythmia, peripheral ischemia, diarrhea, and so forth), and episodes of life-threatening respiratory failure were reported in the CONFIRM trial,[44] which occurred frequently in patients with ACLF Grade 3, a group that is well known to respond poorly to terlipressin and to have poor benefit even in case of response.[48] A randomized trial showed that the administration of terlipressin by continuous infusion (starting dose 2–3 mg/d) was as effective as boluses (1 mg every 6 hours) but had lower rates of side effects.[49] Response to treatment with terlipressin and albumin responders to terlipressin and albumin have a better survival than nonresponders, but liver transplant remains the best treatment of HRS-AKI.[50] On clinical ground, the use of terlipressin and albumin frequently precedes transplant, and the resolution of HRS-AKI is associated with lower needs for renal replacement therapy and lower incidence of chronic kidney disease after transplant.[51]

SUMMARY

In conclusion, ascites is the most common complication of cirrhosis. Preventing further decompensation and ACLF is a key in the management of these patients. Treatment of ascites should be based on the grade of ascites and the presence of complications of ascites.

CLINICS CARE POINTS

- In all patients with first onset of Grade 2–3 ascites or hospitalized due to complications of ascites, a diagnostic paracentesis should be carried out to rule out spontaneous bacterial peritonitis (SBP).
- All patients with ascites should receive etiologic treatment for their liver disease if available.
- All patients with ascites should be referred to a liver transplant unit for checking the eligibility for liver transplant.

- Antimineralocorticoids with/without loop diuretics is still the treatment of choice in patients with ascites.
- In Grade 3 ascites, large-volume paracentesis plus albumin infusion is recommended.
- Transjugular intrahepatic portosystemic shunt should be considered in patients with recurrent/refractory ascites.
- Early administration of antibiotic treatment and albumin is recommended in patients with SBP.
- Antibiotic prophylaxis of SBP should be reserved to evidence-based indications.
- Terlipressin and albumin are the medical treatment of choice for HRS-AKI.

DISCLOSURE

M. Tonon has nothing to disclose. S. Piano received advisory board fees from Mallinckrodt and advises Plasma Protein Therapeutics Association and Resolution Therapeutics.

REFERENCES

1. D'Amico G, Morabito A, D'Amico M, et al. New concepts on the clinical course and stratification of compensated and decompensated cirrhosis. Hepatol Int 2018;12(Suppl 1):34–43.
2. Ratib S, Fleming KM, Crooks CJ, et al. 1- and 5-year survival estimates for people with cirrhosis of the liver in England, 1998–2009: a large population study. J Hepatol 2017;60:282–9.
3. Gines P, Quintero E, Arroyo V, et al. Compensated cirrhosis: natural history and prognostic factors. Hepatology 1987;7:122–8.
4. D'Amico G, Garcia-Tsao G, Pagliaro L. Natural history and prognostic indicators of survival in cirrhosis: a systematic review of 118 studies. J Hepatol 2006;44: 217–31.
5. Moore KP, Wong F, Ginès P, et al. The management of ascites in cirrhosis: Report on the consensus conference of the International Ascites Club. Hepatology 2003; 38:258–66.
6. Arroyo V, Gines P, Gerbes AL, et al. Definition and diagnostic criteria of refractory ascites and hepatorenal syndrome in cirrhosis. International Ascites Club. Hepatology 1996;23:164–76.
7. European Association for the Study of the Liver. EASL Clinical Practice Guidelines for the management of patients with decompensated cirrhosis. J Hepatol 2018; 69:406–60.
8. Salerno F, Borroni G, Moser P, et al. Survival and prognostic factors of cirrhotic patients with ascites: a study of 134 outpatients. Am J Gastroenterol 1993;88: 514–9.
9. Tonon M, Piano S, Gambino CG, et al. Outcomes and Mortality of Grade 1 Ascites and Recurrent Ascites in Patients With Cirrhosis. Clin Gastroenterol Hepatol 2021 Feb;19(2):358–66, e8.
10. Schrier RW, Arroyo V, Bernardi M, et al. Peripheral arterial vasodilation hypothesis: a proposal for the initiation of renal sodium and water retention in cirrhosis. Hepatology 1988;8(5):1151–7.
11. Wiest R, Lawson M, Geuking M. Pathological bacterial translocation in liver cirrhosis. J Hepatol 2014;60:197–209.

12. Albillos A, Lario M, Álvarez-Mon M. Cirrhosis-associated immune dysfunction: distinctive features and clinical relevance. J Hepatol 2014;61:1385–96.
13. Arroyo V, Angeli P, Moreau R, et al. The systemic inflammation hypothesis: Towards a new paradigm of acute decompensation and multiorgan failure in cirrhosis. J Hepatol 2021;74:670–85.
14. Piano S, Angeli P. Bacterial Infections in Cirrhosis as a Cause or Consequence of Decompensation? Clin Liver Dis 2021;25:357–72.
15. Balcar L, Tonon M, Semmler G, et al. Risk of further decompensation/mortality in patients with cirrhosis and ascites as the first single decompensation event. JHEP Rep 2022;4:100513.
16. Piano S, Tonon M, Vettore E, et al. Incidence, predictors and outcomes of acute-on-chronic liver failure in outpatients with cirrhosis. J Hepatol 2017;67:1177–84.
17. Villanueva C, Albillos A, Genescà J, et al. β blockers to prevent decompensation of cirrhosis in patients with clinically significant portal hypertension (PREDESCI): a randomised, double-blind, placebo-controlled, multicentre trial. Lancet 2019; 393:1597–608.
18. de Franchis R, Bosch J, Garcia-Tsao G, et al, Baveno VII Faculty. Baveno VII - Renewing consensus in portal hypertension. J Hepatol 2022;76:959–74.
19. Reynolds TB, Lieberman FL, Goodman AR. Advantages of treatment of ascites without sodium restriction and without complete removal of excess fluid. Gut 1978;19:549–53.
20. Morando F, Rosi S, Gola E, et al. Adherence to a moderate sodium restriction diet in outpatients with cirrhosis and ascites: A real-life cross-sectional study. Liver Int 2015;35:1508–15.
21. Angeli P, Fasolato S, Mazza E, et al. Combined vs. sequential diuretic treatment of ascites in non-azotaemic patients with cirrhosis: Results of an open randomised clinical trial. Gut 2010;59:98–104.
22. Ginès P, Tító L, Arroyo V, et al. Randomized comparative study of therapeutic paracentesis with and without intravenous albumin in cirrhosis. Gastroenterology 1988;94:1493–502.
23. Gines A, Fernandez-Esparrach G, Monescillo A, et al. Randomized trial comparing albumin, dextran 70, and polygeline in cirrhotic patients with ascites treated by paracentesis. Gastroenterology 1996;111:1002–10.
24. Bernardi M, Caraceni P, Navickis RJ, et al. Albumin infusion in patients undergoing large-volume paracentesis: a meta-analysis of randomized trials. Hepatology 2012;55:1172–81.
25. Kim JJ, Tsukamoto MM, Mathur AK, et al. Delayed paracentesis is associated with increased in-hospital mortality in patients with spontaneous bacterial peritonitis. Am J Gastroenterol 2014;109:1436–42.
26. Salerno F, Cammà C, Enea M, et al. Transjugular intrahepatic portosystemic shunt for refractory ascites: a meta-analysis of individual patient data. Gastroenterology 2007;133:825–34.
27. Bureau C, Thabut D, Oberti F, et al. Transjugular Intrahepatic Portosystemic Shunts With Covered Stents Increase Transplant-Free Survival of Patients With Cirrhosis and Recurrent Ascites. Gastroenterology 2017;152:157–63.
28. Bureau C, Thabut D, Jezequel C, et al. The Use of Rifaximin in the Prevention of Overt Hepatic Encephalopathy After Transjugular Intrahepatic Portosystemic Shunt : A Randomized Controlled Trial. Ann Intern Med 2021;174:633–40.
29. Lepida A, Marot A, Trépo E, et al. Systematic review with meta-analysis: Automated low-flow ascites pump therapy for refractory ascites. Aliment Pharmacol Ther 2019;50:978–87.

30. Bernardi M, Angeli P, Claria J, et al. Albumin in decompensated cirrhosis: new concepts and perspectives. Gut 2020;69:1127–38.

31. Caraceni P, Riggio O, Angeli P, et al. Long-term albumin administration in decompensated cirrhosis (ANSWER): an open-label randomised trial. Lancet 2018;391: 2417–29.

32. Di Pascoli M, Fasolato S, Piano S, et al. Long-term administration of human albumin improves survival in patients with cirrhosis and refractory ascites. Liver Int 2019;39:98–105.

33. Solà E, Solé C, Simón-Talero M, et al. Midodrine and albumin for prevention of complications in patients with cirrhosis awaiting liver transplantation. A randomized placebo-controlled trial. J Hepatol 2018;69:1250–9.

34. China L, Freemantle N, Forrest E, et al. A randomized trial of albumin infusions in hospitalized patients with cirrhosis. N Engl J Med 2021;384:808–17.

35. Piano S, Singh V, Caraceni P, et al. Epidemiology and Effects of Bacterial Infections in Patients With Cirrhosis Worldwide. Gastroenterology 2019;156: 1368–80, e10.

36. Fernandez J, Piano S, Bartoletti M, et al. Management of bacterial and fungal infections in cirrhosis: the MDRO challenge. J Hepatol 2021;75:S101–17.

37. Piano S, Fasolato S, Salinas F, et al. The empirical antibiotic treatment of nosocomial spontaneous bacterial peritonitis: results of a randomized, controlled clinical trial. Hepatology 2016;63:1299–309.

38. Sort P, Navasa M, Arroyo V, et al. Effect of Intravenous Albumin on Renal Impairment and Mortality in Patients with Cirrhosis and Spontaneous Bacterial Peritonitis. N Engl J Med 1999;341:403–9.

39. Fernandez J, del Arbol LR, Gomez C, et al. Norfloxacin vs ceftriaxone in the prophylaxis of infections in patients with advanced cirrhosis and hemorrhage. Gastroenterology 2006;131:1049–56.

40. Angeli P, Gines P, Wong F, et al. Diagnosis and management of acute kidney injury in patients with cirrhosis: revised consensus recommendations of the International Club of Ascites. J Hepatol 2015;62:968–74.

41. Fagundes C, Pepin MN, Guevara M, et al. Urinary neutrophil gelatinase-associated lipocalin as biomarker in the differential diagnosis of impairment of kidney function in cirrhosis. Hepatol 2012;57:267–73.

42. Gambino C, Piano S, Stenico M, et al. Diagnostic and prognostic performance of urinary neutrophil gelatinase-associated lipocalin in patients with cirrhosis and acute kidney injury. Hepatology 2022. https://doi.org/10.1002/hep.32799.

43. Martin-Llahì MM, Pepin MN, Guevara M, et al. Terlipressin and albumin versus albumin in patients with cirrhosis and hepatorenal syndrome: a randomized study. Gastroenterology 2008;134:1352–9.

44. Wong F, Pappas SC, Curry MP, et al. Terlipressin plus Albumin for the Treatment of Type 1 Hepatorenal Syndrome. N Engl J Med 2021;384:818–28.

45. Cavallin M, Kamath PS, Merli M, et al. Terlipressin plus albumin versus midodrine and octreotide plus albumin in the treatment of hepatorenal syndrome: a randomized trial. Hepatology 2015;62:567–74.

46. Singh V, Ghosh S, Singh B, et al. Noradrenaline vs. terlipressin in the treatment of hepatorenal syndrome: a randomized study. J Hepatol 2012;56:1293–8.

47. Arora V, Maiwall R, Rajan V, et al. Terlipressin Is Superior to Noradrenaline in the Management of Acute Kidney Injury in Acute on Chronic Liver Failure. Hepatology 2020;71:600–10.

48. Piano S, Schmidt HH, Ariza X, et al. Association Between Grade of Acute on Chronic Liver Failure and Response to Terlipressin and Albumin in Patients With Hepatorenal Syndrome. Clin Gastroenterol Hepatol 2018;16:1792–800.e3.

49. Cavallin M, Piano S, Romano A, et al. Terlipressin given by continuous intravenous infusion versus intravenous boluses in the treatment of hepatorenal syndrome: A randomized controlled study. Hepatology 2016;63:983–92.

50. Boyer TD, Sanyal AJ, Garcia-Tsao G, et al. Impact of liver transplantation on the survival of patients treated for hepatorenal syndrome type 1. Liver Transpl 2011; 17:1328–32.

51. Piano S, Gambino C, Vettore E, et al. Response to Terlipressin and Albumin Is Associated With Improved Liver Transplant Outcomes in Patients With Hepatorenal Syndrome. Hepatology 2021;73:1909–19.

Hepatic Encephalopathy
Diagnostic Tools and Management Strategies

Bryan D. Badal, MD, MS, Jasmohan S. Bajaj, MD*

KEYWORDS

- Covert hepatic encephalopathy • Overt hepatic encephalopathy • Ammonia
- Diagnosis • Management • Treatments

KEY POINTS

- Hepatic encephalopathy (HE) is a common complication of cirrhosis and is associated with decreased quality of life and increased mortality.
- Covert hepatic encephalopathy (CHE) is associated with increased admissions, decreased quality of life, and increased likelihood of progression to overt hepatic encephalopathy (OHE), which needs specialized testing to diagnose.
- OHE is a clinical diagnosis and is supported by the presence of asterixis and should be graded by the West Haven Criteria or Glasgow Coma Scale if decreased consciousness is present. Evaluation should seek to identify precipitants or alternative diagnoses.
- Management of OHE should occur in parallel to the assessment. Patients should be stabilized with particular attention paid to the ability to protect the airway from aspiration and triaged to either the intensive care unit or the general hospital ward. Medical management consists of lactulose administration and rifaximin is recommended in cases of recurrent or persistent HE.
- Recurrence of HE is a common cause of hospital readmission and many aspects (avoiding unnecessary polypharmacy, oral health), multi-disciplinary care and checklists may mitigate the risk of readmission.

INTRODUCTION

Hepatic encephalopathy (HE) is defined as brain dysfunction secondary to liver insufficiency and/or portosystemic shunting. HE is a common manifestation of decompensation in patients with cirrhosis and can present on a spectrum of symptoms ranging from subclinical neurologic abnormalities to coma.[1,2] Development of HE is associated with increased risk of mortality,[3] as well as decreased quality of life.[4] Multiple hospital readmissions are common in HE and can represent a significant economic

Division of Gastroenterology, Hepatology, and Nutrition, Virginia Commonwealth University and Central Virginia Veterans Healthcare System, 1201 Broad Rock Boulevard, Richmond, VA, 23249, USA
* Corresponding author.
E-mail address: jasmohan.bajaj@vcuhealth.org

Med Clin N Am 107 (2023) 517–531
https://doi.org/10.1016/j.mcna.2023.01.003
0025-7125/23/© 2023 Elsevier Inc. All rights reserved.
medical.theclinics.com

burden to patients, caregivers, families, and the health care system.[5-7] Even after effective treatment and resolution of acute episodes of overt HE (OHE), patients may continue to have persistent cognitive deficits.[8] There are three major aspects of the natural history of HE, covert or minimal HE (MHE), the acute confusional state, and the post-OHE recovery stage, where the focus is to prevent a recurrence.

PATHOPHYSIOLOGY

HE occurs in the setting of a complex interplay among multiple organs beyond the liver and brain. Ammonia, which has long been understood as a critical driver of HE, is produced in the gut as a byproduct of bacterial metabolism. Small intestine bacterial overgrowth (SIBO) is common in cirrhosis due to decreased gut motility, producing an environment that not only increases ammonia production but also increases its absorption in the gut.[9] Ammonia enters the liver via the portal vein, where it is normally metabolized via the urea cycle. However, metabolism is decreased in the cirrhotic liver, and thus ammonia enters the systemic circulation, gaining access to the blood-brain barrier. This process can be further exacerbated by the presence of portosystemic shunts resulting from portal hypertension. Widespread inflammation in the setting of cirrhosis increases the permeability of the blood-brain barrier, and once through, ammonia is taken up by astrocytes and converted to glutamine, inducing astrocyte swelling and edema through osmosis.[10] Ammonia also induces gamma-aminobutyric acid (GABA), a major neuro-inhibitory peptide, resulting in a further decrease in neurologic function.[11]

Other organs that normally assist with ammonia clearance, including the kidneys and skeletal muscle, are often concomitantly affected in patients with cirrhosis. In the setting of comorbid renal dysfunction, the kidneys have an impaired ability to excrete ammonia as urea. In addition, when the kidneys are overburdened with excess ammonia, they excrete ammonia back into circulation. Skeletal muscle normally clears and stores ammonia in the form of glutamine. However, sarcopenia is common in patients with cirrhosis, and thus they lack muscle mass that can serve as an important reservoir of ammonia.[12]

Microbiome: Alterations in the microbiome have been noted in patients with cirrhosis and HE. Patients with cirrhosis have more dysbiosis, resulting in a decreased ratio of autochthonous bacteria such as *Firmicutes* to non-autochthonous bacteria such as *Bacteroidetes*.[13] Patients with cirrhosis have also been found to have a higher prevalence of pathogenic bacteria such as *Streptococcaceae* and *Enterobacteriaceae*.[14] Multiple studies have documented that patients with cirrhosis who develop HE have alterations in gut microbial composition and function than those who do have not developed HE.[15-18] Higher microbial dysbiosis is associated with endotoxemia which increases during HE development.[19,20] Microbiome studies also give us insight into which bacteria may be protective against HE. Patients who develop HE have lower amounts of short-chain fatty acids (SCFA) producing bacteria such as *Lachnospiraceae* and *Ruminococcaceae*.[14,19,21] SCFAs are responsible for maintaining healthy colonocytes, as well as lowering colonic pH and decreasing ammonia absorption in the gut (**Fig. 1**).[22,23]

Covert Hepatic Encephalopathy

Identification of CHE in patients with cirrhosis is important, as patients with CHE are at increased risk of developing OHE, higher hospitalization rate, and increased mortality. However, diagnosis of CHE can be challenging and time-consuming, requiring multiple approaches to accurately make the diagnosis.[24] Listed below are different

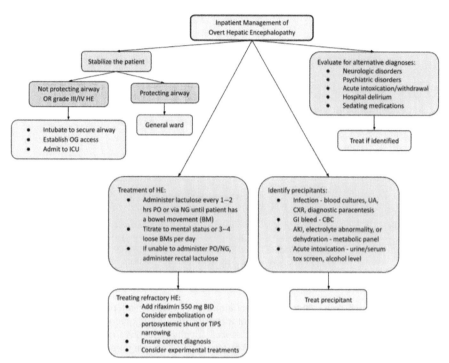

Fig. 1. Four pronged approach to inpatient management of OHE. Stabilization, treatment of OHE, identifying precipitants, and evaluation of alternative diagnoses should occur in parallel. AKI, acute kidney injury; BM, bowel movement; CXR, chest x-ray, GI, gastrointestinal; HE, hepatic encephalopathy; NG, nasogastric; OG, orogastric; OHE, overt hepatic encephalopathy; PO, by mouth; UA, urinalysis.

methods for testing for CHE. Testing should be considered for those without OHE and who are employed, driving, or endorsing a decreased quality of life (**Fig. 2**).[25]

COVERT HEPATIC ENCEPHALOPATHY DIAGNOSIS

Paper-and-Pencil Tests: The psychometric hepatic encephalopathy scale (PHES) is considered the gold standard for the diagnosis of CHE.[26] The PHES involves an array of timed paper-and-pencil tests including line tracing, serial-dotting, digit-symbol, and number connections.[27] Drawbacks to the PHES include the requirement of trained personnel for administration and its time-consuming length, which have limited its uptake in clinical practice.[28] The one-minute animal naming test (ANT), has also been used to diagnose CHE and can be applied without the need for equipment in a clinic population.[29]

    Computer-Based Tests: The Inhibitory Control Test (ICT) is a computer-based test that displays a series of numbers to patients, who are then instructed to respond to targets of alternating X and Y letters, and to ignore lures of non-alternating X and Y letters. The individuals being tested are scored based on the number of targets, avoidance of lures, and target reaction time. Advantages of the ICT include its sensitivity and ability to be administered in the absence of trained personnel.[30]

    Digital Apps: EncephalApp, a digitally based platform developed in 2013, uses the Stroop test to assess the psychomotor speed and cognitive flexibility. The test has "off" and "on" states. In the "off" state, patients are presented with red, blue, or green

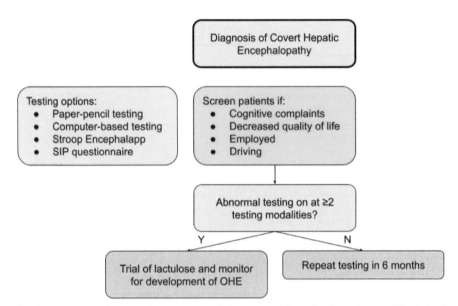

Fig. 2. Diagnosis of covert hepatic encephalopathy. Although all patients with cirrhosis should be considered for screening, special attention should be given to those with cognitive complaints, decreased quality-of-life scores. Ideally, two different testing modalities would be used to make diagnosis, with SIP questionnaire, Animal naming test and EncephalApp/Quickstroop simplest to implement. Patients with abnormal testing on 2 or more modalities should be considered for lactulose therapy.

pound signs (###), and the patient selects the correct text color as fast as possible. In the more difficult "on" state, the patient is presented with a word color in discordantly colored text, for example, the word green in blue text. The test evaluates the patient's time to complete the individual tasks and five runs in both states, providing a diagnosis of CHE in approximately 5 min.[31] The app has been validated and tested in a multicenter study in the United States enrolling over 400 patients with cirrhosis, as well as internationally.[32,33] If the length of the Stroop test prohibits incorporation into routine clinical care, the QuickStroop is available as an abbreviated version. QuickStroop uses just two runs in the above-mentioned "off" state and can be performed in as little as 40 seconds, allowing for an even quicker diagnosis.[34]

Speech Patterns: Evaluations of speech patterns in patients with cirrhosis have found that those with low PHES scores had lower speech rates, longer word duration, and less use of particles compared with those with normal PHES scores.[35] With standardization or artificial intelligence assistance, speech pattern analysis could potentially be developed into a useful screening tool for CHE.

Sickness Impact Profile (SIP): The Sickness Impact Profile is a battery of questions related to patient-related outcomes, and patients fill out a questionnaire of yes/no questions. Higher scores are associated with the increasing prevalence of CHE. One study was able to decrease the number of questions to four domains: balance, irritability, recreation, and eating and still able to screen for patients with CHE with good accuracy.[36]

Treatment of Covert Hepatic Encephalopathy

Most treatments for CHE start with a treatment trial with lactulose as the first line. This can be followed for longer as needed. US-based guidelines state that these treatments can be initiated on a case-by-case basis.

Lactulose: Patients found to have CHE should be considered for treatment with lactulose as this can improve cognition and quality of life scores.[37] Patients should be monitored within 6 months for the development of OHE regardless of lactulose administration as they are at increased risk for the development of OHE than those without CHE.[38,39]

Rifaximin: Rifaximin has been shown to improve cognitive performance as well as driving performance on a simulator compared with a placebo.[40–42] Treatment of CHE patients with cirrhosis can also improve bacterial function and endotoxemia. However, the expense of rifaximin and the lack of larger trials have precluded this from clinical practice.

Albumin: There is evidence that the addition of albumin infusions to lactulose therapy may be beneficial in the treatment of OHE.[43] In a randomized controlled trial, patients with prior OHE, but with continued CHE despite standard therapy, and hypoalbuminemia, were given infusions of albumin 1.5 g/kg or saline placebo for 5 weeks. Patients receiving albumin saw an improvement in their CHE based on PHES and Stroop scores.[44] This was also associated with a decrease in inflammatory markers and endothelial dysfunction markers.[43,44]

Golexanolone: Golexanolone is an investigational drug with the potential for treating HE in a manner independent of ammonia reduction. It is currently the only HE therapy that directly targets the central nervous system through GABA receptor inhibition, reversing the effects of high GABA activity and associated neuro-depression seen in HE.[45]

Overt Hepatic Encephalopathy

Diagnosis and prediction of overt hepatic encephalopathy

Unlike covert HE, overt HE is a clinically evident stage of HE. OHE is a clinical diagnosis,[46] and alternative etiologies of encephalopathy such as intoxication, withdrawal, or neurologic disorders should be investigated.[47] Staging by the West Haven Criteria is considered the gold standard, with disorientation and asterixis distinguishing OHE from CHE.[48] The Glasgow Coma Scale (GCS) is useful when evaluating a patient with decreased consciousness and assessing the need to secure the airway due to the risk of aspiration.[48,49] It is recommended that patients with GCS ≤ 8 be intubated.[46]

Ammonia: Although HE is associated with hyperammonemia, normal serum ammonia levels may vary widely by laboratory and among individuals.[50,51] Variables that may affect the accuracy of measurements include fasting or fed state, time from sample collection to analysis, and storage temperature of samples before analysis.[52] Measurement of serum ammonia is not recommended for the diagnosis of HE.[46] However, if measured, normal serum ammonia levels should prompt clinicians to investigate for alternative diagnoses.[53]

Microbiome: Given the microbiome differences in patients with and without HE, microbiome analysis has been identified as a potential method of screening out those with low risk of CHE risk and will not need testing. Patients with low amounts of *Streptococcus* and high amounts of *Ruminococcus* and *Clostridium* are less likely to test positive for CHE using the PHES or Stroop test.[17] Microbiome analysis could also be used to predict those having grade 3 or 4 encephalopathy during a hospital stay as patients with higher Proteobacteria and lower Firmicutes have been found to be more prone to encephalopathy.[54]

Serum Markers: Reliable serum markers for predicting the development of HE are lacking. A large multicenter study identified metabolite differences associated with the development of grade 3 or 4 HE during the hospital stay, including elevated methyl-4-hydroxybenzoate sulfate and 3 to 4 dihydroxy butyrate, as well as decreased maltose and thyroxine.[55] Although tests for these metabolite levels are not readily accessible for many clinicians, thyroxine testing is more widely available and may therefore be more practical for identifying those at risk for developing HE.

Management of overt hepatic encephalopathy. Initial steps for the management of OHE should include medical stabilization and appropriate triage of the patient. During the physical examination, clinicians should determine the ability of the patient to protect their airway from aspiration, and also grade encephalopathy. Endotracheal intubation should be considered for patients with Grade III/IV encephalopathy or GCS <8, and medications should be administered either intravenously (IV) or via nasogastric (NG) tube to reduce the risk of aspiration. Patients with hypotension or shock should be treated appropriately with IV fluids and may require vasopressors in the event of refractory hypotension despite fluid resuscitation. Ultimately, a decision needs to be made as to where to admit the patient and whether they require an intensive level of care. Patients with grades III/IV encephalopathy are best cared for in an intensive care setting.

After medical stabilization, patients should be evaluated for precipitants and alternative diagnoses. Common precipitants to be ruled out with physical examination and laboratory evaluation include gastrointestinal bleeding, infection, electrolyte abnormalities, and dehydration. Chemistry and complete blood count should be reviewed for abnormalities. Infectious workup should include urinalysis with culture, blood cultures, chest x-ray, and ascites cell count and culture. Prompt paracentesis should be performed as culture data can be used to tailor antibiotics and delay in initiation of appropriate antimicrobial therapy is associated with increased mortality. Brain imaging should be pursued if any focal neurologic examination findings are present. Although HE is associated with changes seen on an electroencephalogram (EEG) its primary clinical utility is in ruling out alternative pathologies such as nonconvulsive status epilepticus.[56] Intoxication or alcohol withdrawal can result in acute encephalopathy and evaluation should include alcohol and drug screens in appropriate patients.

Medical Therapies

Nonabsorbable disaccharides

Nonabsorbable disaccharides, such as lactulose and lactitol, are recommended as first-line therapy in patients with OHE, as well as the prevention of OHE recurrence.[57] As nonabsorbable disaccharides are metabolized by gut bacteria, they create an acidic environment inhospitable for the growth of ammonia-producing bacteria. The low pH also enhances the conversion of ammonia to ionized ammonium, preventing its diffusion into the systemic circulation, as well as creating an osmotic effect that increases peristalsis and thus the elimination of ammonia-producing bacteria.[58] Therapy should be adjusted based on the number of stools, as well as aiming for a stool quality of 3 to 4 on the Bristol Stool Scale (BSS). If patients reach BSS type 5, additional lactulose should be avoided.[59]

Rifaximin. Rifaximin is a broad-spectrum antibiotic with minimal systemic absorption, which treats HE by decreasing the amount of ammonia-producing bacteria in the gut.[60] Treatment with rifaximin plus lactulose has been shown to be superior in the prevention of HE recurrence compared with lactulose alone.[61] It is recommended that patients with more than one episode of HE be started on rifaximin in addition to lactulose for the prevention of HE.[46]

Zinc. Zinc is an important cofactor in nitrogen metabolism, and zinc deficiency decreases the efficiency of the urea cycle.[62] Trials using zinc have reported mixed results regarding efficacy, although the treatment appears safe and has not been associated with adverse outcomes.[63] It is likely beneficial to treat patients with zinc deficiency and HE but should not be used as monotherapy.

L-ornithine L-Aspartate. LOLA consists of two amino acids that can lead to a reduction in serum ammonia via two mechanisms: induction of the urea cycle in hepatocytes, and glutamine synthesis in hepatocytes and skeletal muscles.[64] In clinical trials LOLA has not only been found to decrease serum ammonia but lead to faster recovery and decreased hospital stay, in patients admitted with OHE.[65]

Investigational: rifaximin soluble dispersion tablets. Rifaximin SSD is an experimental formulation of rifaximin with higher water solubility than currently available formulations, which are minimally water soluble and require the presence of bile acids for optimal effect. Although still under investigation, rifaximin SSD may prove useful in the acute inpatient therapy of OHE, as well as reduce the time to resolution of OHE, especially in patients with altered or insufficient bile acids.[66] However, further studies are needed (**Fig. 3**).

Fecal Microbial Transplant

Two small-scale randomized controlled trials have evaluated fecal microbial transplant (FMT) in the prevention of HE. The first study administered FMT via enema to patients with recurrent HE, using donors with high amounts of fecal *Lachnospiraceae* and *Ruminococcaceae*, and found improvements in cognition and intestinal dysbiosis, as well as decreased hospital admissions.[67] The second study administered capsules with donor-enriched *Lachnospiraceae* and *Ruminococcaceae*, and found improvement in HE based on EncephalApp testing in patients with recurrent HE.[68]

Recurrent Hepatic Encephalopathy and Prevention

As mentioned above, HE is one of the major reasons for recurrence and rehospitalization in patients with cirrhosis.[46] Logistic approaches such as checklists

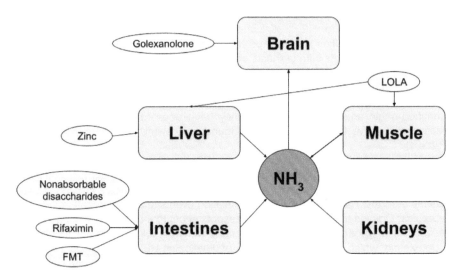

Fig. 3. HE. Treatment is more than just the liver and the brain. Multiple organs including brain, liver, intestines, skeletal muscle, and kidneys participate in nitrogen balance and many of these are targets for HE therapy.

ensure that patients are given adequate treatment as well as medical, radiological, and supportive treatment. After the first HE episode, lactulose is considered standard of care and after that rifaximin should be prescribed. There may be a role for additional therapies such as branched-chain amino acids and L-ornithine L-aspartate but the evidence basis is not strong[69]

Multi-Disciplinary Approach and Checklists

HE management requires a multidisciplinary team approach among a multidisciplinary health care team, the patient, and family members or caregivers. At the time of discharge, interruptive reminders to take lactulose, rifaximin, and follow-up appointments being set could reduce HE[6] Recurrence of HE represents the most common complication of cirrhosis associated with readmission.[5] Checklists may be helpful for patients and caregivers to keep track of treatments and subtle clinical changes that may be signs of impending OHE. Use of smartphone applications may be another method of streamlining checklists and providing quicker access to the health care team as clinical status changes. One such app, the patient buddy app, was tested in a small group of patients and their caregivers and showed promising results in the prevention of HE-related admissions through the use of remote checklist entries that alerted providers for missed entries or abnormal results.[70]

Supportive and Interventional Approaches

Portosystemic Shunts: In patients with recurrent or refractory HE despite optimal lactulose and rifaximin therapy, either spontaneous portosystemic shunts or even created shunts such as transjugular intrahepatic portosystemic shunts should be considered as being the reasons. Spontaneous shunt closure in appropriate patients may decrease the risk of further episodes of HE.[71] In a multicenter study, half of the patients remained free of HE 2 years after the closure of a spontaneously evolved portosystemic shunt.[72] For patients post TIPS with multiple episodes of unprovoked recurrent HE shunt reduction should be considered after risk–benefit discussion as a return of portal hypertension-related symptoms are likely.[73]

Nutrition: Malnutrition and sarcopenia are common in patients with cirrhosis, as well as known risk factors for HE.[74] Clinicians should ensure that patients with cirrhosis receive adequate nutrition including protein which should not be restricted. It is recommended that patients with cirrhosis consume 35 to 45 kcal/kg/d as well as 1.2 to 1.5 g/kg of protein daily.[75] It is recommended that the patient should have small meals throughout the day including a late-evening snack.[75] Consultation with nutrition services is recommended and has been found to prevent hospital readmissions.[76] Branched-chain amino acids although they have been found to improve muscle mass and improve CHE have not been found to prevent the occurrence of OHE (**Table 1**).[77]

Proton Pump Inhibitors (PPIs): Unnecessary PPI use should be avoided in patients with cirrhosis. PPI use is a risk factor for developing HE, and the risk increases with higher doses of PPI.[78,79] PPIs have also been implicated in worsening dysbiosis, placing patients at further risk of hepatic decompensation events and hospitalization.[80,81]

Opioids: Opioids and other neuro-depressants should be avoided when possible in patients with cirrhosis. Opioid use is associated with microbiome changes that induce endotoxemia, which may increase the risk of developing HE. Opioid use is also associated with an increased risk of all-cause readmission in patients with cirrhosis.[82]

Oral Health: Oral hygiene is an important aspect of care for patients with cirrhosis. Periodontitis is common and can lead to systemic inflammation, predisposing patients to the development of HE.[83] Prior periodontitis can also be associated with HE and

Table 1
Classification using the four axes: hepatic encephalopathy diagnosis should be made in the context of the underlying liver disease, severity, time course, and presence of precipitating factor

1	2		3		4	
Type of Underlying Disease		Grade/Severity		Time Course		Presence of Precipitating Factor
A Acute Liver Failure	0 Covert	Psychomotor or executive function decline on psychometric or neuropsychological testing without clinical manifestations	Episodic	Episodes fully resolve for at least 6 mo	Precipitated	Specific factor identified
B Portosystemic shunt/bypass without cirrhosis	1	Shortened attention span; lack of awareness; Cognitive impairment; inability to add or subtract; Anxiety, irritability, or euphoria; Altered sleep rhythm	Recurrent	Episodes recur within 6 mo or less	Spontaneous	No specific precipitating factor identified
C Cirrhosis	2 Overt	Lethargic or apathetic; Disoriented to time; Personality changes; inappropriate behavior; Dyspraxia or asterixis	Persistent	Episodes never fully resolve		
	3	Somnolent or semi-stuporous, but responsive to stimuli; Confusion; Disoriented to time and place; grossly disoriented; Bizarre behavior				
	4	Coma; unresponsive to noxious or painful stimuli				

Underlying liver disease will lead to different treatments. Presence of recurrent HE should prompt the escalation of therapy to rifaximin in addition to lactulose. Precipitating factors should be evaluated and corrected if feasible.

admissions at 3 months in a new multi-center cohort.[84] The effect of periodontal care has been studied in patients with cirrhosis and periodontal disease, and patients are given periodontal care had improvements in oral and gut dysbiosis, systemic inflammation, and CHE scores.[85]

SUMMARY

HE remains an important complication of cirrhosis and is associated with increased mortality, and hospital readmissions, with negative impacts on both patient and caregiver quality of life. Significant pitfalls remain in currently used methods of identifying those with CHE and those at risk for developing OHE. Despite the therapies available, readmission rates in patients with cirrhosis continue to be unacceptably high. Further work is necessary to develop and improve testing, therapies, and systems factors to more effectively identify and manage patients at high risk for HE and associated morbidity and mortality.

CLINICS CARE POINTS

- To make a diagnosis of CHE, patients should have a positive result in at least two testing modalities. Testing modalities include traditional paper-pencil testing such as psychometric HE scale, Computer-based testing such as inhibitory control test, app-based platforms such as Encephalapp, or questionnaires such as Sickness Impact Profile.

- Patients diagnosed with CHE should be trialed on lactulose and monitored for progression to OHE. Other therapies need additional studies to determine effectiveness in the treatment of CHE.

- Preliminary data suggest that differences in microbiome as well as serologic markers such as thyroxine may allow for the identification of at-risk patients for developing OHE.

- Measurements of serum ammonia is not recommended for the diagnosis/prognostication of HE.

- Recurrent or persistent HE despite adequate treatment with lactulose or rifaximin should prompt evaluation of portosystemic shunts and consideration of shunt closure if identified.

- Malnutrition and sarcopenia are risk factors for HE. Patients with cirrhosis should consume 35-45 kcal/kg/d, as well as 1.2-1.5 g/k/d of protein of ideal body weight.

DISCLOSURE

These authors have nothing to disclose.

REFERENCES

1. Poordad FF. Review article: the burden of hepatic encephalopathy. Aliment Pharmacol Ther 2007;25(Suppl 1):3–9.
2. Sanyal AJ, Van Natta ML, Clark J, et al. Prospective Study of Outcomes in Adults with Nonalcoholic Fatty Liver Disease. N Engl J Med 2021;385(17):1559–69.
3. Bustamante J, Rimola A, Ventura PJ, et al. Prognostic significance of hepatic encephalopathy in patients with cirrhosis. J Hepatol 1999;30(5):890–5.
4. Bajaj JS, Duarte-Rojo A, Xie JJ, et al. Minimal Hepatic Encephalopathy and Mild Cognitive Impairment Worsen Quality of Life in Elderly Patients With Cirrhosis. Clin Gastroenterol Hepatol 2020;18(13):3008–16 e2.

5. Tapper EB, Halbert B, Mellinger J. Rates of and Reasons for Hospital Readmissions in Patients With Cirrhosis: A Multistate Population-based Cohort Study. Clin Gastroenterol Hepatol 2016;14(8):1181–1188 e2.

6. Bajaj JS. The Three Villages of Hepatic Encephalopathy. Am J Gastroenterol 2021;116(6):1184–6.

7. Fabrellas N, Moreira R, Carol M, et al. Psychological Burden of Hepatic Encephalopathy on Patients and Caregivers, Clin Transl Gastroenterol, 11(4), 2020, e00159.

8. Bajaj JS, Schubert CM, Heuman DM, et al. Persistence of cognitive impairment after resolution of overt hepatic encephalopathy. Gastroenterology 2010;138(7): 2332–40.

9. Bauer TM, Bauer TM, Steinbruckner B, et al. Small intestinal bacterial overgrowth in patients with cirrhosis: prevalence and relation with spontaneous bacterial peritonitis. Am J Gastroenterol 2001;96(10):2962–7.

10. Dabrowska K, Skowronska K, Popek M, et al. Roles of Glutamate and Glutamine Transport in Ammonia Neurotoxicity: State of the Art and Question Marks. Endocr Metab Immune Disord Drug Targets 2018;18(4):306–15.

11. Llansola M, Montoliu C, Agusti A, et al. Interplay between glutamatergic and GABAergic neurotransmission alterations in cognitive and motor impairment in minimal hepatic encephalopathy. Neurochem Int 2015;88:15–9.

12. Shawcross DL, Davies NA, Williams R, et al. Systemic inflammatory response exacerbates the neuropsychological effects of induced hyperammonemia in cirrhosis. J Hepatol 2004;40(2):247–54.

13. Acharya C, Bajaj JS. Gut Microbiota and Complications of Liver Disease. Gastroenterol Clin North Am 2017;46(1):155–69.

14. Chen Y, Yang F, Lu H, et al. Characterization of fecal microbial communities in patients with liver cirrhosis. Hepatology 2011;54(2):562–72.

15. Bajaj JS, Betrapally NS, Hylemon PB, et al. Salivary microbiota reflects changes in gut microbiota in cirrhosis with hepatic encephalopathy. Hepatology 2015; 62(4):1260–71.

16. Zhang Z, Zhai H, Geng J, et al. Large-scale survey of gut microbiota associated with MHE Via 16S rRNA-based pyrosequencing. Am J Gastroenterol 2013; 108(10):1601–11.

17. Bajaj JS, Fagan A, White MB, et al. Specific Gut and Salivary Microbiota Patterns Are Linked With Different Cognitive Testing Strategies in Minimal Hepatic Encephalopathy. Am J Gastroenterol 2019;114(7):1080–90.

18. Hylemon PB, Ridlon JM, et al. Colonic mucosal microbiome differs from stool microbiome in cirrhosis and hepatic encephalopathy and is linked to cognition and inflammation. Am J Physiol Gastrointest Liver Physiol 2012;303(6):G675–85.

19. Bajaj JS, Heuman DM, Hylemon PB, et al. Altered profile of human gut microbiome is associated with cirrhosis and its complications. J Hepatol 2014;60(5): 940–7.

20. Jain L, Sharma BC, Srivastava S, et al. Serum endotoxin, inflammatory mediators, and magnetic resonance spectroscopy before and after treatment in patients with minimal hepatic encephalopathy. J Gastroenterol Hepatol 2013;28(7):1187–93.

21. Pryde SE, Duncan SH, Hold GL, et al. The microbiology of butyrate formation in the human colon. FEMS Microbiol Lett 2002;217(2):133–9.

22. Wong JM, de Souza R, Kendall CW, et al. Colonic health: fermentation and short chain fatty acids. J Clin Gastroenterol 2006;40(3):235–43.

23. Peng L, Zhai H, Geng J, et al. Butyrate enhances the intestinal barrier by facilitating tight junction assembly via activation of AMP-activated protein kinase in Caco-2 cell monolayers. J Nutr 2009;139(9):1619–25.

24. Patidar KR, Thacker LR, Wade JB, et al. Covert hepatic encephalopathy is independently associated with poor survival and increased risk of hospitalization. Am J Gastroenterol 2014;109(11):1757–63.

25. Acharya C, Bajaj JS. Current Management of Hepatic Encephalopathy. Am J Gastroenterol 2018;113(11):1600–12.

26. Duarte-Rojo A, Estradas J, Hernandez-Ramos R, et al. Validation of the psychometric hepatic encephalopathy score (PHES) for identifying patients with minimal hepatic encephalopathy. Dig Dis Sci 2011;56(10):3014–23.

27. Weissenborn K, Amodio P, Bajaj J, et al. Neuropsychological characterization of hepatic encephalopathy. J Hepatol 2001;34(5):768–73.

28. Saleh ZM, Tapper EB. Predicting which patients with cirrhosis will develop overt hepatic encephalopathy: Beyond psychometric testing, Metab Brain Dis, 2022. Epub ahead of print.

29. Campagna F, Montagnese S, Ridola L, et al. The animal naming test: An easy tool for the assessment of hepatic encephalopathy. Hepatology 2017;66(1):198–208.

30. Bajaj JS, Hafeezullah M, Franco J, et al. Inhibitory control test for the diagnosis of minimal hepatic encephalopathy. Gastroenterology 2008;135(5):1591–600 e1.

31. Bajaj JS, Heuman DM, Sterling RK, et al. Validation of EncephalApp, Smartphone-Based Stroop Test, for the Diagnosis of Covert Hepatic Encephalopathy. Clin Gastroenterol Hepatol 2015;13(10):1828–35 e1.

32. Allampati S, Duarte-Rojo A, Thacker LR, et al. Diagnosis of Minimal Hepatic Encephalopathy Using Stroop EncephalApp: A Multicenter US-Based, Norm-Based Study. Am J Gastroenterol 2016;111(1):78–86.

33. Zeng X, Li XX, Shi PM, et al. Utility of the EncephalApp Stroop Test for covert hepatic encephalopathy screening in Chinese cirrhotic patients. J Gastroenterol Hepatol 2019;34(10):1843–50.

34. Acharya C, Shaw J, Duong N, et al. QuickStroop, a Shortened Version of EncephalApp, Detects Covert Hepatic Encephalopathy With Similar Accuracy Within One Minute. Clin Gastroenterol Hepatol 2022;21(1):136–42.

35. Bloom PP, Robin J, Xu M, et al. Hepatic Encephalopathy is Associated With Slow Speech on Objective Assessment. Am J Gastroenterol 2021;116(9):1950–3.

36. Nabi E, Thacker LR, Wade JB, et al. Diagnosis of covert hepatic encephalopathy without specialized tests. Clin Gastroenterol Hepatol 2014;12(8):1384–9 e2.

37. Prasad S, Dhiman RK, Duseja A, et al. Lactulose improves cognitive functions and health-related quality of life in patients with cirrhosis who have minimal hepatic encephalopathy. Hepatology 2007;45(3):549–59.

38. Hartmann IJ, Groeneweg M, Quero JC, et al. The prognostic significance of subclinical hepatic encephalopathy. Am J Gastroenterol 2000;95(8):2029–34.

39. Kappus MR, Bajaj JS. Covert hepatic encephalopathy: not as minimal as you might think. Clin Gastroenterol Hepatol 2012;10(11):1208–19.

40. Bajaj JS, Heuman DM, Wade JB, et al. Rifaximin improves driving simulator performance in a randomized trial of patients with minimal hepatic encephalopathy. Gastroenterology 2011;140(2):478–87 e1.

41. Bajaj JS, Heuman DM, Sanyal AJ, et al. Modulation of the metabiome by rifaximin in patients with cirrhosis and minimal hepatic encephalopathy. PLoS One 2013; 8(4):e60042.

42. Sidhu SS, Goyal O, Mishra BP, et al. Rifaximin improves psychometric performance and health-related quality of life in patients with minimal hepatic encephalopathy (the RIME Trial). Am J Gastroenterol 2011;106(2):307–16.
43. Sharma BC, Singh J, Srivastava S, et al. Randomized controlled trial comparing lactulose plus albumin versus lactulose alone for treatment of hepatic encephalopathy. J Gastroenterol Hepatol 2017;32(6):1234–9.
44. Fagan A, Gavis EA, Gallagher ML, et al. A double-blind randomized placebo-controlled trial of albumin in outpatients with hepatic encephalopathy: HEAL study. J Hepatol, S0168-8278 2022;22:03116–26.
45. Montagnese S, Lauridsen M, Vilstrup H, et al. A pilot study of golexanolone, a new GABA-A receptor-modulating steroid antagonist, in patients with covert hepatic encephalopathy. J Hepatol 2021;75(1):98–107.
46. Vilstrup H, Amodio P, Bajaj J, et al. Hepatic encephalopathy in chronic liver disease: 2014 Practice Guideline by the American Association for the Study of Liver Diseases and the European Association for the Study of the Liver. Hepatology 2014;60(2):715–35.
47. Cordoba J, Ventura-Cots M, Simón-Talero M, et al. Characteristics, risk factors, and mortality of cirrhotic patients hospitalized for hepatic encephalopathy with and without acute-on-chronic liver failure (ACLF). J Hepatol 2014;60(2):275–81.
48. Bajaj JS, Cordoba J, Mullen KD, et al. Review article: the design of clinical trials in hepatic encephalopathy–an International Society for Hepatic Encephalopathy and Nitrogen Metabolism (ISHEN) consensus statement. Aliment Pharmacol Ther 2011;33(7):739–47.
49. Teasdale G, Jennett B. Assessment of coma and impaired consciousness. A practical scale. Lancet 1974;2(7872):81–4.
50. Ong JP, Aggarwal A, Krieger D, et al. Correlation between ammonia levels and the severity of hepatic encephalopathy. Am J Med 2003;114(3):188–93.
51. Bajaj JS, Bloom PP, Chung RT, et al. Variability and Lability of Ammonia Levels in Healthy Volunteers and Patients With Cirrhosis: Implications for Trial Design and Clinical Practice. Am J Gastroenterol 2020;115(5):783–5.
52. Bajaj JS, Lauridsen M, Tapper EB, et al. Important Unresolved Questions in the Management of Hepatic Encephalopathy: An ISHEN Consensus. Am J Gastroenterol 2020;115(7):989–1002.
53. Drolz A, Jäger B, Wewalka M, et al. Clinical impact of arterial ammonia levels in ICU patients with different liver diseases. Intensive Care Med 2013;39(7):1227–37.
54. Bajaj JS, Vargas HE, Reddy KR, et al. Association Between Intestinal Microbiota Collected at Hospital Admission and Outcomes of Patients With Cirrhosis. Clin Gastroenterol Hepatol 2019;17(4):756–65 e3.
55. Bajaj JS, Tandon P, O'Leary JG, et al. Admission Serum Metabolites and Thyroxine Predict Advanced Hepatic Encephalopathy in a Multicenter Inpatient Cirrhosis Cohort. Clin Gastroenterol Hepatol, S1542-3565 2022;22:00388–93.
56. Wijdicks EF. Hepatic Encephalopathy. N Engl J Med 2016;375(17):1660–70.
57. Sharma BC, Sharma P, Agrawal A, et al. Secondary prophylaxis of hepatic encephalopathy: an open-label randomized controlled trial of lactulose versus placebo. Gastroenterology 2009;137(3):885–91, 891 e1.
58. Elwir S, Rahimi RS. Hepatic Encephalopathy: An Update on the Pathophysiology and Therapeutic Options. J Clin Transl Hepatol 2017;5(2):142–51.
59. Duong NK, Shrestha S, Park D, et al. Bristol Stool Scale as a Determinant of Hepatic Encephalopathy Management in Patients With Cirrhosis. Am J Gastroenterol 2022;117(2):295–300.

60. Sharma BC, Sharma P, Lunia MK, et al. A randomized, double-blind, controlled trial comparing rifaximin plus lactulose with lactulose alone in treatment of overt hepatic encephalopathy. Am J Gastroenterol 2013;108(9):1458–63.

61. Bass NM, Mullen KD, Sanyal A, et al. Rifaximin treatment in hepatic encephalopathy. N Engl J Med 2010;362(12):1071–81.

62. Sundaram V, Shaikh OS. Hepatic encephalopathy: pathophysiology and emerging therapies. Med Clin North Am 2009;93(4):819–36, vii.

63. Shen YC, Chang YH, Fang CJ, et al. Zinc supplementation in patients with cirrhosis and hepatic encephalopathy: a systematic review and meta-analysis. Nutr J 2019;18(1):34.

64. Kircheis G, Luth S. Pharmacokinetic and Pharmacodynamic Properties of L-Ornithine L-Aspartate (LOLA) in Hepatic Encephalopathy. Drugs 2019;79(Suppl 1):23–9.

65. Sidhu SS, Sharma BC, Goyal O, et al. L-ornithine L-aspartate in bouts of overt hepatic encephalopathy. Hepatology 2018;67(2):700–10.

66. Bajaj JS, Hassanein TI, Pyrsopoulos NT, et al. Dosing of Rifaximin Soluble Solid Dispersion Tablets in Adults With Cirrhosis: 2 Randomized, Placebo-controlled Trials. Clin Gastroenterol Hepatol, S1542-3565 2022;2022(00595):X.

67. Bajaj JS, Kassam Z, Fagan A, et al. Fecal microbiota transplant from a rational stool donor improves hepatic encephalopathy: A randomized clinical trial. Hepatology 2017;66(6):1727–38.

68. Bajaj JS, Salzman NH, Acharya C, et al. Fecal Microbial Transplant Capsules Are Safe in Hepatic Encephalopathy: A Phase 1, Randomized, Placebo-Controlled Trial. Hepatology 2019;70(5):1690–703.

69. Alvares-da-Silva MR, de Araujo A, Vicenzi JR, et al. Oral l-ornithine-l-aspartate in minimal hepatic encephalopathy: A randomized, double-blind, placebo-controlled trial. Hepatol Res 2014;44(9):956–63.

70. Ganapathy D, Acharya C, Lachar J, et al. The patient buddy app can potentially prevent hepatic encephalopathy-related readmissions. Liver Int 2017;37(12):1843–51.

71. Sakurabayashi S, Sezai S, Yamamoto Y, et al. Embolization of portal-systemic shunts in cirrhotic patients with chronic recurrent hepatic encephalopathy. Cardiovasc Intervent Radiol 1997;20(2):120–4.

72. Laleman W, Simon-Talero M, Maleux G, et al. Embolization of large spontaneous portosystemic shunts for refractory hepatic encephalopathy: a multicenter survey on safety and efficacy. Hepatology 2013;57(6):2448–57.

73. Boike JR, Thornburg BG, Asrani SK, et al. North American Practice-Based Recommendations for Transjugular Intrahepatic Portosystemic Shunts in Portal Hypertension. Clin Gastroenterol Hepatol 2022;20(8):1636–62 e36.

74. Merli M, Giusto M, Lucidi C, et al. Muscle depletion increases the risk of overt and minimal hepatic encephalopathy: results of a prospective study. Metab Brain Dis 2013;28(2):281–4.

75. Amodio P, Bemeur C, Butterworth R, et al. The nutritional management of hepatic encephalopathy in patients with cirrhosis: International Society for Hepatic Encephalopathy and Nitrogen Metabolism Consensus. Hepatology 2013;58(1):325–36.

76. Reuter B, Shaw J, Hanson J, et al. Nutritional Assessment in Inpatients With Cirrhosis Can Be Improved After Training and Is Associated With Lower Readmissions. Liver Transpl 2019;25(12):1790–9.

77. Les I, Doval E, García-Martínez R, et al. Effects of branched-chain amino acids supplementation in patients with cirrhosis and a previous episode of hepatic encephalopathy: a randomized study. Am J Gastroenterol 2011;106(6):1081–8.
78. Tsai CF, Chen MH, Wang YP, et al. Proton Pump Inhibitors Increase Risk for Hepatic Encephalopathy in Patients With Cirrhosis in A Population Study. Gastroenterology 2017;152(1):134–41.
79. Dam G, Vilstrup H, Watson H, et al. Proton pump inhibitors as a risk factor for hepatic encephalopathy and spontaneous bacterial peritonitis in patients with cirrhosis with ascites. Hepatology 2016;64(4):1265–72.
80. Bajaj JS, Cox IJ, Betrapally NS, et al. Systems biology analysis of omeprazole therapy in cirrhosis demonstrates significant shifts in gut microbiota composition and function. Am J Physiol Gastrointest Liver Physiol 2014;307(10):G951–7.
81. Bajaj JS, Acharya C, Fagan A, et al. Proton Pump Inhibitor Initiation and Withdrawal affects Gut Microbiota and Readmission Risk in Cirrhosis. Am J Gastroenterol 2018;113(8):1177–86.
82. Acharya C, Betrapally NS, Gillevet PM, et al. Chronic opioid use is associated with altered gut microbiota and predicts readmissions in patients with cirrhosis. Aliment Pharmacol Ther 2017;45(2):319–31.
83. Hajishengallis G. Periodontitis: from microbial immune subversion to systemic inflammation. Nat Rev Immunol 2015;15(1):30–44.
84. Bajaj JS, Lai JC, Tandon P, et al. Role of Oral Health, Frailty, and Minimal Hepatic Encephalopathy in the Risk of Hospitalization: A Prospective Multi-Center Cohort of Outpatients With Cirrhosis. Clin Gastroenterol Hepatol, S1542-3565 2022;22: 01012–6.
85. Bajaj JS, Matin P, White MB, et al. Periodontal therapy favorably modulates the oral-gut-hepatic axis in cirrhosis. Am J Physiol Gastrointest Liver Physiol 2018; 315(5):G824–37. Classification of HE in Four Axes.

Alcoholic Hepatitis
The Rising Epidemic

Pranav Penninti, DO[a], Ayooluwatomiwa D. Adekunle, MD, MPH[b],
Ashwani K. Singal, MD, MS[c,d,e],*

KEYWORDS

- Alcoholic hepatitis • Alcohol use disorder • Alcohol-associated liver disease • AH
- AUD • ALD

KEY POINTS

- Alcoholic hepatitis is characterized by new onset or worsening jaundice in the setting of heavy alcohol use and has significant short-term and long-term morbidity and mortality.
- Over the last decade, health care burden from alcoholic hepatitis has been increasing, and this has accelerated in the last 2 to 3 years during the COVID-19 pandemic.
- Corticosteroids, the mainstay of treatment for severe alcoholic hepatitis, are a suboptimal treatment, and there is a need for novel therapeutic agents.
- The long-term prognosis of alcoholic hepatitis is determined by alcohol abstinence, and the treatment for the second pathology of alcohol use disorder is critical.

DISEASE BURDEN AND RISING EPIDEMIC OF ALCOHOLIC HEPATITIS

Alcohol-associated liver disease (ALD) encompasses a spectrum of disease from alcohol-associated steatosis to cirrhosis. Alcohol-associated hepatitis (AH), a unique manifestation on this spectrum, is characterized by new onset or worsening jaundice in the setting of heavy alcohol use with less than 60 days of abstinence before the onset of jaundice.[1] Among patients with severe forms, mortality approaches 20% to 30% at 30 days and 30% to 40% at 6 months.[2] In addition, there is an increased risk of progression to cirrhosis, especially in the setting of continued alcohol use.[3,4]

Over the last decade, since the availability of effective therapy for hepatitis C virus infection, ALD-related hospitalizations and disease burden have been increasing, with ALD currently being the leading indication for liver transplantation (LT). A retrospective study of hospitalized patients in the United States showed a 28.3% increase in AH

[a] Division of Gastroenterology and Hepatology, University of Texas Health San Antonio, TX, USA; [b] Department of Medicine, University of Kentucky, KY, USA; [c] University of South Dakota Sanford School of Medicine, Sioux Falls, SD, USA; [d] Avera Transplant Institute and University Hospital, Avera McKennan University Hospital; [e] VA Medical Center, Sioux Falls, SD 57105, USA
* Corresponding author. University of South Dakota Sanford School of Medicine, Sioux Falls, SD, USA
E-mail address: ashwanisingal.com@gmail.com

Med Clin N Am 107 (2023) 533–554
https://doi.org/10.1016/j.mcna.2022.12.005
0025-7125/23/© 2022 Elsevier Inc. All rights reserved.

hospitalizations between 2007 and 2014.[5] Taken together, this increasing disease burden results in increased health care utilization, costs, morbidity, and mortality.[6] In 2011 alone, the average cost of a hospitalization for AH was $37,769 with an average length of hospitalization of 6.5 days.[7] More recently, between 2012 and 2016, alcohol-associated cirrhosis accounted for $22.7 billion in hospitalizations costs and an increasing trend has been observed.[6]

These increasing trends are disproportionately increasing in specific demographic populations of young adults, females, and minorities.[5,7,8] For example, a study of 14,547 adolescents and young adults aged 15 to 39 years enrolled in the National Health and Nutrition Examination Survey between 1988 to 2012 showed an increase in the prevalence of ALD from 2.3% between 1988 and 1994 to 5.1% between 2007 and 2012 period.[9] Another similar study of 1,319 adolescents and young adults between 2017 and 2018 showed 8.5% prevalence of excessive alcohol intake in the overall study population and a 56.59% prevalence of ALD among those with excessive drinking.[10] In another study using population-level vital statistics data, the highest average annual increase in cirrhosis-related deaths was observed among individuals aged 25 to 34 years (10.5% during 2009–2016), which was entirely driven by ALD.[11] Similarly, disease burden related to hospitalizations due to AH was shown to be increased by 37.6% among females compared with 22.3% increase among males during the same time period.[5] This and other studies have also shown disproportionate increase in disease burden among Native Americans and Hispanics compared with whites.[5]

The COVID pandemic has further exacerbated the problem by increasing excessive alcohol consumption, alcohol use disorder (AUD), and ALD, particularly among patients younger than 40 years (**Table 1**).[18] A Canadian retrospective study revealed a significant increase in average monthly admissions for AH during the pandemic (22.1/10,000 admissions) compared with the pre-pandemic period (11.6/10,000 admissions).[21] These trends have been corroborated by other studies and are expected to continue, with effects persisting over the coming years.[6,22] For example, a modeling study projected additional 8000 ALD-related deaths and 18,700 cases of decompensated cirrhosis from a 1-year increase in alcohol consumption during the COVID-19 pandemic.[16]

Clearly, physicians, internists, gastroenterologists, and hepatologists will continue to face these patients with advanced ALD and AH over the years to come. Hence, there is a need for an improved understanding on how to evaluate and manage these patients, and this review is timely to meet this educational need. From here on, the authors discuss and provide recent updates on the pathophysiology, diagnosis, and treatment of patients with AH.

DIAGNOSIS

The clinical syndrome of AH includes a constellation of jaundice, malaise, fever, tender hepatomegaly, and anorexia in the setting of heavy and often active alcohol use.[4] The clinical presentation can vary from mild jaundice, hepatic decompensation, and acute on chronic liver failure with failure of one or more organs in most severe forms. The NIAAA Alcoholic Hepatitis Consortia has proposed clinical criteria (**Fig. 1**) for a probable diagnosis of AH.[1] Patients not meeting one or more of these criteria (possible AH) would need a liver biopsy for diagnosis (definite AH).[23] When a liver biopsy is performed, a transjugular liver biopsy is recommended given frequent coexistence of coagulopathy and/or ascites in these sick patients. The histologic features of AH include hepatocellular ballooning, neutrophilic lobular inflammation, Mallory–Denk bodies, and megamitochondria.[3] Sclerosing hyaline necrosis characterized by

Table 1
Studies assessing the effect of COVID-19 on alcohol consumption, alcohol use disorder, alcohol-associated liver disease, and alcoholic hepatitis

Author	Outcome	Study Design	Study Findings
Alcohol use disorder			
Yeo et al,[12] 2022	AUD-related mortality	Modeling	Outcome increased by 24.7% in 2020 and 21.95% in 2021 vs projected rates.
White et al,[13] 2022	Alcohol-related deaths	Cross-sectional	Outcome increased by 25.9% in 2020 vs 2019.
Sharma et al,[14] 2021	Alcohol withdrawal hospitalizations	Retrospective single-center cohort	34% increase in hospitalizations related to alcohol withdrawal in 2020 vs same period in 2019.
Barbosa et al,[15] 2021	Alcohol consumption	Cross-sectional survey	20% increase in harmful alcohol use and 21% increase in binge drinking between 02/2020 and 04/2020.
Alcohol-associated liver disease			
Julien et al,[16] 2021	ALD-related outcomes	Modeling	Projected 18,700 additional decompensated cirrhosis (including 1000 HCC cases) with 8000 additional deaths between 2020 and 2040 from 1-y increase in alcohol use.
Deutsch-Link et al,[17] 2022	ALD-related mortality	Cross-sectional	Outcomes increased by 21% in males and 27% in females in 2020 vs 2019.
Alcoholic hepatitis			
Sohal et al,[18] 2022	AH hospitalizations	Retrospective multicenter cohort	Increased AH hospitalizations by 51% in 2020 vs 2019 (100% increase in <40 y age and 125% increase in females).
Damjanovska et al,[19] 2022	AH incidence	Retrospective national database study on over 8 million patients between 06/2020 and 06/2021, and over 6.5 million before 06/2020	AH diagnosis in 98.5/100,000 between 06/2020 and 06/2021 vs 35.6/100,000 before 06/2020 with highest increase in black patients.
Gonzalez et al,[20] 2022	AH hospitalizations	Retrospective single-center cohort	AH hospitalizations increased by more than 50% in 2020 vs 2016–2019

Abbreviations: AH, alcoholic hepatitis; ALD, alcohol-associated liver disease; AUD, alcohol use disorder; HCC, hepatocellular carcinoma.
Adapted from Deutsch-Link S, Jiang Y, Peery AF, Barritt AS, Bataller R, Moon AM. Alcohol-Associated Liver Disease Mortality Increased From 2017 to 2020 and Accelerated During the COVID-19 Pandemic. Clin Gastroenterol Hepatol. 2022 Sep;20(9):2142-2144.e2. https://doi.org/10.1016/j.cgh.2022.03.017. Epub 2022 Mar 19. PMID: 35314353; PMCID: PMC8933289.

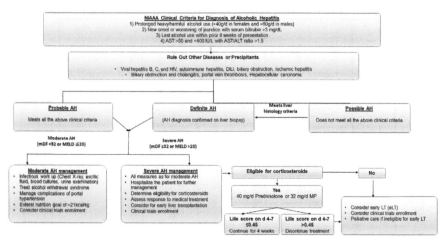

Fig. 1. NIAAA Alcoholic Hepatitis Consortia. ALT, alanine aminotransferase; AST, aspartate aminotransferase; AUD, alcohol use disorder; CXR, chest X-ray; DILI, drug-induced liver injury; HCC, hepatocellular carcinoma; LT, liver transplant; mDF, Maddrey Discriminant Function; MELD, Model for End-Stage Liver Disease; UA, urinalysis; UC, urine culture.

perivenular hepatocyte necrosis and pericellular fibrosis with chicken wire appearance is characteristic findings and is present in most severe cases.[3]

DETERMINING PROGNOSIS
Clinical Models

Maddrey Discriminant Function (mDF) and Model for End-Stage Liver Disease (MELD) score are most commonly used to stratify disease severity and candidacy for cortico-steroid treatment (MELD >20, mDF $\geq$32).[24] Other scores such as Glasgow Alcoholic Hepatitis Score (GAHS) and age, serum bilirubin, International Normalized Ratio (INR), and serum creatinine (ABIC) score have also been used.[25,26] In an international study assessing performance characteristics of prognostication tools, the MELD score demonstrated a higher area under the receiving operating characteristic curve (AUROC) in predicting mortality at 28 and 90 days compared with mDF, MELD-Na, GAHS, and ABIC scores.[27]

Among corticosteroid-treated patients, Lille score at 1 week is used to determine treatment response, with the algorithm factoring mainly change in bilirubin along with several pretreatment variables. With the range of Lille score of 0 to 1, a score of $\leq$0.45 at 1 week defines response to treatment, and corticosteroids are discontinued at 1 week in nonre-sponders.[28] It has been further stratified to define complete responders (Lille <0.16), partial responders (Lille 0.16–0.56), and null responders (Lille >0.56) with 28-day survival strongly correlated to this stratification (91%, 79%, and 53%, respectively).[29] The Lille score at day 4 can be used if patients are ready for discharge, and its accuracy in deter-mining treatment response is similar to day-7 Lille with a 91.1% agreement ($\kappa = 0.82$, $P < .001$).[30] A combination of a static model with baseline MELD score and a dynamic model with day-7 Lille score is better than mDF + Lille or ABIC + Lille in determining mor-tality at 2 and at 6 months.[31] As none of the clinical scores is an ideal model with limitations of all scores (**Table 2**),[32] the search for an ideal score continues for an improved diag-nostic and prognostic biomarkers.

Several noninvasive biomarkers have been assessed aiming to improve the accu-racy of diagnosis and in predicting prognosis of AH (**Table 3**). However, none of these is currently available for routine use in clinical practice.[40]

Table 2
Comparison of prognostic models for alcoholic hepatitis

Model	Type of Model	Components / Link to online calculator	Advantages	Disadvantages
mDF	Static	PT, total bilirubin https://www.mdcalc.com/calc/56/maddreys-discriminant-function-alcoholic-hepatitis	• Oldest validated model to assess the disease severity • Commonly used in clinical trials • Simple bedside calculation	• Use of PT, which is not standardized across laboratories • Low specificity (62%)[32]
MELD	Static	Total bilirubin, INR, creatinine https://www.mayoclinic.org/medical-professionals/transplant-medicine/calculators/meld-model/itt-20434705	• Best validated score to predict disease severity • Can be used to determine need for corticosteroids	• Requires online calculator.
GAHS	Static	Age, total bilirubin, PT, BUN, WBC https://www.mdcalc.com/calc/680/glasgow-alcoholic-hepatitis-score	• Better performance than mDF • Simple bedside use in clinical practice	• Use of PT, which is not standardized across laboratories • Not validated outside of the United Kingdom.
ABIC	Static	Age, total bilirubin, creatinine https://www.mdcalc.com/calc/10136/abic-score-alcoholic-hepatitis	• Uses INR as opposed to PT	• Not frequently used • Not validated outside of Spain
AHHS	Static	Fibrosis, bilirubinostasis, PMN infiltration, mega mitochondria https://globalrph.com/medcalcs/alcoholic-hepatitis-histological-score-ahhs/	• Can help rule out alternative disease processes. • Can highlight features associated with favorable prognosis such as mega mitochondria and marked PMN infiltration	• Biopsy rarely performed • Poor inter-provider reliability on interpretation of overall and different histologic findings. • Accuracy in predicting disease severity lower than clinical scores.
Lille	Dynamic	Age, albumin, PT, creatinine, day 1 total bilirubin, day 7 total bilirubin http://www.lillemodel.com/score.asp	• A validated dynamic model to determine response to medical treatment.	• Use of PT, which is not standardized across laboratories • Complex score which requires an online calculator.

Abbreviations: ABIC, age, bilirubin, INR, and creatinine; AHHS, alcoholic hepatitis histologic score; BUN, blood urea nitrogen; GAHS, Glasgow Alcoholic Hepatitis Score; mDF, Maddrey Discriminant Function; MELD, Model for End-Stage Liver Disease; PMN, polymorphonuclear neutrophils; PT, prothrombin time; WBC, white blood count.

Table 3
Emerging biomarkers for alcoholic hepatitis diagnosis, prognosis, and assessment of treatment response

Biomarker	Summary	Test Characteristics
Biomarkers for Diagnosis of AH		
Breath TAP (triethylamine, acetone, and pentane)	Volatile compounds in breath samples, measured by mass spectrometry	97% sensitivity and 72% specificity for a TAP score of 28%; 80% sensitivity and 86% specificity for a score of 51.[33]
Cytokeratin-18 M65 level	Cytokeratin-18 is an intermediate filament protein released from damaged hepatocytes. Measured by ELISA for M65 and M30, which are circulating fragments of cytokeratin-18.	67% sensitivity and 92% specificity at an M65 > 2000 IU/L; 93% sensitivity and 62% specificity at M65 < 641 IU/L.[34]
miRNA-192	MicroRNAs are small, non-coding segments of RNA involved in regulation of gene expression. Measured by quantitative PCR.	AUC of 0.95 for diagnosis of AH.[35]
Biomarkers to predict prognosis of AH patients		
Cytokeratin-18 M30 and M65 level	Measured by ELISA for M65 and M30, which are circulating fragments of cytokeratin-18.	AUROC for M30 was 0.616 and AUROC for M65 was 0.627 for 90-d mortality.[36]
Total and conjugated bile acids	Total bile acids and conjugated acids increase in AH due to cholestasis and further propagate liver injury. Measured by mass spectrometry.	Correlates with MELD (P = .06).[37]
FGF19	Negative feedback regulator of bile acid synthesis. Measured by ELISA for serum FGF19.	Correlates with 30-d mortality in patients with MELD $\geq$ 29.[37]
CD163	Marker of inflammatory macrophage activation. Measured by ELISA for serum CD163.	Independent predictor of 84-d mortality. Correlates with MELD and GAHS (P < .02).[38]

LPS	Marker of bacterial translocation. Measured by a quantitative chromogenic assay.	3.6% 90-d mortality with serum LPS $\leq$1.3 EU/mL compared with 50% mortality with serum LPS >1.3 EU/mL (P < .001).[39]
Treatment response		
Cytokeratin-18 M30 level	Cytokeratin-18 is an intermediate filament protein released from damaged hepatocytes. Measured by ELISA for M65 and M30, which are circulating fragments of cytokeratin-18.	Improved 90-d survival in patients treated with corticosteroids when M30 > 5000 U/L (Odds Ratio [OR] 0.433, P = .0398).[36]
LPS	Marker of bacterial translocation. Measured by a quantitative chromogenic assay.	100% of patients with serum LPS $\leq$1.3 EU/mL responded to corticosteroids, whereas 61.1% of patients with serum LPS >1.3 EU/mL were nonresponder (P = .006).[39]

Abbreviations: AUC, area under curve; AUROC, area under receiver operating curve; CD163, Cluster of Differentiation 163; ELISA, enzyme-linked immunosorbent assay; FGF19, fibroblast growth factor 19; LPS, lipopolysaccharide; MELD, Model for End-Stage Liver Disease; miRNA, microribonucleic acid; PCR, polymerase chain reaction.

TREATMENT
Nutrition

Malnutrition is a frequent complication in AH patients as this is a catabolic condition due to systemic inflammation. In an observational study among hospitalized veterans with AH, an in-hospital mortality of over 90% was observed with a daily caloric intake of below 1000 kilocalories (kcal) and everyone survived the hospitalization if the daily caloric intake was over 3000 kilocalories. A randomized trial comparing corticosteroids vs. enteral nutrition supplementation of 2000 kcal/d via nasogastric did not show any significant difference in 28-day mortality.[41] In another randomized controlled trial, 174 patients with biopsy-proven severe AH were randomized to enteral nutrition for 14 days as an adjunct to corticosteroid therapy versus corticosteroids alone. Although there was no difference in mortality at 1 or 6 months in this study, daily caloric intake below 21.5 kcal/kg/d, irrespective of the study arm, was associated with higher 6-month mortality (65.8% vs 33.1%, $P < .001$).[42] In addition, almost half of the patients were unable to tolerate the nasogastric tube for the entirety of the planned 14-day treatment duration. Clearly, a daily caloric intake should be monitored among hospitalized patients who are suspected of poor oral intake and nutritional supplementation recommended for those with daily intake below 1200 calories. Oral route is preferred, and a parenteral route is used if oral route is not possible.[43]

Pharmacological Therapies

Corticosteroid (prednisolone 40 mg/d or methylprednisolone 32 mg/d) is recommended as the first-line treatment of severe AH patients.[43–45] However, the efficacy of corticosteroids in AH has remained conflicting across studies since the first report of a randomized controlled trial in 1971.[46] The Steroids or Pentoxifylline for Alcoholic Hepatitis (STOPAH) study randomized 1103 severe AH patients but could only demonstrate a modest 28-day survival benefit of prednisolone of 86.2% compared with 82% survival among placebo-treated patients, $P = .056$.[47] Two separate meta-analyses, including the STOPAH study confirmed that prednisolone improves the 28-day survival by 46% and 36%, respectively. However, none of these meta-analyses showed any benefit of corticosteroids at 3 or 6 months.[29,48]

Apart from the limited survival benefit, 30% to 40% of patients remain ineligible for corticosteroids due to relative contraindications such as active bacterial infection, gastrointestinal bleeding, and hepatorenal syndrome. Further, only 40% to 50% of those treated with corticosteroids can complete the full 28-day regimen, as the treatment has to be discontinued in 40% to 50% of nonresponders at 1 week of treatment due to increased risk of bacterial and fungal infections in these with continuation of treatment without any benefit and unpredictable response to treatment in 50% to 60% patients.[28,49] Moreover, corticosteroids are not recommended for patients with moderate AH (MELD score 11–20), a disease with up to 10% 3-month mortality.[50] These limitations of corticosteroid therapy result in their heterogeneous use, with only 25% of providers reported to use these drugs in severe AH patients.[51,52]

The use of corticosteroids can be optimized with simple biomarkers with personalized use in those likely to respond to these medications. For example, serum levels of bacterial DNA at baseline among patients enrolled in the STOPAH study were associated with a risk of bacterial infection after exposure to corticosteroids. In a retrospective, multicenter international cohort of 3,380 patients with severe AH, benefit of corticosteroids was observed between MELD scores of 21 and 51, with the maximum benefit among those with MELD scores between 25 and 39 (Hazard Ratio [HR] 0.61;

95% CI 0.39–0.95; $P = .027$).[24] Based on these data, corticosteroids can be personalized in eligible patients with MELD scores between 25 and 39 for the maximum survival benefit.

Pentoxifylline, a phosphodiesterase inhibitor has historically been used for the treatment of severe AH based on its documented survival benefit in the initial seminal study.[53] However, based on the lack of benefit in the STOPAH study and subsequent meta-analyses, this is currently not recommended as a treatment option for patients with severe AH.[54] Antagonists of Tumor Necrosis Factor-Alpha (TNF-α) such as infliximab and etanercept also failed and in fact were associated with worse survival in the intervention arm due to the development of infection with these drugs. Extracorporeal cellular therapy (ELAD), which uses hepatoblastoma-derived C3A cells expressing anti-inflammatory proteins in addition to growth factors, has been studied as an ancillary treatment modality for severe AH. In a trial randomizing patients with standard of care therapy (corticosteroids or pentoxifylline) versus standard of care therapy in addition to 3 days of ELAD, overall survival was not different between the two groups at 91 days with a 47.9% mortality rate in the ELAD group and 47.7% mortality rate in the control group (HR 1.03; 95% CI 0.69–1.53).[55]

Emerging Therapies

Given the limitations of currently existing treatment options, treatment strategies focusing on multiple targets (**Fig. 2**) are currently being investigated as potential therapies for patients with AH.[56,57]

Therapies targeting gut dysbiosis

Alcohol consumption is associated with intestinal bacterial overgrowth with reduced alpha diversity, disruption of the intestinal tight junctions with bacterial translocation to the portal circulation, and impaired Kupffer cell clearance of lipopolysaccharide (LPS).[58] Pathogen-associated molecular patterns such as LPS are recognized by toll-like receptor 4 on the surface of Kupffer cells and other hepatic cells leading to cytokine signaling and activation of inflammatory pathways.

Fecal microbiota transplant (FMT) is a promising tool for modulating the gut-liver axis and improving the alpha diversity of the gut microbiome. In a pilot study of 195 patients with ALD, the use of FMT among eight steroid ineligible patients was associated with improved survival compared with historical controls treated with standard of care (87.5% vs 33.3%; $P = .018$).[59] In a phase 1 double-blinded randomized control trial, the use of FMT was associated with a significant reduction in alcohol craving among a higher proportion of treated patients compared with placebo (90% vs 30%).[60] Another retrospective analysis comparing long-term outcomes in patients with corticosteroid-responsive severe AH receiving healthy-donor FMT via nasoduodenal tube for 7 days compared with corticosteroids found a significantly lower incidence of alcohol relapse was in the FMT group (28.6% vs 53.8%; $P = .04$).[61] In addition, FMT treatment was associated with significantly lower incidence of hepatic encephalopathy, ascites, infections, and reduced risk of hospitalization.

Therapies targeting inflammatory pathways

Anakinra is an interleukin (IL)-1 receptor antagonist that targets IL-1, a major cytokine in the pathogenesis of AH. Randomized controlled trial from the Defeat Alcoholic Steatohepatitis compared combination of Anakinra (IL-1 receptor antagonist), pentoxifylline, and zinc oxide against corticosteroids alone in severe AH. This was a negative trial with no survival benefit at 28, 90, or 180 days in the intervention arm.[62] However, the risk of fungal infection was lower in the intervention arm (0% vs 5%, $P = .02$).

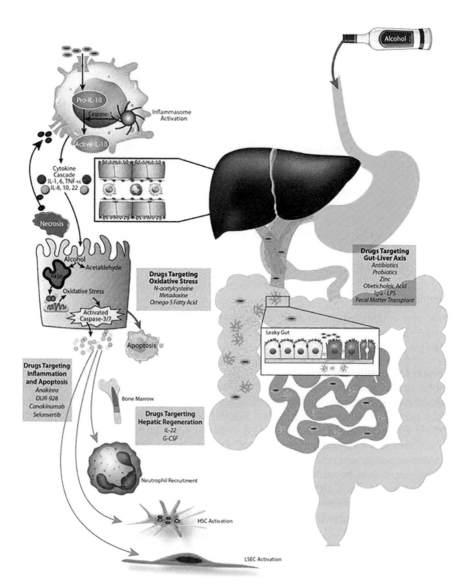

Fig. 2. Diagnosis and treatment of alcoholic hepatitis.

Another double-blind randomized placebo-controlled trial of adults with severe AH (MELD 20–35) compared anakinra combined with zinc with prednisone. This trial was terminated early due to reduced survival and higher occurrence of acute kidney injury in the active arm of anakinra (69.9% vs 91%, $P = .003$ and 41% vs 21%, $P = .005$, respectively).[63]

DUR-928 is an endogenous sulfated oxysterol which reduces the expression of proinflammatory cytokines, regulates lipid metabolism, and stimulates cell survival. In a Phase 2a study on 18 patients with moderate and severe AH, there was an 89% response rate as reflected by a Lille score on day 7 of treatment.[57] There was a significant decrease in MELD at Day 28 in all patients ($P = .005$) and in those with baseline

MELD 21 to 30 (P = .051). None of the enrolled patients died during the study period of 28 days. DUR-928 was also found to be safe and well-tolerated.[64]

Therapies targeting oxidative stress
N-acetylcysteine (NAC) is an antioxidant that replenishes glutathione levels and attenuates free radical-induced injury. NAC combined with corticosteroids in one study reduced mortality at 1 month (8% vs 24%; P = .006), however, failed to meet the primary outcome of 6-month survival.[65] However, NAC was beneficial in reducing the risk of infection and of hepatorenal syndrome.

Metadoxine, an antioxidant, increases hepatic glutathione and adenosine triphosphate levels. In a randomized controlled trial, metadoxine in combination with prednisolone versus prednisolone alone improved patient survival in severe AH patients at 3 months (68.6% vs 20%, P = .0001) and at 6 months (48.6% vs 20%, P = .003).[66] Interestingly, patients receiving metadoxine maintained greater abstinence compared with those receiving placebo (74.5% vs 59.4%, P = .02). Larger trials are needed to validate these results.

Therapies enhancing liver regeneration
IL-22, a cytokine of IL-10 family, is known to provide hepatoprotective effects to improve oxidative stress and fibrosis, in turn promoting liver repair and regeneration.[56,67] A phase 2 trial in 24 patients with moderate and severe AH (MELD 11–28) showed an excellent safety profile of two infusions on days 1 and 7 of F-652, a recombinant fusion protein combining IL-22 and immunoglobulin G2. This was a dose-escalating study of 10, 30, and 45 mcg/kg of the active drug, with three patients enrolled with moderate and three with severe AH at each of three different doses. The drug significantly improved the MELD score and serum aminotransferases at days 28 and 42 from baseline, P < .005. A total of 83% patients enrolled in the study responded as determined by Lille score at day 7 of treatment, as compared with 6% to 12% of untreated cohorts and 56% in a prospective cohort treated with corticosteroids.[68] The drug was associated with reduction in the levels of circulating extracellular vesicles at 28 days and of cytokine levels at days 28 and 42[68].

Granulocyte-colony stimulating factor (G-CSF) is a glycoprotein which stimulates the bone marrow to release neutrophils and stem cells into the circulation, subsequently stimulating hepatocyte regeneration as well as proliferation of hepatocyte progenitor cells. A meta-analysis pooling data from seven randomized controlled trials (five from Asia and two from Europe) demonstrated an overall 90-day survival benefit in the G-CSF treated group (OR 0.28; 95% CI 0.09–0.88).[69] However, there was a high degree of heterogeneity with the Asian cohort demonstrating the majority of the benefit, whereas there was a trend toward worse outcomes in the G-CSF group in the European cohort (OR 1.89; 95% CI 0.90–3.98). Studies are in progress to substantiate the role of G-CSF in the United States, in the management of patients with severe AH (**Table 4**).

Early Liver Transplantation

Traditionally, transplant centers until a decade ago required a minimum 6-month abstinence period before consideration for LT.[70,71] However, several studies have shown that minimum abstinence period of 6 months to be a poor predictor of recurrence of alcohol use after LT.[72,73] More consistent and accurate predictors are younger age, psychosomatic status, psychiatric comorbidities, failed previous rehabilitation attempts, and family history of alcoholism.[74,75] The 6-month rule was challenged in a prospective study from the Franco-Belgian group, with the use of early LT (eLT) in

Table 4
Active or recently completed trials of emerging therapeutic agents for alcoholic hepatitis

Therapeutic Agent	Mechanism	Study Design	Disease Severity	Primary Endpoint	Trial Identifier	Current Status
Therapies Targeting Oxidative Stress						
N-acetylcysteine (NAC)	Antioxidant	• RCT: NAC + CS vs CS • RCT: NAC + CS vs CS	• mDF ≥32 • mDF ≥32	• All-cause mortality at 6 mo • Improvement in monocyte oxidative burst	• NCT05294744 • NCT03069300	• Not yet recruiting • Phase 3 recruiting
Metadoxine	Antioxidant	RCT: CS, PTX, metadoxine + CS, metadoxine + PTX	mDF ≥32	Survival at 30 d	NCT02161653	Phase 4 completed, improved survival at 3 and at 6 mo as well as improved abstinence
Omega 5 fatty acid	Peroxisome Proliferator Activated-Receptor (PPAR) gamma agonist	Placebo controlled RCT: Omega 5 fatty acid + SOC vs placebo + SOC	mDF ≥32	30-d survival	NCT03732586	Recruiting
Therapies Targeting Hepatic Inflammation						
DUR-928 (endogenous sulfated oxysterol)	Hepatic regeneration, inflammatory response, cell survival	Placebo-controlled RCT: DUR-928 30 mg vs DUR 928 90 mg vs placebo + SOC	MELD 21–30 and mDF ≥32	Difference in 90-d mortality or liver transplant	NCT04563026	Phase 2 recruiting
Anakinra	IL-1 receptor antagonist	RCT: anakinra + zinc + pentoxifylline vs CS	mDF ≥32 and MELD >20	Survival at 6 mo	NCT04072822	Phase 2 completed, no difference in survival, but lower rate of fungal infection in the active arm

Canakinumab	IL-1β antagonist	Placebo controlled RCT: canakinumab vs placebo	mDF ≥32 and MELD ≦27	Improvement in AHHS after 28 d	NCT03775109	Phase 2 completed, no improvement in survival
Selonsertib	ASK-1 antagonist	Placebo-controlled RCT: selonsertib + CS vs selonsertib + placebo	mDF ≥32	Safety and SAE at 28 d + 30 d	NCT02854631	Phase 2 completed, no improvement in survival or in liver function
Emricasan	Pan-caspase inhibitor	Placebo controlled RCT: Emricasan vs placebo	MELD 21–34 or MELD 35–40 if SOFA <10	Survival at 28 d	NCT01912404	Phase 2 terminated due to concerns of Pharmacokinetics / Pharmacodynamics (PK/PD) concerns
Therapies Enhancing Hepatic Regeneration						
G-CSF	Hepatic regeneration	Placebo-controlled RCT: prednisolone + G-CSF vs prednisolone vs G-CSF	mDF≥ 32	Survival at 90 d	NCT04066179	Unknown recruitment status
IL-22/F-652	Regeneration, antioxidant, anti-inflammatory	Open-label, dose-escalating trial	MELD 11–28	Safety and SAE at 42 d	NCT02655510	Phase 2 completed, demonstrated safety
Therapies Targeting Gut-Liver Axis						
FMT	Modulation of gut microbiome	• Placebo-controlled RCT: FMT + SOC vs placebo + SOC • RCT: FMT vs SOC (steroid-ineligible patients)	• MELD >15 and/ or mDF ≥32 • mDF ≥32 and MELD ≥20	• Survival at 12 mo, change in microbiome at different time points • Survival at 3 mo and transplant-free survival	• NCT05006430 • NCT05285592	• Phase 1 recruiting • Recruiting

(continued on next page)

Table 4
(continued)

Therapeutic Agent	Mechanism	Study Design	Disease Severity	Primary Endpoint	Trial Identifier	Current Status
Purified bovine colostrum	Immunoglobulin G (IgG) antibodies against LPS	Placebo-controlled RCT: bovine colostrum vs placebo	mDF ≥32 and MELD ≥21	Survival at 3 mo	NCT02473341	Phase 3 recruiting
Augmentin	Antibiotic	Placebo-controlled RCT: augmentin + CS vs CS	mDF ≥32 and MELD ≥21	Survival at 2 mo	NCT02281929	Phase 3 completed, pending final results
Rifaximin	Antibiotic	Case control: rifaximin + SOC vs SOC	mDF ≥32	Development of any bacterial infection	NCT02116556	Phase 2 completed, significant decrease in infection and liver-related complications
Lactobacillus rhamnosus GG	Probiotic	Placebo-controlled RCT: Lactobacillus vs placebo	MELD<20	Change in MELD	NCT01922895	Phase 2 terminated due to lack of funding
Obeticholic acid (OCA)	FXR agonist; bile acid agonist, anti-inflammatory	Placebo-controlled RCT: OCA vs placebo	MELD 12–19	Change in MELD at 6 wk	NCT02039219	Phase 2 terminated due to post-marketing reports of hepatotoxicity

Abbreviations: AHHS, alcoholic hepatitis histologic score; ASK, apoptosis signaling kinase; CS, corticosteroid; FMT, fecal microbiota transplant; FXR, Farnesoid X receptor; G-CSF, granulocyte-colony stimulating factor; IL, interleukin; LPS, lipopolysaccharide; mDF, Maddrey discriminant function; MELD, Model for End-Stage Liver Disease; NCT, clinical trial identifier; PTX, pentoxifylline; RCT, randomized-controlled trial; SAE, serious adverse event; SOC, standard of care; SOFA, sequential organ failure assessment.

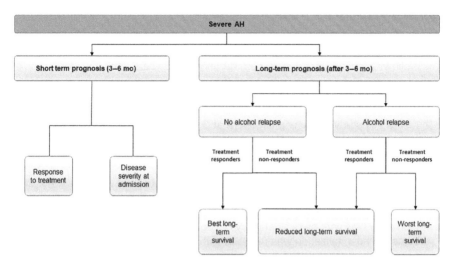

Fig. 3. Determinants of short-term and long-term prognosis in severe alcoholic hepatitis.

selected 26 severe AH patients with their first AH episode who did not respond to corticosteroids and had excellent psychosocial status. Compared with matched 26 patients who did not meet the selection criteria, eLT provided survival benefit with patient survival of 77% at 6 months compared with 23% survival among non-transplanted patients at same time points. Recurrence of alcohol use was acceptable in three patients at 2 years, two of these patients engaging in harmful alcohol use. Further, all the deaths in the patients in the study were within first 6 months, confirming that these patients cannot afford to wait for 6 months to meet with the requirement of minimum of 6 months abstinence.[50] Since then, other studies have shown similar benefit with eLT in severe AH patients.[76–79] In a retrospective study of patients who underwent eLT for severe AH, 1-year survival (94%) and 3-year survival (84%) were found to be similar to LT for other indications. The cumulative incidence of alcohol use post-LT was 25% at 1 year and 34% at 3 years with the only predictor for alcohol use post-LT being younger age on multivariable analysis.[76] In a meta-analysis including 11 studies, similar rates of relapse were observed between patients with severe AH undergoing eLT compared with those with cirrhosis undergoing elective transplantation (OR = 1.68, 95%CI = 0.79–3.58, P = .2). Furthermore, 6-month survival rates were similar between both groups (OR = 2.00, 95% CI = 0.95–4.23).[80] Currently, eLT is recommended among highly selected patients with severe AH.[43–45]

The awareness on benefits of eLT has increased enthusiasm within the transplant community with an increasing use of eLT for severe AH patients. However, the fairness of allocating organs to patients with AH has been questioned, as these patients may be perceived as having played a role in the evolution of their disease by some individuals, whereas others consider a more empathetic approach to them and consider dual pathology in these patients of liver disease and of AUD.[81,82] However, ethical implications of using a scarce resource for AH, risk of recurrent alcohol use questioning the utility of LT, and lack of accurate objective scores in predicting candidates at high risk for alcohol recurrence after LT have resulted in a significant heterogeneous use of eLT across providers and transplant centers.[83–85] Clearly, multicenter prospective studies are needed to refine selection criteria and develop a protocol which can be uniformly followed across centers for candidate selection for eLT in AH patients.

Treatment of Alcohol Use Disorder

Alcohol abstinence is the single most important determinant of long-term patient survival among patients surviving the initial AH episode (**Fig. 3**).[86–88] In a prospective study following patients for a maximum duration of 12 years after a diagnosis of AH, alcohol relapse of greater than 30 g per day was associated with an increased risk of death (HR 3.9, 95% CI 2.61–5.82) 6 months after the time of initial AH diagnosis.[89] However, maintaining abstinence is difficult with only 45% and 37% patients enrolled in the STOPAH study remaining abstinent at 3 months and at 1 year respectively.[47] Clearly, treatment of comorbid AUD becomes crucial in ALD patients using behavioral therapies (cognitive behavioral therapy, motivational interviewing, and support groups such as Alcoholics Anonymous) and/or pharmacologic therapies. FDA-approved medications (disulfiram, naltrexone, and acamprosate) to treat AUD have not been studied in randomized studies among patients with ALD. In a retrospective study on 160 (100 with liver disease of which 47 had decompensated cirrhosis) patients, naltrexone use was safe as evaluated by changes in liver aminotransferases. Further, 2 years risk of hospitalization was reduced with naltrexone use of 30 days or more.[90] Of the non-FDA-approved therapies, baclofen has been studied in the context of ALD and AH. In a retrospective study, the use of baclofen in 35 AH patients once serum bilirubin level has reduced to below 10 mg/dL and encephalopathy has resolved was safe with 97% of patients remaining abstinent over a mean follow-up period of 5.8 months.[91] Currently, baclofen and gabapentin are recommended treatment options for advanced ALD patients including those with AH.[43–45,92]

However, in the real world, AUD treatment is rarely used.[93] In a large study of 35,682 veterans with a diagnosis of AUD and cirrhosis, only 14% received AUD treatment, with pharmacotherapy used in only 1.4%.[93] Several barriers at the level of patients (reduced awareness, perception of stigma with ALD diagnosis, focus on liver disease and not on AUD), clinicians (lack of time and training in addiction medicine), and administration (lack of initiative, focus on other drug and substance use disorders, and siloed practices of addiction and hepatology specialists) limit addressing AUD in ALD patients.[94,95] Further, several administrative and system wide barriers related to billing, cost, and resources limit establishing multidisciplinary integrated care models to address the dual pathology of liver disease by hepatologists and AUD by addiction team under one roof in a collocated clinic.[94,96] Strategies are needed to overcome these barriers are needed to promote and establish integrated care of ALD patients with hepatology and addiction teams during pre-transplant as well as post-transplant care, with improvement in long-term outcomes and survival of patients with ALD and AH.

SUMMARY

The rising health care burden related to AH during the last decade and acceleration during the COVID-19 era has resulted in this disease entity emerging as an epidemic, especially in young individuals at the prime of their life. Further, in the background, there is a potential for high short-term mortality in most severe forms, whereas there is a lack of effective therapies, AH currently is an area of urgent attention from researchers to develop effective therapies, and from public health officials to derive strategies targeting to reduce the availability of alcohol in the community, especially through increase prices and higher taxation on alcohol. Several therapeutic targets are being examined, with some of these such as FMT, interleukin-22, DUR-928, and G-CSF being of potential promise. Early LT, in select cases, is emerging as an acceptable form of life-saving intervention. Although efforts are ongoing to develop newer pharmacotherapies and strategies targeting alcohol use, it is critical to promote integrated multidisciplinary care models for control of alcohol use and improvement in long-term outcomes of patients with ALD and AH.

CLINICS CARE POINTS

- Alcoholic hepatitis is characterized by new onset or worsening jaundice in the setting of heavy alcohol use and has significant short-term and long-term morbidity and mortality.
- Over the last decade, health care burden from alcoholic hepatitis has been increasing, and this has accelerated in the last 2 to 3 years during the COVID-19 pandemic.
- Corticosteroids, the mainstay of treatment for severe alcoholic hepatitis, is a suboptimal treatment, and there is a need for novel therapeutic agents.
- Several therapeutic targets are being examined, with some of these especially fecal microbiota transplant, interleukin-22, DUR-928, and granulocyte-colony stimulating factor (G-CSF) being of potential promise.
- Long-term prognosis of alcoholic hepatitis is determined by alcohol abstinence, and the treatment of the dual entities of liver disease and alcohol use disorder is critical.
- Integrated multidisciplinary care models with hepatology and addiction teams should be promoted to control alcohol use and improve long-term outcomes of patients with alcohol-associated liver disease and alcoholic hepatitis.

DISCLOSURES

None of the authors have any financial or any other disclosures.

REFERENCES

1. Crabb DW, Bataller R, Chalasani NP, et al. Standard Definitions and Common Data Elements for Clinical Trials in Patients With Alcoholic Hepatitis: Recommendation From the NIAAA Alcoholic Hepatitis Consortia. Gastroenterology 2016; 150(4):785–90.
2. Maddrey WC, Boitnott JK, Bedine MS, et al. Corticosteroid therapy of alcoholic hepatitis. Gastroenterology 1978;75(2):193–9.
3. Philips CA, Augustine P, Yerol PK, et al. Severe alcoholic hepatitis: current perspectives. HMER 2019;11:97–108.
4. Basra S. Definition, epidemiology and magnitude of alcoholic hepatitis. WJH 2011;3(5):108.
5. Shirazi F, Singal AK, Wong RJ. Alcohol-associated Cirrhosis and Alcoholic Hepatitis Hospitalization Trends in the United States. J Clin Gastroenterol 2021;55(2):174–9.
6. Hirode G, Saab S, Wong RJ. Trends in the Burden of Chronic Liver Disease Among Hospitalized US Adults. JAMA Netw Open 2020;3(4):e201997.
7. Liangpunsakul S. Clinical Characteristics and Mortality of Hospitalized Alcoholic Hepatitis Patients in the United States. J Clin Gastroenterol 2011;45(8):714–9.
8. Mandayam S, Jamal MM, Morgan TR. Epidemiology of Alcoholic Liver Disease. Semin Liver Dis 2004;24(03):217–32.
9. Doycheva I, Watt KD, Rifai G, et al. Increasing Burden of Chronic Liver Disease Among Adolescents and Young Adults in the USA: A Silent Epidemic. Dig Dis Sci 2017;62(5):1373–80.

10. Alkhouri N, Almomani A, Le P, et al. The prevalence of alcoholic and nonalcoholic fatty liver disease in adolescents and young adults in the United States: analysis of the NHANES database. BMC Gastroenterol 2022;22:366.

11. Tapper EB, Parikh ND. Mortality due to cirrhosis and liver cancer in the United States, 1999-2016: observational study. BMJ 2018;362:k2817.

12. Yeo YH, He X, Ting PS, et al. Evaluation of Trends in Alcohol Use Disorder-Related Mortality in the US Before and During the COVID-19 Pandemic. JAMA Netw Open 2022;5(5):e2210259.

13. White AM, Castle IJP, Powell PA, et al. Alcohol-Related Deaths During the COVID-19 Pandemic. JAMA 2022;327(17):1704-6.

14. Sharma RA, Subedi K, Gbadebo BM, et al. Alcohol Withdrawal Rates in Hospitalized Patients During the COVID-19 Pandemic. JAMA Netw Open 2021;4(3): e210422.

15. Barbosa C, Cowell AJ, Dowd WN. Alcohol Consumption in Response to the COVID-19 Pandemic in the United States. J Addict Med 2021;15(4):341-4.

16. Julien J, Ayer T, Tapper EB, et al. Effect of increased alcohol consumption during COVID-19 pandemic on alcohol-associated liver disease: A modeling study. Hepatology 2022;75(6):1480-90.

17. Deutsch-Link S, Jiang Y, Peery AF, et al. Alcohol-Associated Liver Disease Mortality Increased From 2017 to 2020 and Accelerated During the COVID-19 Pandemic. Clin Gastroenterol Hepatol 2022;20(9):2142-4, e2.

18. Sohal A, Khalid S, Green V, et al. The Pandemic Within the Pandemic. J Clin Gastroenterol 2022;56(3):e171-5.

19. Damjanovska S, Karb DB, Cohen SM. Increasing Prevalence and Racial Disparity of Alcohol-Related Gastrointestinal and Liver Disease During the COVID-19 Pandemic: A Population-Based National Study. J Clin Gastroenterol 2022. Publish Ahead of Print.

20. Gonzalez HC, Zhou Y, Nimri FM, et al. Alcohol-related hepatitis admissions increased 50% in the first months of the COVID-19 pandemic in the USA. Liver Int 2022;42(4):762-4.

21. Shaheen AA, Kong K, Ma C, et al. Impact of the COVID-19 Pandemic on Hospitalizations for Alcoholic Hepatitis or Cirrhosis in Alberta, Canada. Clin Gastroenterol Hepatol 2022;20(5):e1170-9.

22. Marlowe N, Lam D, Krebs W, et al. Prevalence, co-morbidities, and in-hospital mortality of patients hospitalized with alcohol-associated hepatitis in the United States from 2015 to 2019. Alcohol Clin Exp Res 2022;46(8):1472-81.

23. Dhanda AD. Is liver biopsy necessary in the management of alcoholic hepatitis? WJG 2013;19(44):7825.

24. Arab JP, Díaz LA, Baeza N, et al. Identification of optimal therapeutic window for steroid use in severe alcohol-associated hepatitis: A worldwide study. J Hepatol 2021;75(5):1026-33.

25. Rahimi E, Pan JJ. Prognostic models for alcoholic hepatitis. Biomark Res 2015; 3:20.

26. Dominguez M, Rincón D, Abraldes JG, et al. A New Scoring System for Prognostic Stratification of Patients With Alcoholic Hepatitis. Am J Gastroenterol 2008;103(11):2747-56. https://doi.org/10.1111/j.1572-0241.2008.02104.x.

27. Morales-Arráez D, Ventura-Cots M, Altamirano J, et al. The MELD Score Is Superior to the Maddrey Discriminant Function Score to Predict Short-Term Mortality in Alcohol-Associated Hepatitis: A Global Study. Am J Gastroenterol 2022;117(2): 301-10.

28. Louvet A, Naveau S, Abdelnour M, et al. The Lille model: A new tool for therapeutic strategy in patients with severe alcoholic hepatitis treated with steroids. Hepatology 2007;45(6):1348–54.

29. Mathurin P, O'Grady J, Carithers RL, et al. Corticosteroids improve short-term survival in patients with severe alcoholic hepatitis: meta-analysis of individual patient data. Gut 2011;60(2):255–60.

30. Garcia-Saenz-de-Sicilia M, Duvoor C, Altamirano J, et al. A Day-4 Lille Model Predicts Response to Corticosteroids and Mortality in Severe Alcoholic Hepatitis. Am J Gastroenterol 2017;112(2):306–15.

31. Louvet A, Labreuche J, Artru F, et al. Combining Data From Liver Disease Scoring Systems Better Predicts Outcomes of Patients With Alcoholic Hepatitis. Gastroenterology 2015;149(2):398–406, e8.

32. Kulkarni K, Tran T, Medrano M, et al. The Role of the Discriminant Factor in the Assessment and Treatment of Alcoholic Hepatitis. J Clin Gastroenterol 2004; 38(5):453–9.

33. Hanouneh IA, Zein NN, Cikach F, et al. The Breathprints in Patients with Liver Disease Identify Novel Breath Biomarkers in Alcoholic Hepatitis. Clin Gastroenterol Hepatol 2014;12(3):516–23.

34. Bissonnette J, Altamirano J, Devue C, et al. A prospective study of the utility of plasma biomarkers to diagnose alcoholic hepatitis. Hepatology 2017;66(2): 555–63.

35. Momen-Heravi F, Saha B, Kodys K, et al. Increased number of circulating exosomes and their microRNA cargos are potential novel biomarkers in alcoholic hepatitis. J Transl Med 2015;13:261.

36. Atkinson SR, Grove JI, Liebig S, et al. In Severe Alcoholic Hepatitis, Serum Keratin-18 Fragments Are Diagnostic, Prognostic, and Theragnostic Biomarkers. ACG 2020;115(11):1857–68.

37. Brandl K, Hartmann P, Jih LJ, et al. Dysregulation of serum bile acids and FGF19 in alcoholic hepatitis. J Hepatol 2018;69(2):396–405.

38. Sandahl TD, Grønbæk H, Møller HJ, et al. Hepatic Macrophage Activation and the LPS Pathway in Patients With Alcoholic Hepatitis: A Prospective Cohort Study. Am J Gastroenterol 2014;109(11):1749–56.

39. Michelena J, Altamirano J, Abraldes JG, et al. Systemic Inflammatory Response and Serum Lipopolysaccharide Levels Predict Multiple Organ Failure and Death in Alcoholic Hepatitis. Hepatology 2015;62(3):762–72.

40. Gala KS, Vatsalya V. Emerging Noninvasive Biomarkers, and Medical Management Strategies for Alcoholic Hepatitis: Present Understanding and Scope. Cells 2020;9(3):524.

41. Cabré E, Rodríguez-Iglesias P, Caballería J, et al. Short- and long-term outcome of severe alcohol-induced hepatitis treated with steroids or enteral nutrition: A multicenter randomized trial. Hepatology 2000;32(1):36–42.

42. Moreno C, Deltenre P, Senterre C, et al. Intensive Enteral Nutrition Is Ineffective for Patients With Severe Alcoholic Hepatitis Treated With Corticosteroids. Gastroenterology 2016;150(4):903–10, e8.

43. Singal AK, Bataller R, Ahn J, et al. ACG Clinical Guideline: Alcoholic Liver Disease. Am J Gastroenterol 2018;113(2):175–94.

44. Crabb DW, Im GY, Szabo G, et al. Diagnosis and Treatment of Alcohol-Associated Liver Diseases: 2019 Practice Guidance From the American Association for the Study of Liver Diseases. Hepatology 2020;71(1):306–33.

45. Thursz M, Gual A, Lackner C, et al. EASL Clinical Practice Guidelines: Management of alcohol-related liver disease. J Hepatol 2018;69(1):154–81.

46. Singal AK, Walia I, Singal A, et al. Corticosteroids and pentoxifylline for the treatment of alcoholic hepatitis: Current status. World J Hepatol 2011;3(8):205–10.

47. Thursz MR, Richardson P, Allison M, et al. Prednisolone or Pentoxifylline for Alcoholic Hepatitis. N Engl J Med 2015;372(17):1619–28.

48. Louvet A, Thursz MR, Kim DJ, et al. Corticosteroids Reduce Risk of Death Within 28 Days for Patients With Severe Alcoholic Hepatitis, Compared With Pentoxifylline or Placebo—a Meta-analysis of Individual Data From Controlled Trials. Gastroenterology 2018;155(2):458–68, e8.

49. Louvet A, Wartel F, Castel H, et al. Infection in patients with severe alcoholic hepatitis treated with steroids: early response to therapy is the key factor. Gastroenterology 2009;137(2):541–8.

50. Philippe M, Christophe M, Didier S, et al. Early Liver Transplantation for Severe Alcoholic Hepatitis. N Engl J Med 2011;365:1790–800.

51. Raff E, Singal AK. Optimal management of alcoholic hepatitis. Minerva Gastroenterol Dietol 2014;60(1):15.

52. Singal AK, Salameh H, Singal A, et al. Management practices of hepatitis C virus infected alcoholic hepatitis patients: A survey of physicians. World J Gastrointest Pharmacol Ther 2013;4(2):16–22.

53. Akriviadis E, Botla R, Briggs W, et al. Pentoxifylline improves short-term survival in severe acute alcoholic hepatitis: A double-blind, placebo-controlled trial. Gastroenterology 2000;119(6):1637–48.

54. Singh S, Murad MH, Chandar AK, et al. Comparative Effectiveness of Pharmacological Interventions for Severe Alcoholic Hepatitis: A Systematic Review and Network Meta-analysis. Gastroenterology 2015;149(4):958–70, e12.

55. Thompson J, Jones N, Al-Khafaji A, et al. Extracorporeal cellular therapy (ELAD) in severe alcoholic hepatitis: A multinational, prospective, controlled, randomized trial. Liver Transpl 2018;24(3):380–93.

56. Singal AK, Shah VH. Current trials and novel therapeutic targets for alcoholic hepatitis. J Hepatol 2019;70(2):305–13.

57. Thanda Han MA, Pyrsopoulos N. Emerging Therapies for Alcoholic Hepatitis. Clin Liver Dis 2021;25(3):603–24.

58. Purohit V, Bode JC, Bode C, et al. Alcohol, Intestinal Bacterial Growth, Intestinal Permeability to Endotoxin, and Medical Consequences. Alcohol 2008;42(5):349–61.

59. Philips CA, Pande A, Shasthry SM, et al. Healthy Donor Fecal Microbiota Transplantation in Steroid-Ineligible Severe Alcoholic Hepatitis: A Pilot Study. Clin Gastroenterol Hepatol 2017;15(4):600–2.

60. Bajaj JS, Gavis EA, Fagan A, et al. A Randomized Clinical Trial of Fecal Microbiota Transplant for Alcohol Use Disorder. Hepatology 2021;73(5):1688–700.

61. Philips CA, Ahamed R, Rajesh S, et al. Long-term Outcomes of Stool Transplant in Alcohol-associated Hepatitis—Analysis of Clinical Outcomes, Relapse, Gut Microbiota and Comparisons with Standard Care. J Clin Exp Hepatol 2022;12(4):1124–32.

62. Szabo G, Mitchell M, McClain CJ, et al. IL-1 receptor antagonist plus pentoxifylline and zinc for severe alcohol-associated hepatitis. Hepatology 2022;76(4):1058–68.

63. Gawrieh S, Dasarathy S, Tu W, et al. Anakinra plus Zinc versus Prednisone for Treatment of Severe Alcohol-Associated Hepatitis: A Randomized Controlled Trial. Poster presented at: The Liver Meeting. November 4-8, 2012; Washington D.C.

64. Hassanein T, Stein L, Flamm S. Safety and Efficacy of DUR-928: A Potential New Therapy for Acute Alcoholic Hepatitis. Hepatology 2019;70(6):1483A–4A.

65. Nguyen-Khac E, Thevenot T, Piquet MA, et al. Glucocorticoids plus N -Acetylcysteine in Severe Alcoholic Hepatitis. N Engl J Med 2011;365(19):1781–9.

66. Higuera-de la Tijera F, Servín-Caamaño AI, Serralde-Zúñiga AE, et al. Metadoxine improves the three- and six-month survival rates in patients with severe alcoholic hepatitis. World J Gastroenterol 2015;21(16):4975–85.

67. Brand S, Dambacher J, Beigel F, et al. IL-22-mediated liver cell regeneration is abrogated by SOCS-1/3 overexpression in vitro. Am J Physiology-Gastrointestinal Liver Physiol 2007;292(4):G1019–28.

68. Arab JP, Sehrawat TS, Simonetto DA, et al. An open label, dose escalation study to assess the safety and efficacy of il-22 agonist f-652 in patients with alcoholic hepatitis. Hepatology 2020;72(2):441–53.

69. Marot A, Singal AK, Moreno C, et al. Granulocyte colony-stimulating factor for alcoholic hepatitis: A systematic review and meta-analysis of randomised controlled trials. JHEP Rep 2020;2(5):100139.

70. Lucey MR, Brown KA, Everson GT, et al. Minimal criteria for placement of adults on the liver transplant waiting list: A report of a national conference organized by the American Society of Transplant Physicians and the American Association for the Study of Liver Diseases. Liver Transplant Surg 1997;3(6):628–37.

71. Everhart JE, Beresford TP. Liver transplantation for alcoholic liver disease: A survey of transplantation programs in the United States. Liver Transplant Surg 1997;3(3):220–6.

72. Jauhar S, Talwalkar JA, Schneekloth T, et al. Analysis of factors that predict alcohol relapse following liver transplantation. Liver Transplant 2004;10(3):408–11.

73. Are preoperative patterns of alcohol consumption predictive of relapse after liver transplantation for alcoholic liver disease?. Available at: https://onlinelibrary.wiley.com doi:10.1111/j.1432-2277.2005.00208.x. Accessed November 20, 2022.

74. Mccallum S, Masterton G. Liver transplantation for alcoholic liver disease: a systematic review of psychosocial selection criteria. Alcohol Alcohol 2006;41(4):358–63.

75. Lim J, Curry MP, Sundaram V. Risk factors and outcomes associated with alcohol relapse after liver transplantation. World J Hepatol 2017;9(17):771–80.

76. Lee BP, Mehta N, Platt L, et al. Outcomes of Early Liver Transplantation for Patients With Severe Alcoholic Hepatitis. Gastroenterology 2018;155(2):422–30.e1.

77. Lee BP, Chen PH, Haugen C, et al. Three-year Results of a Pilot Program in Early Liver Transplantation for Severe Alcoholic Hepatitis. Ann Surg 2017;265(1):20–9.

78. Carrique L, Quance J, Tan A, et al. Results of Early Transplantation for Alcohol-Related Cirrhosis: Integrated Addiction Treatment With Low Rate of Relapse. Gastroenterology 2021;161(6):1896–906, e2.

79. Herrick-Reynolds KM, Punchhi G, Greenberg RS, et al. Evaluation of Early vs Standard Liver Transplant for Alcohol-Associated Liver Disease. JAMA Surg 2021;156(11):1026–34.

80. Marot A, Dubois M, Trépo E, et al. Liver transplantation for alcoholic hepatitis: A systematic review with meta-analysis. PLoS One 2018;13(1):e0190823.

81. Mellinger JL, Volk ML. Transplantation for Alcohol-related Liver Disease: Is It Fair? Alcohol Alcohol 2018;53(2):173–7.

82. Glannon W. Responsibility and Priority in Liver Transplantation. Camb Q Healthc Ethics 2009;18(1):23–35.

83. Bangaru S, Pedersen MR, MacConmara MP, et al. Survey of Liver Transplantation Practices for Severe Acute Alcoholic Hepatitis: Survey of Liver Transplantation. Liver Transpl 2018;24(10):1357–62.

84. Cotter TG, Sandıkçı B, Paul S, et al. Liver transplantation for alcoholic hepatitis in the United States: Excellent outcomes with profound temporal and geographic variation in frequency. Am J Transpl 2021;21(3):1039–55.

85. Bittermann T, Mahmud N, Weinberg EM, et al. Rising Trend in Waitlisting for Alcoholic Hepatitis With More Favorable Outcomes Than Other High Model for End-stage Liver Disease in the Current Era. Transplantation 2022;106(7):1401–10.

86. Altamirano J, López-Pelayo H, Michelena J, et al. Alcohol abstinence in patients surviving an episode of alcoholic hepatitis: Prediction and impact on long-term survival: Altamirano, López-Pelayo, et al. Hepatology 2017;66(6):1842–53.

87. Elfeki MA, Abdallah MA, Leggio L, et al. Simultaneous management of alcohol use disorder and of liver disease: a systematic review and meta-analysis. J Addict Med 2022. https://doi.org/10.1097/ADM.0000000000001084. Publish Ahead of Print.

88. Evans MD, Diaz J, Adamusiak AM, et al. Predictors of Survival After Liver Transplantation in Patients With the Highest Acuity (MELD $\geq$40). Ann Surg 2020;272(3): 458–66.

89. Louvet A, Labreuche J, Artru F, et al. Main drivers of outcome differ between short term and long term in severe alcoholic hepatitis: A prospective study. Hepatology 2017;66(5):1464–73.

90. Ayyala D, Bottyan T, Tien C, et al. Naltrexone for alcohol use disorder: Hepatic safety in patients with and without liver disease. Hepaol Commun 2022;6: 3433–42.

91. Yamini D, Lee SH, Avanesyan A, et al. Utilization of Baclofen in Maintenance of Alcohol Abstinence in Patients with Alcohol Dependence and Alcoholic Hepatitis with or without Cirrhosis. Alcohol Alcohol 2014;49(4):453–6.

92. Reus VI, Hilty DM, Pasic J, et al. The American Psychiatric Association Practice Guideline for the Pharmacological Treatment of Patients With Alcohol Use Disorder. Am J Psychiatry 2018;175(1):86–90.

93. Rogal S, Youk A, Zhang H, et al. Impact of Alcohol Use Disorder Treatment on Clinical Outcomes among Patients with Cirrhosis. Hepatology 2020;71(6): 2080–92.

94. DiMartini AF, Leggio L, Singal AK. Barriers to the management of alcohol use disorder and alcohol-associated liver disease: strategies to implement integrated care models. Lancet Gastroenterol Hepatol 2022;7(2):186–95.

95. Lucey MR, Singal AK. Integrated Treatment of Alcohol Use Disorder in Patients With Alcohol-Associated Liver Disease: An Evolving Story. Hepatology 2020; 71(6):1891–3.

96. Mellinger JL, Scott Winder G, DeJonckheere M, et al. Misconceptions, preferences and barriers to alcohol use disorder treatment in alcohol-related cirrhosis. J Substance Abuse Treat 2018;91:20–7.

Inpatient Hepatology Consultation

A Practical Approach for Clinicians

Luis Antonio Díaz, MD[a], Josefina Pages, MD[b],
Victoria Mainardi, MD[c], Manuel Mendizabal, MD[b],*

KEYWORDS

- Cirrhosis • Decompensated cirrhosis • Spontaneous bacterial peritonitis
- Hepatic encephalopathy • Acute variceal bleeding • Esophagogastroduodenoscopy
- Serum-ascites albumin gradient • Clinically significant portal hypertension

KEY POINTS

- Complications related to portal hypertension frequently cause hospitalizations due to decompensated cirrhosis. Those patients admitted are also vulnerable to developing new onset or recurrence of liver-related complications.
- Potential precipitants of hepatic decompensation should be carefully addressed and prevented in every hospitalized patient with cirrhosis. Most decompensations might not have specific clinical symptoms, and a high clinical suspicion is fundamental.
- Once acute variceal bleeding is suspected, administration of crystalloids and blood products is essential. Esophagogastroduodenoscopy (EGD) is a diagnostic and therapeutic procedure and should be performed during the first 12 hours before admission.
- A diagnostic paracentesis should be performed in all patients with cirrhosis admitted for ascites and new onset decompensation. An absolute neutrophil count of 250/mm^3 or greater confirms spontaneous bacterial peritonitis and should prompt antibiotic therapy.
- In acute episodes of hepatic encephalopathy, a search and treatment of precipitant factors and alternative/coexisting causes should be done properly.

INTRODUCTION

Cirrhosis is the end-stage of chronic liver disease and constitutes a leading cause of potential years of working life lost, especially in the Americas and Europe.[1] Its natural history is characterized by an asymptomatic phase called compensated cirrhosis, followed by a rapidly progressive phase characterized by liver-related complications

---

[a] Department of Gastroenterology, Escuela de Medicina, Pontificia Universidad Católica de Chile, Santiago, Chile; [b] Hepatology and Liver Transplant Unit, Hospital Universitario Austral, Pilar, Provincia de Buenos Aires, Argentina; [c] Hepatology and Liver Transplant Unit, Hospital Central de Las Fuerzas Armadas, Montevideo, Uruguay
* Corresponding author. Unidad de Hígado y Trasplante Hepático, Hospital Universitario Austral, Av. Presidente Perón 1500, Pilar (B1629HJ), Buenos Aires, Argentina.
E-mail address: mmendiza@cas.austral.edu.ar

Med Clin N Am 107 (2023) 555–565
https://doi.org/10.1016/j.mcna.2023.01.006
0025-7125/23/© 2023 Elsevier Inc. All rights reserved.

termed decompensated cirrhosis. This is a nontrivial distinction because the long-term prognosis is highly different between both stages.[2] Complications could be related to portal hypertension and/or liver dysfunction, including ascites, portal hypertensive gastrointestinal (GI) bleeding, encephalopathy, and jaundice. Most of these decompensating factors might also trigger other complications such as sepsis, spontaneous bacterial peritonitis (SBP), refractory ascites, and hepatorenal syndrome.

Decompensated cirrhosis poses a great challenge in clinical practice and represents around 2% of hospital admissions in the United States.[3] These complications are associated with high economic costs, length of stay, and mortality.[4] A study conducted in the United States showed that related costs were estimated at US$ 7.37 billion in 2014.[3] Approximately 70% of discharged patients could suffer a readmission but 22% of them could be preventable with proper management after discharge.[5] Moreover, the model for end-stage liver disease (MELD) score, serum sodium, and the number of medications on discharge were significant risk factors for readmission.[5] Thus, early targeting of key pathogenic events could prevent cirrhosis progression and complications, constituting the cornerstone for managing inpatients with cirrhosis.[4] Based on 3 clinical cases, this review will discuss some of the most important precipitants of hepatic decompensation, including acute variceal bleeding (AVB), SBP, and hepatic encephalopathy (HE; **Figs. 1** and **2**).

MANAGEMENT OF ACUTE GASTROINTESTINAL BLEEDING IN HOSPITALIZED PATIENTS WITH CIRRHOSIS
Case Presentation

A 69-year-old female patient was admitted to the hospital with a hip fracture, having been recently diagnosed with alcohol-associated cirrhosis with no history of liver-related decompensations. The patient was receiving non-steroidal anti-inflammatory drugs (NSAIDs) and proton pump inhibitors. Two days after the admission, the patient presented with melena. On examination, there was no asterixis or clinically evident ascites. Vital signs were all within normal limits. Serum chemical tests were remarkable for

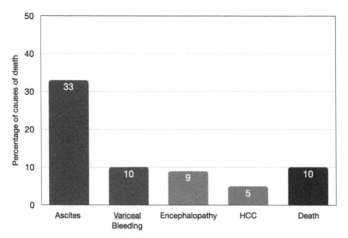

Fig. 1. Twenty-year proportions of patients presenting a first decompensating event in 377 patients with compensated cirrhosis at the diagnosis. (*Data from* D'Amico et.al. Competing risks and prognostic stages of cirrhosis: a 25-year inception cohort study of 494 patients. Aliment Pharmacol Ther. 2014 May;39(10):1180-93. https://doi.org/10.1111/apt.12721. Epub 2014 Mar 24. PMID: 24654740.)

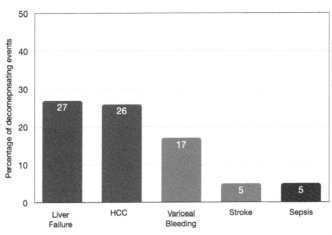

Fig. 2. Twenty-year proportions of causes of death in 377 patients presenting a first decompensating event. (*Data from* D'Amico et.al. Competing risks and prognostic stages of cirrhosis: a 25-year inception cohort study of 494 patients. Aliment Pharmacol Ther. 2014 May;39(10):1180-93. https://doi.org/10.1111/apt.12721. Epub 2014 Mar 24. PMID: 24654740.)

platelets 95,000/mm^3, hemoglobin 7.4 g/dL, international normalized ratio (INR) 1.7, creatinine 1.1 mg/dL, sodium 133 meq/L, albumin 3.2 g/dL, and bilirubin 2.5 mg/dL.

Clinical question
What is the differential diagnosis of a patient with cirrhosis who presents with melena?

DISCUSSION

Upper and lower GI bleeding is a common complication in hospitalized patients. Differential diagnoses of melena in patients with cirrhosis should include peptic ulcer, portal hypertensive gastropathy, Mallory Weiss syndrome, and AVB from esophageal and/or gastric varices. In patients with clinically significant portal hypertension (CSPH), AVB represents 70% of all upper GI bleeding events and remains one of the most severe and immediate life-threatening complications.[6] Patients with CSPH are at high risk of developing gastroesophageal varices. Moreover, 42% of patients with Child-Pugh A have gastro-esophageal varices, whereas more than 72% of patients with Child-Pugh class B/C do.[7] In this case, according to the patient's blood tests and physical examination, the patient had a Child-Pugh class B, so the chances of having gastroesophageal varices were high.

Acute GI bleeding in cirrhosis is a medical emergency with an elevated incidence of complications, and with associated high mortality. In this scenario, the main goals are maintaining hemodynamic stability, controlling bleeding, and preventing complications.[8,9] In this case, AVB must be suspected promptly and treatment should be started as soon as bleeding is clinically confirmed, regardless of the lack of confirmation by EGD.[10] General resurrection and supportive measures should be initiated immediately to maintain hemodynamic stability and ensure adequate tissue perfusion and oxygen delivery. Two peripheral intravenous catheters (14G or 16G) should be placed to guide facilitate resuscitation. Volume expansion with crystalloids should be performed conservatively monitoring volemic status.[8-10] A restrictive transfusion strategy is adequate in most patients with acute GI bleeding, starting when hemoglobin reaches a threshold of around 7 g/dL to maintain it between 7 and 9 g/dL.

Exceptions to this threshold include cardiovascular diseases, wherein we would prefer to avoid overexpansion and trigger acute heart failure or acute pulmonary edema. In patients with cirrhosis, conventional measures of clotting, such as prothrombin time, may not reflect the bleeding risk. Although there is no currently available data regarding the management of thrombocytopenia and coagulopathy, a proper evaluation including other modalities such as thromboelastography is desirable.[10,11] EGD should be performed within 12 hours of suspicion of bleeding but those with massive bleeding and hemodynamic instability would require it as soon as possible. Orotracheal intubation is reserved to protect the airway if the patient presents with HE grade III/IV, massive hematemesis, or hemodynamic instability. Abdominal imaging to rule out hepatocellular carcinoma and portal or splanchnic thrombosis should be performed in patients with AVB.[8,9]

Variceal hemorrhage is due to CSPH rather than coagulation abnormalities; thus, treatment should focus on lowering portal pressure.[9,12] Vasoactive drug therapy should be initiated as soon as AVB is suspected and before EGD. Either somatostatin, octreotide, or terlipressin is accepted option. After AVB is confirmed, vasoactive drug therapy should be administered for 2 to 5 days to avoid early rebleeding. Endoscopic band ligation is the recommended treatment presenting fewer adverse effects and achieving more effective control of bleeding than sclerotherapy, whereas cyanoacrylate injection is reserved for patients bleeding from gastric varices.[10,13,14] Antibiotic prophylaxis is recommended to reduce the incidence of infections, variceal rebleeding, and death. The choice of antibiotic should be based on the severity of liver disease and the local prevalence of quinolone-resistance bacterial infections. It is recommended to initiate quinolones (norfloxacin 400 mg bid) or ceftriaxone (1 g/daily i.v.) at presentation of bleeding and administered for 7 days.[13-15]

Despite all the recommended measures, up to 10% to 15% of patients with AVB have persistent bleeding or early rebleeding. In such cases, transjugular intrahepatic portosystemic shunt (TIPS) should be considered. Early TIPS insertion within 72 hours may be ideal in patients bleeding from esophageal or gastro-oesophageal varices who meet any of the following criteria: Child-Pugh class C less than 14 points or Child-Pugh class B greater than 7 with active bleeding at initial endoscopy. In case of massive bleeding, balloon tamponade should be used as a temporary "bridge" until definitive treatment can be instituted and can be used for a maximum of 24 hours.[10] Recurrence of variceal hemorrhage reaches around 60%; thus, patients should be placed on nonselective beta blockers and continue with endoscopic variceal ligation every 3 to 4 weeks until varices are eradicated.[14,16]

SUMMARY

In this patient, EGD was performed without the presence of active bleeding but large esophageal varices with red wall signs were present. Endoscopic band ligation was performed during the same procedure. The patient was admitted to the intensive care unit. Terlipressin and ciprofloxacin were administered for 5 and 7 days, respectively. The patient was discharged on day 7 on carvedilol 12.5 mg bid, with plans for follow-up endoscopy and band ligation.

A Patient with Cirrhosis Admitted for New Onset of Ascites and Suspected Infection

Case presentation

A 62-year-old man with cirrhosis due to nonalcoholic fatty liver disease (NAFLD) and a baseline Child-Pugh class B (7) was admitted for increased abdominal distention, diffuse abdominal pain, peripheral edema, nausea, bloating, and chills. He had a recent EGD and was noted to have small esophageal varices. The patient presented a mean arterial pressure of 70 mm Hg, HR 83/min, 101°F (axillary temperature), without supplemental oxygen requirement, and was oriented in space and time. Abdominal ultrasonography revealed moderate-to-severe ascites, and a Doppler study noted patency of the portal vein. Serum chemistry tests were remarkable for a creatinine 1.2 mg/dL and C reactive protein of 4.2 mg/dL (normal upper limit of 0.5 mg/dL). Diagnostic paracentesis was performed, and the ascitic fluid demonstrated a serum-ascites albumin gradient (SAAG) of 2.4 g/dL with an absolute neutrophil count of 650/mm^3.

Clinical question
How to address a patient with cirrhosis and with new onset of ascites and fever?

DISCUSSION

Ascites is the leading cause of decompensation in cirrhosis and occurs in up to 10% of patients with compensated cirrhosis annually.[17] Although cirrhosis is the cause for ascites in around 80%, other causes should be ruled out, including malignancy, heart failure, tuberculosis, and pancreatic disease.[4] Diagnostic paracentesis is mandatory in all the patients with cirrhosis admitted for worsening ascites (grade 2 or 3) or new onset of hepatic decompensation event such as HE, and the analysis should include at least the absolute neutrophil count, total protein and albumin concentration, and culture of ascitic fluid.[4,18] The primary assessment of patients with ascites should also include liver and renal function, serum and urine electrolytes, and abdominal Doppler ultrasound. The SAAG is the best method to determine if ascitic fluid is secondary to portal hypertension and is calculated by subtracting the ascitic fluid albumin from the serum albumin in simultaneously obtained samples. A SAAG of 1.1 g/dL or greater has an accuracy of 97% in differentiating portal hypertension from other causes.[19] In our clinical case, a SAAG of 2.4 g/dL confirmed that the ascites was due to portal hypertension.

On hospitalization, up to 34% of patients with decompensated cirrhosis present with bacterial infections.[20] In this scenario, the most frequent infection is SBP accounting for 27% of cases, followed by urinary tract infections (22%), pneumonia (19%), bacteremia (8%), and skin and soft tissue infections (8%).[21] A careful examination should be undertaken, seeking for fever, hypothermia, chills, and other specific symptoms from potential sources. In particular, SBP is a bacterial infection of ascitic fluid without any intra-abdominal evident treatable source of infection. Most patients report abdominal pain, tenderness, or ileus; however, around one-third of them can be asymptomatic.[18] The absolute neutrophil count in ascitic fluid constitutes the cornerstone for diagnosing SBP. A neutrophil count of 250/mm^3 or greater has high sensitivity but the highest specificity is achieved with a count of 500/mm^3 or greater.[22] Thus, there is consensus on using an absolute neutrophil count 250/mm^3 or greater to avoid delayed antibiotic use. This latter aspect is not trivial because an observational study showed that delayed diagnosis is associated with a 2.7-fold increased mortality.[23] Ascites culture is also relevant to guide antibiotic therapy and should be included in all patients. Despite traditional cultures having a yield of close to 40%, an inoculum of 10 mL or greater of ascitic fluid into blood culture bottles could notably improve its sensitivity (up to 90%).[24] Less than 5% of cirrhotic patients present with secondary bacterial peritonitis. The key clues in the ascitic fluid are the presence of a very high ascitic neutrophil count, high ascitic protein concentration, or multiple organisms on ascitic culture.[4] All patients with suspected secondary bacterial peritonitis should undergo prompt abdominal imaging and assessment by the surgery team.

Most episodes of SBP are monomicrobial and are due to gram-negative bacteria in around 60%, whereas fungi are observed in less than 5% of cases but are associated with a worse prognosis.[25] The most frequent pathogens are enteric, including *Escherichia coli*, *Klebsiella pneumoniae*, *Staphylococcus aureus*, *Enterococcus faecalis*, and *Enterococcus faecium*.[21] However, there is an increasing prevalence of multidrug-resistant (MDR) bacteria, reaching 34% of infections. This finding is higher in Asia, especially in India, and the main risk factors are the use of antibiotics in the 3 months before hospitalization and prior health-care exposure.[21] Intravenous antibiotic therapy is the primary treatment of SBP. Third-generation cephalosporins have been traditionally recommended as a first-line treatment (ceftriaxone and cefotaxime).[4,18] However, antibiotics should be carefully chosen due to the increasing prevalence of MDR bacteria. Thus, treatment should be selected according to patient's earlier infections and local epidemiology in those with risk factors for MDR infections. Due to the excess mortality in patients with septic shock due to SBP and inappropriate initial antimicrobial therapy, the use of carbapenems with or without a glycopeptide should be considered, with a proper adjustment using cultures. A new diagnostic paracentesis after 48 hours is highly recommended, and a decrease of absolute neutrophil count by more than 25% is considered a successful response to treatment. This strategy could be helpful to shorten antibiotic therapy in adequate responders or adjust antibiotic treatment properly in those who do not meet response criteria. Conversely, asymptomatic patients with an absolute neutrophil count less than 250/mm^3 and a positive bacteriologic culture (bacterascites) might not benefit from antibiotics.[4,18] In such patients, a repeat paracentesis is recommended to see if they have onto classic SBP or if bacterascites has resolved.

Infections frequently precipitate acute kidney injury (AKI) among patients with cirrhosis, whereas AKI is the leading cause of death in patients with SBP. Early identification of patients at risk, expansion of the intravascular volume, and avoiding nephrotoxic drugs are the keys to preventing and managing AKI.[26] Notably, albumin has several mechanisms beyond oncotic properties, including antioxidant, scavenging, immune-modulating, and endothelium protective functions.[27] Prior evidence has shown that albumin administration could decrease mortality in decompensated cirrhosis, especially in those who already have renal dysfunction (blood urea nitrogen >30 mg/dL or creatinine >1.0 mg/dL) or severe hepatic decompensation (bilirubin >5 mg/dL).[18] The standard dose of albumin recommended by clinical guidelines in SBP has been arbitrarily set at 1.5 g/kg on day 1 and 1 g/kg on day 3.[28] Further evidence is necessary to explore different doses of albumin in SBP.

Long-term prophylactic antibiotics are a helpful strategy to prevent SBP recurrence. An earlier study based on norfloxacin 400 mg daily versus placebo demonstrated a significant decrease in recurrence at 1 year (20% vs 68%, respectively).[29] Because several countries (including the United States) do not have norfloxacin widely available, the use of ciprofloxacin seems a good alternative in clinical practice.

SUMMARY

In this clinical case, SBP was diagnosed early, and ceftriaxone was promptly initiated in the emergency room. Albumin was also administered with a consequent improvement in renal function. A new diagnostic paracentesis was performed, demonstrated a decrease of 37% in the absolute neutrophil count at 48 hours, and the patient completed a 5-day course of intravenous antibiotics and was discharged on an oral antibiotic, as secondary prophylaxis against SBP.

A Patient with Cirrhosis and Sensory Impairment

Case presentation

A 59-year-old woman with NAFLD compensated cirrhosis, and CSPH characterized by small esophageal varices, without a history of earlier decompensations, underwent urgent surgery for a strangulated inguinal hernia. After 48 hours of surgery, she developed sensory impairment. Physical examination revealed HR of 102, mild dehydration, lethargy, disorientation to time, and asterixis. The patient was diagnosed with grade II HE. There were no other neurologic signs, fever, or evidence of surgical site infection. In particular, the abdominal examination was normal. Serum chemistries were notable for creatinine 0.9 mg/dL, sodium 128 mmol/L, potassium 3.2 mmol/L, glucose 67 mg/dL, total bilirubin 1.2 mg/dL, INR 1.3, and IU/L albumin 3.2 mg/dL.

Clinical question

How should we manage a patient with cirrhosis and an acute altered consciousness?

DISCUSSION

The postoperative period is a vulnerable time for patients with cirrhosis. In this case, the patient developed abnormal behavior and compromised cognition. In patients with advanced liver disease and portosystemic shunting, the alterations of brain functioning are usually due to HE. This decompensation is a common and modifiable cause of postoperative delirium associated with inpatient morbidity and mortality. HE interferes with the patient's capacity to follow postoperative instructions and nutritional goals, increasing the risk of nosocomial complications, such as falls.[30] Risk factors associated with their development include history of HE, high MELD-Na, GI bleeding, postoperative state, electrolyte disorders, infections, and exposure to some medications such as benzodiazepines.[30]

HE occurs in 30% to 40% of patients with cirrhosis during the course of their disease, reaching a recurrence rate of up to 40% during a 30-day period.[31] Its development, as well as other complications related to CSPH, marks the transition from compensated to decompensated stage of cirrhosis, and which is associated with a substantial worsening of patient prognosis.[2,32] The burden of HE goes beyond morbidity and mortality and directs costs for the health-care system, including indirect costs for patients and families, the inability to work, poor quality of life, and unfitness to drive.[33]

Diagnosis of the first episode of HE can be challenging. HE produces a wide spectrum of nonspecific neurologic and psychiatric manifestations, and it has been graded according to the West Haven criteria. This classification ranges from 0 to 4, including personality changes (apathy, irritability, and disinhibition) and alterations of the sleep–wake cycle (grade 1), disorientation to time and space (grade 2), acute confused state with agitation or somnolence, stupor (grade 3), and finally coma (grade 4). Asterixis is often present in grade 2 but other neurologic signs such as hypertonia, hyperreflexia, and Babinski sign are less frequent.[31,34] Patients with no particular symptoms beyond abnormal behavior on psychometric tests have been identified as covert HE. Although covert HE is mild, it is associated with distraction, incompetent driving, and frequent falls. HE remains a diagnosis of exclusion of other neuro-psychiatric diseases and relevant differential diagnoses should be ruled out. Therefore, these patients should undergo the same standardized diagnostic evaluation as any other patient with altered consciousness, especially when diagnosing the first episode of HE.[31,35] The diagnostic workup varies according to the degree of impairment and the clinical suspicion of other diagnoses[33] and includes blood tests for glucose, liver and kidney function, electrolytes, inflammatory markers, complete blood count, vitamin B12, and thyroid-stimulating hormone levels.[35,36] Brain imaging should be performed in case of clinical suspicion of a cerebral lesion or hemorrhage. Lumbar puncture may be necessary to rule out meningitis, and an electroencephalogram to exclude nonconvulsive seizures in more severe cases. Screening for alcohol levels and psychoactive drugs in outpatients, who present with altered mental status. Measurement of plasma ammonia levels has a high-negative predictive value, and a normal ammonia level in a patient with cirrhosis and delirium should prompt further differential diagnostic workup for other causes of delirium.[35]

The main aims of treatment of an episode of overt HE are reducing its duration, limiting its consequences, preventing recurrence, and limiting the impact on quality of life. Therefore, treatment of an acute episode of overt HE includes.

1. Airway management. Patients with HE grades III-IV of West Haven classification should be treated in an intensive care setting. If the Glasgow Coma Score is 8 or less, the airway should be secured with orotracheal intubation in order to prevent aspiration.[33–35]
2. Identify and eventually treat alternative and coexisting causes. Include a computed tomography (CT) scan of the head for first episode of HE, if there is a history of fall, headache, or if physical examination reveals a focal deficit.[33,35]
3. Identify and correct precipitating factors. In some cases, multiple precipitating events may coexist. Infections represent the most common precipitating event (31%), followed by constipation (29.4%), dehydration/diuretic overdose (17.7%), hyponatremia (11.2%), or GI bleeding (12.6%).[33] Identifying and treating any of these factors is of paramount importance in reversing an acute episode of HE. If used, sedatives (opioids or benzodiazepines) should be discontinued.[31,34,35]
4. Specific treatment of HE. Most of the therapies for HE target ammonia. The majority of ammonia is produced in the gut, and the liver is not efficiently able to detoxify ammonia into urea. Thus, reducing ammonia production and absorption from the gut is the strategy to reduce circulating ammonia levels. Nonabsorbable disaccharides are effective in treating and preventing HE and are the recommended first-line treatment of HE. Lactulose is the most extensive agent used to treat acute episodes of HE. If the patient can swallow, it is administered orally but it can also be administered through oro/nasogastric tube and rectally. The dose is 25 mL every 1 to 2 hours until loose bowel movements are produced, and subsequently titrated to maintain 2 to 3 bowel movements per day.[31] Other alternatives include antimicrobial agents, such as rifaximin, which act against enteric bacteria and reduce ammonia production. Rifaximin should be used as an add-on to lactulose to treat acute episodes of HE and to prevent recurrence. Individuals who recover from an episode of HE are at higher risk of developing recurrent episodes of overt HE. Lactulose is also effective in preventing subsequent episodes of overt HE. Rifaximin as an add-on to lactulose is more effective than lactulose alone in reducing the risk of hospitalizations in those with overt HE.[34]

In patients with a history of overt HE and with improvement of liver function and nutritional status and in whom precipitant factors have been controlled and not likely to recur (ie, a patient with a history of overt HE precipitated by GI bleeding in whom varices have been obliterated), discontinuation of secondary HE prophylaxis can be considered on an individual basis.[34]

SUMMARY

The patient had correction of electrolyte disturbance and hypoglycemia, and a CT scan revealed no brain lesions. Lactulose was initiated, and on the following day,

HE resolved. The patient was discharged 3 days later with lactulose as secondary prophylaxis for recurrent HE.

CLINICS CARE POINTS

- Acute GI bleeding in cirrhosis is a medical emergency with an elevated incidence of complications.
- Variceal bleeding must be suspected promptly and treatment should be started as soon as bleeding is clinically confirmed.
- Cirrhosis is the most common cause of ascites representing around 80% of the cases.
- Ascites is the leading cause of decompensation in patients with cirrhosis.
- Spontaneous bacterial peritonitis is the most frequent nfection in hospitalized patients with decompensated cirrhosis.
- Alterations of brain functioning in patients with cirrhosis are usually due to hepatic encephalopathy.
- The main aims of treatment of an episode of overt HE are reducing its duration, preventing recurrence, and limiting the impact on quality of life.

CONFLICT OF INTEREST

The authors declare no conflict of interest.

FINANCIAL SUPPORT/ACKNOWLEDGMENTS

None.

AUTHORS' CONTRIBUTIONS

M. Mendizabal conceived the article. L.A. Diaz and M. Mendizabal designed the figure. All authors participated in drafting the article and revising it critically. All authors gave final approval of the version submitted.

REFERENCES

1. Karlsen TH, Sheron N, Zelber-Sagi S, et al. The EASL–Lancet Liver Commission: protecting the next generation of Europeans against liver disease complications and premature mortality. Lancet 2022;399(10319):61–116.
2. D'Amico G, Garcia-Tsao G, Pagliaro L. Natural history and prognostic indicators of survival in cirrhosis: a systematic review of 118 studies. J Hepatol 2006;44(1):217–31.
3. Desai AP, Mohan P, Nokes B, et al. Increasing Economic Burden in Hospitalized Patients With Cirrhosis: Analysis of a National Database. Clin Transl Gastroenterol 2019;10(7):e00062.
4. European Association for the Study of the Liver. Electronic address: easloffice@easloffice.eu, European Association for the Study of the Liver. EASL Clinical Practice Guidelines for the management of patients with decompensated cirrhosis. J Hepatol 2018;69(2):406–60.
5. Volk ML, Tocco RS, Bazick J, et al. Hospital readmissions among patients with decompensated cirrhosis. Am J Gastroenterol 2012;107(2):247–52.

6. Sanyal AJ, Bosch J, Blei A, et al. Portal hypertension and its complications. Gastroenterology 2008;134(6):1715–28.

7. Kovalak M, Lake J, Mattek N, et al. Endoscopic screening for varices in cirrhotic patients: data from a national endoscopic database. Gastrointest Endosc 2007; 65(1):82–8.

8. Garcia-Tsao G, Bosch J, Groszmann RJ. Portal hypertension and variceal bleeding–unresolved issues. Summary of an American Association for the study of liver diseases and European Association for the study of the liver single-topic conference. Hepatology 2008;47(5):1764–72.

9. Garcia-Tsao G, Bosch J. Management of varices and variceal hemorrhage in cirrhosis. N Engl J Med 2010;362(9):823–32.

10. de Franchis R, Bosch J, Garcia-Tsao G, et al. Baveno VII Faculty. Baveno VII - Renewing consensus in portal hypertension. J Hepatol 2022;76(4):959–74.

11. Villanueva C, Colomo A, Bosch A, et al. Transfusion strategies for acute upper gastrointestinal bleeding. N Engl J Med 2013;368(1):11–21.

12. García-Pagán JC, Gracia-Sancho J, Bosch J. Functional aspects on the pathophysiology of portal hypertension in cirrhosis. J Hepatol 2012;57(2):458–61.

13. Garcia-Tsao G, Abraldes JG, Berzigotti A, et al. Portal hypertensive bleeding in cirrhosis: Risk stratification, diagnosis, and management: 2016 practice guidance by the American Association for the study of liver diseases. Hepatology 2017;65(1):310–35.

14. Bernard B, Grangé JD, Khac EN, et al. Antibiotic prophylaxis for the prevention of bacterial infections in cirrhotic patients with gastrointestinal bleeding: a metaanalysis. Hepatology 1999;29(6):1655–61.

15. Chavez-Tapia NC, Barrientos-Gutierrez T, Tellez-Avila F, et al. Meta-analysis: antibiotic prophylaxis for cirrhotic patients with upper gastrointestinal bleeding - an updated Cochrane review. Aliment Pharmacol Ther 2011;34(5):509–18.

16. García-Pagán JC, Caca K, Bureau C, et al. Early use of TIPS in patients with cirrhosis and variceal bleeding. N Engl J Med 2010;362(25):2370–9.

17. Ginés P, Quintero E, Arroyo V, et al. Compensated cirrhosis: natural history and prognostic factors. Hepatology 1987;7(1):122–8.

18. Biggins SW, Angeli P, Garcia-Tsao G, et al. Diagnosis, Evaluation, and Management of Ascites, Spontaneous Bacterial Peritonitis and Hepatorenal Syndrome: 2021 Practice Guidance by the American Association for the Study of Liver Diseases. Hepatology 2021;74(2):1014–48.

19. Runyon BA, Montano AA, Akriviadis EA, et al. The serum-ascites albumin gradient is superior to the exudate-transudate concept in the differential diagnosis of ascites. Ann Intern Med 1992;117(3):215–20.

20. Tandon P, Garcia-Tsao G. Bacterial infections, sepsis, and multiorgan failure in cirrhosis. Semin Liver Dis 2008;28(1):26–42.

21. Piano S, Singh V, Caraceni P, et al. Epidemiology and Effects of Bacterial Infections in Patients With Cirrhosis Worldwide. Gastroenterology 2019;156(5): 1368–80, e10.

22. Wong CL, Holroyd-Leduc J, Thorpe KE, et al. Does this patient have bacterial peritonitis or portal hypertension? How do I perform a paracentesis and analyze the results? JAMA 2008;299(10):1166–78.

23. Kim JJ, Tsukamoto MM, Mathur AK, et al. Delayed paracentesis is associated with increased in-hospital mortality in patients with spontaneous bacterial peritonitis. Am J Gastroenterol 2014;109(9):1436–42.

24. Runyon BA, Canawati HN, Akriviadis EA. Optimization of ascitic fluid culture technique. Gastroenterology 1988;95(5):1351–5.

25. Gravito-Soares M, Gravito-Soares E, Lopes S, et al. Spontaneous fungal perito-nitis: a rare but severe complication of liver cirrhosis. Eur J Gastroenterol Hepatol 2017;29(9):1010–6.
26. Angeli P, Garcia-Tsao G, Nadim MK, et al. News in pathophysiology, definition and classification of hepatorenal syndrome: A step beyond the International Club of Ascites (ICA) consensus document. J Hepatol 2019;71(4):811–22.
27. Bernardi M, Angeli P, Claria J, et al. Albumin in decompensated cirrhosis: new concepts and perspectives. Gut 2020;69(6):1127–38.
28. Sort P, Navasa M, Arroyo V, et al. Effect of intravenous albumin on renal impair-ment and mortality in patients with cirrhosis and spontaneous bacterial peritonitis. N Engl J Med 1999;341(6):403–9.
29. Ginés P, Rimola A, Planas R, et al. Norfloxacin prevents spontaneous bacterial peritonitis recurrence in cirrhosis: results of a double-blind, placebo-controlled trial. Hepatology 1990;12(4 Pt 1):716–24.
30. Saleh ZM, Solano QP, Louissaint J, et al. The incidence and outcome of postop-erative hepatic encephalopathy in patients with cirrhosis. United European Gas-troenterol J 2021;9(6):672–80.
31. Vilstrup H, Amodio P, Bajaj J, et al. Hepatic encephalopathy in chronic liver dis-ease: 2014 Practice Guideline by the American Association for the Study of Liver Diseases and the European Association for the Study of the Liver. Hepatology 2014;60(2):715–35.
32. Tapper EB, Aberasturi D, Zhao Z, et al. Outcomes after hepatic encephalopathy in population-based cohorts of patients with cirrhosis. Aliment Pharmacol Ther 2020;51(12):1397–405.
33. Ridola L, Riggio O, Gioia S, et al. Clinical management of type C hepatic enceph-alopathy. United European Gastroenterol J 2020;8(5):536–43.
34. Mendizabal M, Silva MO. Images in clinical medicine. Asterixis. N Engl J Med 2010;363(9):e14.
35. European Association for the Study of the Liver. Electronic address: easloffi-ce@easloffice.eu, European Association for the Study of the Liver. EASL clinical practice guidelines on the management of hepatic encephalopathy. J Hepatol 2022;77(3):807–24.
36. Rose CF, Amodio P, Bajaj JS, et al. Hepatic encephalopathy: Novel insights into classification, pathophysiology and therapy. J Hepatol 2020;73(6):1526–47.

Intensive Care Unit Care of a Patient with Cirrhosis

Mahathi Avadhanam, MBBS[a], Anand V. Kulkarni, MD, DM[b],*

KEYWORDS

- Critical care hepatology • Acute kidney injury • ACLF • Encephalopathy
- Infections in cirrhosis

KEY POINTS

- ICU mortality of a patient with cirrhosis is high.
- Common reasons for ICU admission are infection, organ failure, and variceal bleeding.
- POCUS (Point of Ultrasonography) has revolutionalised the care of a critically ill patient.
- Bristol and SPICT (Supportive and Palliative Care Indicators tool) are objective scores to identify patients who may not benefit from ICU care.

INTRODUCTION

Cirrhosis is an end-stage liver disease due to distortion of liver architecture by varied causes. It is the leading cause of liver-related mortality around the world.[1] The Asia-Pacific region accounts for more than half of the global population and approximately 62.6% of global deaths due to liver diseases.[2] As per data from the United Kingdom, between 1992 and 2012, the number of intensive care unit (ICU) admissions for cirrhosis rose from 1.6% to 3.1%.[3] By 2017, patients with liver cirrhosis comprised up to 15% of all ICU admissions.[4] Common causes of liver cirrhosis are alcohol, nonalcoholic steatohepatitis, and hepatitis B and C viruses.[5,6] Patients with alcohol-associated liver disease admitted to ICU have increased mortality compared with other etiologies.[3] Huang and colleagues conducted a nationwide, population-based propensity score-matched study of reimbursement claims data from Taiwan's National Health Insurance Program, which revealed that cirrhotic patients admitted to the ICU showed significantly higher ICU mortality and increased medical expenditure compared with non-cirrhotic controls.[7] The in-hospital mortality of these patients has been historically very high.[8] However, the crude ICU mortality has reduced from 41% to 31% in the 1992 to 2012 period.[3] Although concluding that cirrhosis is a strong negative predictor of survival for patients admitted to the ICU, Kubesch and

[a] Department of Emergency Medicine, Queen Elizabeth hospital, London, UK; [b] Department of Hepatology, AIG Hospitals, Gachibowli, Hyderabad, India-500032
* Corresponding author. Department of Hepatology, AIG Hospitals, Gachibowli, Hyderabad, India-500032.
E-mail address: anandvk90@gmail.com

Med Clin N Am 107 (2023) 567–587
https://doi.org/10.1016/j.mcna.2022.12.006
0025-7125/23/© 2022 Elsevier Inc. All rights reserved.
medical.theclinics.com

colleagues reported that mortality increased proportionately with Model for End-Stage Liver Disease (MELD) scores in the cirrhosis group, reinforcing the relevance of the MELD score in mortality prediction.[9]

INDICATIONS FOR INTENSIVE CARE UNIT ADMISSION IN A PATIENT WITH CIRRHOSIS

Common indications for ICU admission or in-hospital transfer to ICU of patients with cirrhosis include:

- Infection/sepsis
- Shock due to any cause—hypovolemic, cardiogenic, septic
- Altered sensorium—hepatic encephalopathy (HE), alcohol withdrawal, or uremic encephalopathy
- Variceal and non-variceal bleeding
- Acute kidney injury (AKI)-hepato-renal syndrome progressing to chronic renal failure.
- Acute symptomatic portal vein thrombosis/splanchnic vein thrombosis
- Coagulopathy-related (or spontaneous) intracranial bleed
- Hemoperitoneum (traumatic or spontaneous)
- Rupture of hepatocellular carcinoma
- Post-surgery monitoring for liver failure
- Acute-on-chronic liver failure (ACLF) is a clinical syndrome that is an extreme form of liver disease associated with extrahepatic organ failures and consequently, high short-term mortality.[10,11] ACLF can be triggered by a variety of extrahepatic infections, gastrointestinal (GI) hemorrhage, procedures like transjugular intrahepatic portosystemic shunt (TIPS), or intrahepatic factors (viral hepatitis, alcohol, drug-induced liver injury, autoimmune liver disease).[12] Patients with ACLF require organ support in the form of renal replacement therapy, mechanical ventilation, vasopressor therapy, and plasma exchange. Therefore, most patients with ACLF require prompt referral and appropriate ICU care to modify the course of the disease favourably.[8]

Other indications for ICU admission are listed in **Table 1**.[13]

APPROACH TO MANAGEMENT

The Airway, Breathing, Circulation, Disability, Exposure (ABCDE) approach can be adapted for the care of patients with cirrhosis who need ICU admission.[14]

Airway

- If the patient is able to speak, ensure that the airway is patent.
- If the patient is unconscious or has depressed consciousness (due to hepatic/septic/uremic encephalopathy) Glasgow Coma Scale (GCS) less than 8—consider intubation for airway protection.
- Consider intubation in case of massive acute upper GI hemorrhage to prevent aspiration and in case of dyspnea/respiratory fatigue due to hydrothorax or pneumonia.

Breathing

- Observe breathing pattern, look for any signs of respiratory distress, check respiratory rate, and oxygen saturation using pulse oximeter
- Clubbing can be noted in patients with hepatopulmonary syndrome (other causes: primary biliary cholangitis).

Table 1 Objective indications for intensive care unit admission	
Type of Complication	**Criteria for ICU Admission**
Infection	Septic shock (MAP <65 mm Hg or requirement of vasopressor therapy) Change in SOFA score $\geq$2 Fever and/or qSOFA score $\geq$2 More than >1 extrahepatic organ failure
Variceal bleeding	Hemorrhagic shock (or requirement of vasopressor) Intubation and mechanical ventilation for airway protection Need for balloon tamponade
Encephalopathy	$\geq$2 Grade hepatic encephalopathy Uremic encephalopathy or alcohol intoxication or withdrawal requiring restraint
Renal failure	Development of renal injury not responsive to routine medical management Acute need for renal replacement therapy Requirement of norepinephrine therapy for HRS
Respiratory failure	PaO_2/FiO_2 <200 Persistent tachypnea (>30/min) Impending respiratory failure due to massive hydrothorax or ARDS Respiratory acidosis (pH < 7.2)
Cardiovascular compromise	Hypotension (MAP <65 mm Hg or requirement of vasopressor therapy) Acute ischemic heart disease or arrhythmias requiring monitoring

Abbreviations: FiO_2, fraction of inspired oxygen; ICU, intensive care unit; PaO_2, partial pressure of arterial oxygen; qSOFA, quick SOFA; SOFA, sequential organ failure assessment.

Modified from Dong V, Karvellas CJ. Acute-on-chronic liver failure: Objective admission and support criteria in the intensive care unit. JHEP Reports. 2019;1:44 to 52.

- In case oxygen saturation is less than 93% (after ruling out chronic obstructive pulmonary disease [COPD]), start supplemental oxygen (nasal cannula/face mask/non-rebreathing mask) and investigate the cause of hypoxia.
- Observe chest wall, look for any defects, check jugular venous pressure, look for presence of any chest drains and their patency, and look for abdominal distension
- Check the position of trachea
- Auscultate breath sounds and palpate chest wall
- Consider noninvasive ventilation if indicated, and the patient is cooperative
- Frequent arterial blood gas (ABG) sampling for PaO_2 levels
- In case of severe respiratory distress, consider mechanical ventilation

Differential diagnosis for dyspnea in cirrhosis can be due to pulmonary or extrapulmonary causes. Pulmonary causes include pneumonia, COPD, bronchitis, hepatopulmonary syndrome, pulmonary edema, hepatic hydrothorax, and portopulmonary hypertension. Extrapulmonary causes include tense ascites, anemia, and cardiac failure. Conditions affecting both the lung and liver, which can lead to shortness of breath, include alpha-1 antitrypsin deficiency, cystic fibrosis, and sarcoidosis.

Circulation

- Observe the color of palpebral conjunctiva, nail bed, and hands
- Check temperature of extremities and measure capillary refill time

- Palpate pulse—rate, rhythm, volume, and character (hyperdynamic circulation in cirrhosis)
- Monitor blood pressure (intra-arterial blood pressure monitoring is preferred).
- Auscultate for heart sounds/murmurs (anemic murmurs are common in cirrhosis).
- Look for any signs of bleeding—petechiae/ecchymosis, bleeding gums, hematuria, hematemesis, hematochezia, melena, any open wounds, or trauma.
- Secure intravenous (IV) access with two large bore cannulas (especially in patients with variceal bleeding)
- Secure central line and arterial line
- Order for biochemistry, hematology, and microbiology investigations (consider rapid point-of-care tests to diagnose infections)
- In case of low blood pressure, give a fluid bolus of 500 mL of warmed crystalloid solution within 15 minutes (consider smaller fluid replacement volume in case of known history of heart failure/cardiac disease). Intravenous albumin is also an excellent replacement fluid in patients with sepsis but needs monitoring for fluid overload.[15]
- Reassess response to fluid challenge after 5 minutes. In cirrhotic patients with additional organ failures, the goal mean arterial pressure (MAP) is typically 60 to 65 mm Hg to ensure end-organ perfusion.
- Consider escalation to vasopressor support in case of no improvement. Norepinephrine is the first choice. Terlipressin can be the second drug in the presence of kidney injury to improve renal perfusion.
- In case of chest pain, suspect acute coronary syndrome and perform 12-lead electrocardiogram.

Differential diagnosis for circulatory dysfunction in cirrhosis includes distributive shock due to sepsis, hypovolemic shock due to third spacing of fluid (ascites, pedal edema), GI bleeding, high-output cardiac failure, cardiogenic shock, and arrhythmias due to cirrhotic cardiomyopathy, electrolyte abnormalities, and hyperbilirubinemia (cholecardia).

Disability

- Review ABC to exclude hypoxia and hypotension as causes for unconsciousness
- Review for any drugs that could cause sedation or toxicity
- Measure capillary glucose to rule out hypoglycemia
- Examine pupils (size, equality, and reaction to light)
- Assess consciousness using GCS or AVPU method (Alert, responds to Vocal stimuli, responds to Painful stimuli, or Unresponsive to all stimuli)

Differential diagnosis for impaired consciousness in patients with cirrhosis includes HE, alcohol withdrawal/intoxication, metabolic encephalopathy, administration of sedative or analgesic drugs, stroke, and psychiatric illness.

Exposure

Expose the patient adequately for physical examination while respecting dignity
Examine from head to toe to assess signs of liver cell failure, including alopecia, icterus, loss of axillary hair, gynecomastia, spider nevi, Dupuytren's contracture, palmar erythema, visible abdominal vein collaterals, and testicular atrophy. Look for signs of skin and soft tissue infection, abdominal wall hematoma, and ecchymosis. Cyanosis/discoloration of peripheral limbs is common in patients on terlipressin therapy and needs to be assessed frequently.

POINT-OF-CARE ULTRASONOGRAPHY FOR INITIAL INTENSIVE CARE ASSESSMENT

The use of point-of-care ultrasonography (POCUS) has revolutionized the care of critically ill patients.[16,17] The ultrasonography (USG) machine is now considered an integral part of the ICU. The Society of Critical Care Medicine has proposed guidelines for intensivists using POCUS.[18] From the perspective of managing critically ill cirrhotic patients in the ICU, USG is regularly used for bedside screening, detection of potential emergencies, and performing procedures. Screening of these patients for initial ICU assessment is started with the abdomen and then followed by the lung, heart, lower limbs (to rule out deep vein thrombosis) and lastly transcranial Doppler and optic nerve sheath diameter assessment (when cerebral edema because of HE/acute liver failure is suspected)[19,20] (**Table 2**). Bennet and colleagues recommend a sequential approach while using POCUS for initial evaluation and resuscitation.[21] Most patients in the ICU are on albumin infusions and/or crystalloid infusions (for AKI, shock, and spontaneous bacterial peritonitis [SBP]) and require frequent monitoring for volume overload. This can be done through POCUS assessment of abdominal inferior vena cava (IVC) diameter and pulmonary B lines, which can then guide the therapy and

Table 2
Point -of- care ultrasonography in the liver intensive care unit

Organ/ Site	POCUS Application	Procedural Application
Abdomen	Liver echotexture, space occupying lesions, IVC diameter and volume status, portal vein (thrombosis), presence of free fluid, identification of abdominal aorta, inferior epigastric artery	USG-guided diagnostic and therapeutic paracentesis, liver biopsy
Lung	Presence of lung sliding (normal), loss of lung sliding and barcode sign on M mode (pneumothorax), presence of fluid (pleural effusion, loculated pleural effusion, hepatic hydrothorax), presence of B lines (subpleural consolidation, pulmonary edema, pneumonia), identification of diaphragm	USG-guided diagnostic and therapeutic thoracentesis, placement of intercostal chest drain
Heart	Focused echocardiography to look for contractility of the heart, LV systolic function, RA/RV dilatation (pulmonary embolism), IVC diameter and collapsibility, presence of free fluid in the pericardium (pericardial effusion, cardiac tamponade)	USG-guided pericardial drainage (diagnostic and therapeutic), placement of cannulas for ECMO
Lower Limbs	Compressibility of femoral, popliteal veins (to rule out deep vein thrombosis)	
Head	Pulsatility indices >1.2 on transcranial Doppler and/or optic nerve sheath diameter > 0.5 cm (to rule out cerebral edema)	

Abbreviations: ECMO, extracorporeal membrane oxygenation; IVC, inferior vena cava; LV, left ventricle, RA, right atrium; RV, right ventricle; USG, ultrasonography.

reduce the risk of respiratory failure. USG can also be incorporated at various steps of the ABCD approach to aid with differential diagnosis while performing interventions (like securing vascular access in case of hypotension and placement of central and arterial lines).[22] However, POCUS has limitations.[19] Certain patient-related factors which hinder a good examination include large-volume ascites, obesity, emphysema, and postoperative patients who have large dressings. Last, a major limitation of POCUS is its dependence on the expertise of the operator[19] **(Fig. 1)**.

MANAGEMENT OF SPECIFIC COMPLICATIONS OF CIRRHOSIS IN INTENSIVE CARE UNIT
Infections, Sepsis, and Septic Shock

Infections are common in patients with cirrhosis and ACLF due to altered gut permeability, immune dysfunction, hypocomplementemia, and concomitant comorbidities.[23] Cirrhosis-associated immune dysfunction predisposes these patients to rapid spread of systemic inflammation and consequent sepsis.[24,25] These infections are largely bacterial, especially gram-negative bacilli (like *Klebsiella spp*, pseudomonas, and *Escherichia coli*). However, with growing antimicrobial resistance, the emergence of multidrug-resistant organisms (*Enterococcus spp, Staphylococcus aureus*) has been noted.[26] Treatment of these patients requires a multidisciplinary approach with expertise in critical care hepatology.

Common sites of infection include peritoneum (SBP), followed by urinary tract, lung, skin, and soft tissue (SSTI).[23,27,28] Postprocedure bacteremia (after any therapeutic procedure) and spontaneous bacteremia are also frequent in patients with cirrhosis. Cultures are positive in 50% to 70% of cases.[29] Invasive fungal infections are responsible for approximately 3% to 7% of culture-positive infections in cirrhosis.[30] These

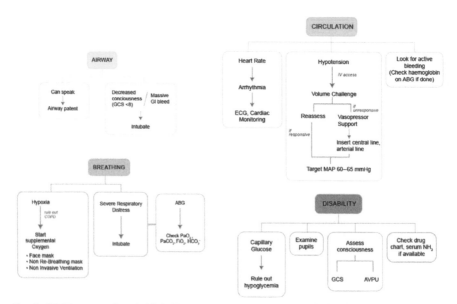

Fig. 1. ABCD approach to initial ICU management. ABG, arterial blood gas; AVPU, Alert, responds to Vocal stimuli, responds to Painful stimuli or Unresponsive to all stimuli; ECG, electrocardiogram; FiO_2, fraction of inspired oxygen; GCS, Glasgow Coma Scale; GI, gastrointestinal; HCO_3, bicarbonate; MAP, mean arterial pressure; NH_3, ammonia; $PaCO_2$, partial pressure of arterial carbon dioxide; PaO_2, partial pressure of arterial oxygen.

are more commonly seen as secondary or hospital-acquired infections complicating ACLF.[31]

Cirrhosis patients with bacterial infections have an abnormally enhanced pro-inflammatory host response. Multiorgan failure is often observed in cirrhotic patients with severe sepsis.[32] Sepsis is known to worsen existing liver failure in cirrhosis. Even in the absence of infection, circulatory disturbances are observed in cirrhosis.[33] This includes hyperdynamic circulation with high cardiac output, relatively lower arterial pressures, and low systemic vascular resistance.[34] In the presence of infections in these patients, the circulation becomes increasingly hyperdynamic and hyporeactive to therapeutic doses of adrenergic drugs. Sepsis can also trigger renal, circulatory, and cerebral failure leading to very high mortality.[12]

Moreau and colleagues noted a higher incidence of septic shock-associated hyper-lactatemia in patients with cirrhosis. Sepsis is associated with in-hospital mortality of 65%, and septic shock in patients with cirrhosis can have an extremely high ICU mortality rate.[35,36] Fever, qSOFA (quick sequential organ failure assessment) score, and rise in SOFA score (2 points) can aid in diagnosing infection in patients with cirrhosis.[23,37,38] Fernandez and colleagues demonstrated that adequate empirical antibiotic strategies are a key factor in the management of infections, especially in ACLF.[39] Inappropriate first-line therapies were associated with increased mortality. It is suggested to initiate broad antibiotic therapy covering all potential pathogens at high doses within the first 48 to 72 hours of diagnosis of infection to improve outcomes.[39] Antibiotic stewardship must be a part of sepsis management in patients with cirrhosis. Therefore, antibiotics should be deescalated as soon as the culture reports are available to minimize the development of resistant strains.

Variceal Bleeding

Acute variceal bleeding is one of the common indications for ICU admission. The 1-year mortality of patients with variceal bleeding is approximately 57%, with nearly half of the deaths occurring within 6 weeks from the first episode of bleeding.[40] The most important risk factors for mortality include liver functional status (Child-Pugh score), bacterial infections, and renal dysfunction (assessed by serum creatinine levels).[41] Patients requiring ICU admission for significant blood loss, liver failure, and variceal bleeding that cannot be controlled endoscopically have been found to have poor outcomes.[42] The Asian Pacific Association for the Study of the Liver (APASL) proposed a severity score for acute variceal bleeding in 2011[43] (**Table 3**). The score has been externally validated to predict treatment failure but not in-hospital mortality or rebleeding rates.[44] A MELD-based model to predict mortality risk among patients with acute variceal bleeding was developed by Reverter and colleagues, whereas we recognize that the MELD-based mortality prediction is more objective and useful in clinical settings[45] (**Table 4**).

For resuscitation, the restoration of MAP to allow adequate tissue perfusion is paramount.[46] Low blood volume increases the risk of renal failure and mortality.[47] A restrictive transfusion strategy with a hemoglobin target of 7 g/dL significantly improved outcomes in patients with acute upper GI bleeding.[48] The use of prophylactic antibiotics (ceftriaxone 1 g/d for 7 days) in this group of patients has been shown to significantly reduce the incidence of bacterial infections, all-cause mortality, the incidence of rebleeding events, and length of hospital stay.[49] These benefits were independent of the choice of antibiotic; therefore, selection should be made by considering local guidelines, resistance patterns, and cost.[50]

Augustin and colleagues reported that a combination of somatostatin, antibiotics, and endoscopic ligation after an acute variceal bleed in a real-world setting was

Table 3
Asian Pacific Association for the Study of the Liver severity score for acute variceal bleeding[43]

Parameter	Value	Point
Systolic blood pressure	>90 mm Hg and no postural drop	0
	>90 mm Hg with postural drop	1
	<90 mm Hg	2
Child–Turcotte–Pugh class	A	0
	B	1
	C	2
Platelet count	≥100,000 mm³	0
	<100,000 mm³	1
Infection	Absent	0
	Present	1
Active bleeding at endoscopy	Absent	0
	Present	1
	Total	Minimum 0, Maximum 7

Data from Sarin SK, Kumar A, Angus PW, Baijal SS, Baik SK, Bayraktar Y, et al. Diagnosis and management of acute variceal bleeding: Asian Pacific Association for Study of the Liver recommendations. Hepatol Int. 2011;5:607-24.

associated with low mortality, even in high-risk patients.[51] Vasoactive agents like somatostatin, octreotide, and terlipressin were found to be comparable in efficacy and safety in the control of variceal hemorrhage[52] **(Table 5)**. A minimum of 48 hours of therapy is suggested, although the drug can be administered for a maximum of 5 days after variceal bleeding.[53] Lin and colleagues analyzed data about proton pump inhibitor (PPI) use in cirrhotic patients with variceal bleeds and found that it can reduce the rate of rebleeding (but not bleed-related mortality) after endoscopic therapy for both urgent treatment and prophylaxis.[54] Initial studies recommended that at least 4 weeks of PPI administration, irrespective of bleeding location could reduce rebleed rate. However, the current BAVENO VII guidelines recommend that PPIs should be stopped after endoscopy and cessation of bleed.[53] Lau and colleagues noted that urgent endoscopy (within 6 hours) was not beneficial in reducing the 30-day mortality for acute

Table 4
Model for End-Stage Liver Disease score-based mortality risk prediction for acute variceal bleeding[45]

MELD Score	% Mortality Risk	Risk Category
≤8	≤2.5%	Low
9–11	3%–5%	Low
12–15	5%–10%	Intermediate
16–19	12%–20%	Intermediate
20–25	23%–46%	High
26–29	52%–66%	High
≥30	≥71%	High

Abbreviations: MELD, Model for End-Stage Liver Disease.
Modified from Reverter E, Tandon P, Augustin S, Turon F, Casu S, Bastiampillai R, et al. A MELD-based model to determine risk of mortality among patients with acute variceal bleeding. Gastroenterology. 2014;146:412-19.e3.

Table 5
Drugs and dosage recommended for acute variceal bleeding

Name of Drug	Dose	Comments
Antibiotic	IV ceftriaxone 1 g/d	In places of high anti-microbial resistance, it is worthwhile to consider local resistance patterns and initiate antibiotics accordingly.
Terlipressin	2 mg IV bolus followed by 1–2 mg IV every 4–6 h (recommended) Or 1 mg bolus followed by 2–4 mg/d infusion	Either of these 3 drugs can be used. Vasoactive agents must be initiated at the earliest and continued for 5 d maximum or at least 24 h after control of bleeding.
Somatostatin	500 mcg IV bolus followed by 250 mcg/hr continuous IV infusion	Terlipressin is contraindicated in patients with hypoxemia, ACLF-3,
Octreotide	50 mcg IV bolus followed by 50 mcg/hr continuous IV infusion	and those with a history of ischemic heart disease and elderly (age>70 y). Monitor sodium levels, as hyponatremia is common in those receiving terlipressin.
Erythromycin	250 mg IV bolus at least 0.5–2 h prior to endoscopy	Electrocardiogram before injection is must to rule out QT prolongation
Packed red cells	As per requirement	Target hemoglobin 7–8 g/dL

variceal bleeds.[55] Similar findings were reported by Guo and colleagues and concluded that early endoscopy (within 24 hours) after adequate resuscitation and medical optimization had good outcomes in patients with acute upper GI bleeds.[56]

Emergency TIPS or preemptive TIPS (pTIPS) can be considered in patients who are at high risk of rebleeding after endoscopy[57] (**Table 6**). Although recommended to perform pTIPS in Child, it is less feasible in clinical practice as patients with Child C are historically considered as a contraindication for TIPS due to increased mortality post-TIPS. Analysis by Majeed and colleagues concluded that the rate of ICU admissions (0.8% in 2005–0.4% in 2016) and mortality (25% in 2005–16% in 2016) of

Table 6
Indications for emergency and preemptive transjugular intrahepatic portosystemic shunt[57]

Types of TIPS	Definitions/Indications
Emergency/rescue TIPS	Recommended in patients with cirrhosis who have been successfully banded but who rebleed at any time during admission (after endoscopy)
Preemptive TIPS	Recommended in patients at high risk of failing standard of care. They should undergo TIPS creation as soon as endoscopic variceal ligation is successfully performed and within 72 h of admission. Patients with CTP Class C (10–13 points) and CTP Class B (8–9 points) with active bleeding at endoscopy are most likely to benefit.
Salvage TIPS	Any patient (independent of CTP Class) with uncontrolled acute variceal hemorrhage at endoscopy or persistent profuse bleeding despite endoscopy should be considered for salvage TIPS.

Abbreviations: CTP, Child–Turcotte–Pugh, TIPS, transjugular intrahepatic portosystemic shunt.

cirrhotic patients with acute variceal bleeding has significantly declined over time when compared with other causes of ICU admissions.[58] These outcomes were found to be comparable between liver transplant centers and non-transplant centers.[58]

Non-Variceal Bleeding

The data on non-variceal bleeding among patients with cirrhosis are scant. Romcea and colleagues reported that the prevalence of non-variceal bleeding in cirrhotic patients is 27% and that non-variceal hemorrhages usually have a comparatively lower mortality rate.[59] The most common causes of non-variceal upper GI bleeds are portal hypertensive gastropathy and gastric vascular ectasia.[59,60] Common lower GI causes include portal hypertensive colopathy and hemorrhoids.[59,61] Gastroduodenal ulcers are an infrequent source of non-variceal bleeding in cirrhotic patients but can be severe and associated with high mortality.[61,62] Marmo and colleagues analyzed data from an Italian registry for Upper Gastrointestinal (UGI) bleeds and concluded that in cirrhotic patients with non-variceal bleeds, the 30-day mortality was low (<5%).[63] Advanced age, low hemoglobin levels at presentation, and comorbidities were strong independent predictors of mortality.[63] They emphasized the need to perform upper GI endoscopy to investigate the etiology of bleeding and to establish proper and focused therapy. Thromboelastography-based correction of coagulopathy has been shown to be superior in the management in of non-variceal upper GI bleeds due to a lower volume of blood products being transfused.[60]

Hepatic Encephalopathy

HE is one of the complications of decompensated cirrhosis which presents with a wide range of neuropsychiatric symptoms from mild alteration of the sleep-wake cycle to coma (**Table 7**). Stewart and colleagues observed that HE is an important component of the natural progression of cirrhosis which can affect the survival of patients.[64] They strongly suggested that it can provide additional prognostic information independent of the MELD criteria. The incidence of overt HE is 40% in patients with cirrhosis.[65] Patients with advanced HE have a 35% ICU mortality rate. However, patients with advanced HE and no other organ dysfunction other than the need for mechanical ventilation have better outcomes in the ICU.[66] A low thyroxine levels at admission has been reported to be an effective marker for predicting advanced HE in patients with cirrhosis.[67] This, however, requires further validation.

Management involves rigorous screening for other differential diagnoses and identification of triggers.[68] Specific therapies for HE includes purging through the use of nonabsorbable disaccharides like lactulose or polyethylene glycol, which are widely regarded as first-line management for cirrhosis-associated HE.[69,70] Oral rifaximin therapy and intravenous administration of L-ornithine L-aspartate are currently not recommended for the management of overt HE due to weak evidence.[71,72] Although few studies have reported excellent efficacy of fecal microbiota transplant as a potential treatment of HE, the treatment, however, is largely limited to clinical trials.[73] If treated adequately, HE is regarded as a reversible condition.

Extracorporeal Liver Assist Devices in Intensive Care Unit

Results from studies on extracorporeal liver assist devices have been variable. Molecular adsorbent recirculating system (MARS), Prometheus (fractionated plasma separation and adsorption system), and single pass albumin dialysis have been extensively evaluated in patients with liver failure. Of these, MARS has been shown to be an effective bridging therapy for liver transplantation. MARS can remove protein-bound substances and decreases the plasma concentrations of bilirubin,

Table 7
West Haven criteria for hepatic encephalopathy

WHC including MHE	ISHEN	Description	Suggested Operative Criteria	Comment
Unimpaired		No encephalopathy at all, no history of HE	Tested and proved to be normal	No universal criteria for diagnosis. Local standards and expertise required
Minimal	Covert	Psychometric or neuropsychological alterations of tests exploring psychomotor speed/executive functions or neurophysiological alterations without clinical evidence of mental change	Abnormal results of established psychometric or neuropsychological tests without clinical manifestations	
Grade I		• Trivial lack of awareness • Euphoria or anxiety • Shortened attention span • Impairment of addition or subtraction • Altered sleep rhythm	Despite oriented in time and space (see below), the patient seems to have some cognitive/behavioral decay with respect to his or her standard on clinical examination or to the caregivers	Clinical findings usually not reproducible
Grade II	Overt	• Lethargy or apathy • Disorientation for time • Obvious personality change • Inappropriate behavior • Dyspraxia • Asterixis	Disoriented for time (at least three of the followings are wrong: day of the month, day of the week, month, season, or year) ± the other mentioned symptoms	Clinical findings variable, but reproducible to some extent
Grade III		• Somnolence to semi-stupor • Responsive to stimuli • Confused • Gross disorientation • Bizarre behavior	Disoriented also for space (at least three of the following wrongly reported: country, state [or region], city, or place) ± the other mentioned symptoms	Clinical findings reproducible to some extent
Grade IV		Coma	Does not respond even to painful stimuli	Comatose state usually reproducible

Abbreviations: ISHEN, International Society for Hepatic Encephalopathy and Nitrogen Metabolism; MHE, minimal hepatic encephalopathy; WHC, West Haven criteria.

urea, bile acids, ammonia, and creatinine.[74] MARS has shown reasonable efficacy in the improvement of HE; however, none of the studies have demonstrated survival benefits till date.[75]

Plasma exchange is also an effective bridging therapy and has been shown to reduce ammonia levels and contain the cytokine storm, especially in patients with acute liver failure.[76–78] Plasma exchange could also prolong the transplant–free survival; however, validation in larger real-world cohorts is needed.

Renal Failure

Renal failure in patients with cirrhosis is due to splanchnic vasodilation and intrarenal vasoconstriction triggered by portal hypertension. In the late stages of cirrhosis, arterial pressures are maintained by activation of vasoconstrictor systems such as the renin–angiotensin system, the sympathetic nervous system, and non-osmotic hypersecretion of antidiuretic hormone. The effect of these systems on sodium and water retention may lead to edema, ascites, and eventually renal failure. Renal failure in cirrhotic patients is frequently associated with ascites and edema.[79] It can be classified broadly into: (a) hepatorenal syndrome (HRS) and (b) AKI due to other factors (sepsis, alcoholic hepatitis, diuretic, and drug-induced). HRS can be further classified as HRS-AKI and HRS-non-AKI (HRS-NAKI). HRS-AKI is defined as a rise in serum creatinine by ≥ 0.3 mg/dL or $\geq 50\%$ from baseline value within 48 hours and/or decrease in urinary output ≤ 0.5 mL/kg in ≥ 6 hours in patients with cirrhosis and ascites[80] (Table 8). HRS is a diagnosis of exclusion after all potential causes of acute kidney injury are ruled out.[81] The probability of HRS in patients with decompensated cirrhosis is estimated to be 18% at 1 year and up to 40% at 5 years.[82] Cirrhotic patients additionally have reduced muscle mass and decreased hepatic conversion of creatine to creatinine.[83,84] Therefore, renal failure can be diagnosed late and greatly

Table 8 International Club of Ascites classification of kidney injury	
Nomenclature	Definition
AKI	Rise in sCr by ≥ 0.3 mg/dL within 48 h or $\geq 50\%$ increase in sCr within prior 7 d
Staging of AKI	
Stage 1	Stage 1a: an increase in sCr by ≥ 0.3 mg/dL or an increase in sCr by ≥ 1.5–2 fold from baseline with final sCr <1.5 mg/dL. Stage 1b: an increase in sCr by ≥ 0.3 mg/dL or an increase in sCr by ≥ 1.5–2 fold from baseline with final sCr ≥ 1.5 mg/dL
Stage 2	An increase in sCr by 2–3 fold from baseline
Stage 3	An increase in sCr >3 fold from baseline or sCr≥ 4 mg/dL with an acute rise by ≥ 0.3 mg/dL or requirement of RRT
Acute kidney disease	GFR<60 mL/min/1.73 m^2 for 3 mo or decrease in GFR $\geq 35\%$ for < 3 mo Or increase in sCr $\geq 50\%$ for < 3 mo
Chronic kidney disease	GFR<60 mL/min/1.73 m^2 for ≥ 3 mo

Abbreviations: AKI, acute kidney injury; GFR, glomerular filtration rate; RRT, renal replacement therapy; sCr, serum creatinine.

Data from European Association for the Study of the Liver. Electronic address: easloffice@easloffice.eu; European Association for the Study of the Liver. EASL Clinical Practice Guidelines for the management of patients with decompensated cirrhosis. J Hepatol. 2018 Aug;69(2):406-460. https://doi.org/10.1016/j.jhep.2018.03.024. Epub 2018 Apr 10. Erratum in: J Hepatol. 2018 Nov;69(5):1207. PMID: 29653741.

underestimated by serum creatinine levels. These patients frequently present with complications of renal failure, including metabolic acidosis, volume overload, and electrolyte abnormalities which may be an indication for ICU admission.[81] Volume expansion with albumin is the first-line of therapy for HRS. Terlipressin, a vasopressin analogue, is an effective drug in a majority of patients with HRS and is used as initial therapy.[85,86] Patients with ACLF-3 and those with hypoxemia are at higher risk of pulmonary failure and are not candidates for terlipressin therapy.[87,88] Patients who do not respond to medical management can be offered renal replacement therapy in the interim while awaiting liver transplantation.[81] Mackle and colleagues reported 55%

Table 9		
Other intensive care unit complications, their diagnosis, prevention, and management		
Complication	**Diagnosis**	**Prevention and Management**
Hemoperitoneum	Ascitic fluid analysis Blood gas analysis of ascitic fluid (compare hemoglobin and electrolyte values of hemorrhagic ascites with blood for rapid identification of bleed)	Z technique of ascitic tapping can prevent hemoperitoneum. Monitor abdominal pressures through intra-abdominal catheters. TEG (thromboelastography)-based coagulopathy correction. CT (computed tomography) angiography and embolization of bleeding source. Avoid tigecycline antibiotic.
Adrenal insufficiency	Delta total cortisol (difference in peak values—baseline early morning value) < 250 nmol/L	Prevalent in 20%–70% of patients admitted to ICU. Treat underlying cause. Low-dose hydrocortisone 50 mg thrice daily.
Ecchymosis	Frequent clinical examination	Intermittent deflation of BP cuff can prevent. Frequent position change. TEG-based correction. Mark the area of ecchymosis for assessment of response.
Bedsores	Frequent clinical examination	Proper nursing care, frequent change of position, early identification and treatment, appropriate dressing of wound, debridement and skin grafting (if needed), vacuum-assisted closure therapy if indicated, adequate antibiotic coverage if infected
Ventilator-acquired pneumonia (VAP)	Based on microbial culture of endotracheal secretions and clinical correlation	Oral hygiene, proper suctioning of oral and endotracheal secretions, maintaining safe cuff pressures, head-end elevation of bed, maintaining VAP bundle, initiating appropriate antibiotic therapy based on culture and sensitivity

(continued on next page)

Table 9 (continued)		
Complication	**Diagnosis**	**Prevention and Management**
Urinary tract infection	Based on microbial culture of urine and clinical correlation	Avoid prolonged catheterization. Aseptic precautions while handling catheters. Immediate change of diapers (in those with encephalopathic/ intubated patients) to prevent prolonged exposure to fecal content. No role of prophylactic antibiotic
Wasting/cachexia	Frequent clinical examination	Adequate calorie and protein intake, liaison with clinical dieticians specializing in nutrition for critically ill patients, encourage enteral feeding wherever feasible
Critical illness neuromyopathy	Nerve conduction studies	Mobilization and physiotherapy

prevalence of renal impairment in those with alcohol-induced cirrhosis patients, and in whom the in-hospital mortality was 87%.[89]

Other complications noted in patients with cirrhosis admitted to ICU and its management are discussed in **Table 9**.

Palliative Care

Although the care of liver disease patients and the availability of newer bridging therapies have improved in recent years, the outcome of these patients in the absence of timely liver transplantation remains dismal. Data analyzed by the commission set up by the Foundation of Liver Research, United Kingdom, noted that standardized mortality rates have shot up by 400% over the last 50 years and most patients with end-stage liver disease die prematurely, especially in the working age group (between 18–65 years).[90] The median cost in the last year of life was significantly greater for patients with end-stage liver disease ($51,235 vs $44,456) than those without end-stage liver disease.[91] The cost for every hospital admission that ended in mortality was £9615 compared with £4598 for each hospice care admission that ended with death.[92] The stress on resources and the financial burden of managing these patients has paved the way toward conversations around the integration of palliative care in patients with end-stage liver disease who are unlikely to benefit from the continuation of multi-organ supportive care or are unfit for liver transplantation. Timely identification of patients who may be candidates for supportive and palliative care is an empathetic approach to providing patient-centric medical care. To objectively identify the patients who will benefit from this, prognostic scoring systems such as Bristol and the Supportive and Palliative Care Indicators Tool (SPICT) have been proposed for use[93,94] (**Table 10**). Research into their effectiveness is still underway. However, clinical judgment of the severity of illness and patient response to treatment are also important considerations in initiating palliative care. This approach recognizes the mental burden of a potentially terminal condition on the patients and their caregivers and provides them with alternative management options which can improve their quality of life and reduce the number of invasive procedures that may ultimately prove to be futile.[95–97]

Table 10 Criteria for initiating palliative care			
Scoring System	Patient Population	Criteria/Indicators	Interpretation
Bristol tool	Inpatients	• Child-Pugh C • ≥2 liver-related admissions in the last 6 mo • On-going alcohol use • Unsuitable for transplant workup • WHO performance status 3–4 Each criteria has one point	Child-Pugh C, a cumulative score of 3 or above, and the presence of Child-Pugh C disease along with at least another poor prognostic criteria has excellent ability to identify at risk patients who may die over the next 12 mo. This can be used to justify the implementation of supportive/palliative care.
SPICT	Any patient	a. Cirrhosis with one or more complications in the last 12 mo • Diuretic resistant ascites • Hepatic encephalopathy • Hepatorenal syndrome • Bacterial peritonitis • Recurrent variceal bleeds b. Patients unfit for liver transplantation	Review current management plan and perform assessment for unmet supportive and palliative care needs

Abbreviations: SPICT, Supportive and Palliative Care Indicators Tool; WHO, World Health Organization.

SUMMARY

Complications of decompensated cirrhosis are often indications for intensive care. The need for organ-supportive care is particularly important in patients who are awaiting a liver transplant and have a survival potential. Septic patients with decompensated cirrhosis have an increased ICU and in-hospital mortality, which is independent of comorbidities and organ dysfunction.[3] Patients with cirrhosis have higher 30-day ICU mortality and increased medical expenditure. However, the patients who survive hospital discharge have better long-term outcomes.[8] Nutrition should be individualized and addressed for each patient in ICU in liaison with dieticians.[98] The use of extracorporeal liver support devices is still restricted to a clinical trial setting. It is important to identify candidates who are not suitable for transplantation, as the continuation of organ-supportive care without clinical improvement has been found to be futile due to the high mortality associated with the condition. Data from UKs Intensive Care National Audit and Research Center have demonstrated that 68% of patients with decompensated cirrhosis will survive to get discharged from the ICU.[36] However, due to differences in the availability of resources and personnel, these data may not be universally applicable. In conclusion, appropriate care of a cirrhosis patient admitted to ICU can improve outcomes lest they are deemed futile.

CLINICS CARE POINTS

- Airway, breathing, circulation, disability, and complete exposure (ABCDE) method of assessement are helpful in treating a cirrhosis patient admitted to ICD.

- Fluid resuscitation should be done judiciously using POCUS (point of care ultrasonography).
- Antibiotic stewardship must be a part of sepsis management in patients with cirrhosis to prevent rise in microbial resistance.

GRANT SUPPORT

None.

FINANCIAL DISCLOSURES

None.

POTENTIAL CONFLICTS OF INTEREST

None.

REFERENCES

1. The global, regional, and national burden of cirrhosis by cause in 195 countries and territories, 1990-2017: a systematic analysis for the Global Burden of Disease Study 2017. Lancet Gastroenterol Hepatol 2020;5:245–66.
2. Sarin SK, Kumar M, Eslam M, et al. Liver diseases in the Asia-Pacific region: a Lancet Gastroenterology & Hepatology Commission. Lancet Gastroenterol Hepatol 2020;5:167–228.
3. McPhail MJW, Parrott F, Wendon JA, et al. Incidence and Outcomes for Patients With Cirrhosis Admitted to the United Kingdom Critical Care Units. Crit Care Med 2018;46:705–12.
4. Warren A, Soulsby CR, Puxty A, et al. Long-term outcome of patients with liver cirrhosis admitted to a general intensive care unit. Ann Intensive Care 2017;7:37.
5. Idalsoaga F, Kulkarni AV, Mousa OY, et al. Non-alcoholic fatty liver disease and alcohol-related liver disease: two intertwined entities. Front Med (Lausanne) 2020;7:448.
6. Kulkarni AV, Duvvuru NR. Management of hepatitis B and C in special population. World J Gastroenterol 2021;27:6861–73.
7. Huang Y-F, Lin C-S, Cherng Y-G, et al. A population-based cohort study of mortality of intensive care unit patients with liver cirrhosis. BMC Gastroenterol 2020; 20:15.
8. Passi NN, McPhail MJ. The patient with cirrhosis in the intensive care unit and the management of acute-on-chronic liver failure. J Intensive Care Soc 2022;23: 78–86.
9. Kubesch A, Peiffer KH, Abramowski H, et al. The presence of liver cirrhosis is a strong negative predictor of survival for patients admitted to the intensive care unit - Cirrhosis in intensive care patients. Z Gastroenterol 2021;59:657–64.
10. Moreau R, Jalan R, Gines P, et al. Acute-on-chronic liver failure is a distinct syndrome that develops in patients with acute decompensation of cirrhosis. Gastroenterology 2013;144:1426–37, 37.e1-9.
11. Sarin SK, Choudhury A, Sharma MK, et al. Acute-on-chronic liver failure: consensus recommendations of the Asian Pacific association for the study of the liver (APASL): an update. Hepatol Int 2019;13:353–90.
12. Hernaez R, Solà E, Moreau R, et al. Acute-on-chronic liver failure: an update. Gut 2017;66:541–53.

13. Dong V, Karvellas CJ. Acute-on-chronic liver failure: objective admission and support criteria in the intensive care unit. JHEP Rep 2019;1:44–52.
14. Thim T, Krarup NHV, Grove EL, et al. Initial assessment and treatment with the airway, breathing, circulation, disability, exposure (ABCDE) approach. Int J Gen Med 2012;5:117.
15. Maiwall R, Kumar A, Pasupuleti SSR, et al. A randomized-controlled trial comparing 20% albumin to plasmalyte in patients with cirrhosis and sepsis-induced hypotension [ALPS trial]. J Hepatol 2022;77:670–82.
16. Guevarra K, Greenstein Y. Ultrasonography in the Critical Care Unit. Curr Cardiol Rep 2020;22:145.
17. Moore CL, Copel JA. Point-of-care ultrasonography. N Engl J Med 2011;364: 749–57.
18. Levitov A, Frankel HL, Blaivas M, et al. Guidelines for the appropriate use of bedside general and cardiac ultrasonography in the evaluation of critically ill patients-part II: cardiac ultrasonography. Crit Care Med 2016;44:1206–27.
19. Kajal K, Premkumar M, Chaluvashetty SB, et al. Point-of-care thoracic ultrasonography in patients with cirrhosis and liver failure. Cureus 2021;13:e15559.
20. Reynolds AS, Liang J, Raiss M, et al. Fatal cerebral edema in patients with decompensated cirrhosis: a case series. J Crit Care 2021;61:115–8.
21. Bennett CE, Samavedam S, Jayaprakash N, et al. When to incorporate point-of-care ultrasound (POCUS) into the initial assessment of acutely ill patients: a pilot crossover study to compare 2 POCUS-assisted simulation protocols. Cardiovasc Ultrasound 2018;16:14.
22. Kameda T, Kimura A. Basic point-of-care ultrasound framework based on the airway, breathing, and circulation approach for the initial management of shock and dyspnea. Acute Med Surg 2020;7:e481.
23. Kulkarni AV, Premkumar M, Arab JP, et al. Early Diagnosis and Prevention of Infections in Cirrhosis. Semin Liver Dis 2022;42:293–312.
24. Bonnel AR, Bunchorntavakul C, Reddy KR. Immune dysfunction and infections in patients with cirrhosis. Clin Gastroenterol Hepatol 2011;9:727–38.
25. Bajaj JS, Kamath PS, Reddy KR. The Evolving Challenge of Infections in Cirrhosis. N Engl J Med 2021;384:2317–30.
26. Cullaro G, Sharma R, Trebicka J, et al. Precipitants of Acute-on-Chronic Liver Failure: An Opportunity for Preventative Measures to Improve Outcomes. Liver Transpl 2020;26:283–93.
27. Kulkarni AV, Tirumalle S, Premkumar M, et al. Primary norfloxacin prophylaxis for APASI-defined acute-on-chronic liver failure: a placebo-controlled double-blind randomized trial. Am J Gastroenterol 2022;117:607–16.
28. Kulkarni AV, Anand L, Vyas AK, et al. Omega-3 fatty acid lipid emulsions are safe and effective in reducing endotoxemia and sepsis in acute-on-chronic liver failure: An open-label randomized controlled trial. J Gastroenterol Hepatol 2021; 36:1953–61.
29. Gustot T, Durand F, Lebrec D, et al. Severe sepsis in cirrhosis. Hepatology 2009; 50:2022–33.
30. Bajaj JS, Reddy RK, Tandon P, et al. Prediction of fungal infection development and their impact on survival using the NACSELD cohort. Am J Gastroenterol 2018;113:556–63.
31. Fernández J, Piano S, Bartoletti M, et al. Management of bacterial and fungal infections in cirrhosis: The MDRO challenge. J Hepatol 2021;75(Suppl 1): S101–s107.

32. Bajaj JS, O'Leary JG, Reddy KR, et al. Survival in infection-related acute-on-chronic liver failure is defined by extrahepatic organ failures. Hepatology 2014; 60:250–6.

33. Simonetto DA, Piccolo Serafim L, Gallo de Moraes A, et al. Management of sepsis in patients with cirrhosis: current evidence and practical approach. Hepatology 2019;70:418–28.

34. Kulkarni AV, Kumar P, Sharma M, et al. Pathophysiology and Prevention of Paracentesis-induced Circulatory Dysfunction: A Concise Review. J Clin Transl Hepatol 2020;8:42–8.

35. Moreau R, Hadengue A, Soupison T, et al. Septic shock in patients with cirrhosis: hemodynamic and metabolic characteristics and intensive care unit outcome. Crit Care Med 1992;20:746–50.

36. Chebl RB, Tamim H, Sadat M, et al. Outcomes of septic cirrhosis patients admitted to the intensive care unit: a retrospective cohort study. Medicine (Baltimore) 2021;100:e27593.

37. Piano S, Bartoletti M, Tonon M, et al. Assessment of Sepsis-3 criteria and quick SOFA in patients with cirrhosis and bacterial infections. Gut 2018;67:1892–9.

38. Augustinho FC, Zocche TL, Borgonovo A, et al. Applicability of Sepsis-3 criteria and quick Sequential Organ Failure Assessment in patients with cirrhosis hospitalised for bacterial infections. Liver Int 2019;39:307–15.

39. Fernández J, Acevedo J, Wiest R, et al. Bacterial and fungal infections in acute-on-chronic liver failure: prevalence, characteristics and impact on prognosis. Gut 2018;67:1870–80.

40. D'Amico G, Garcia-Tsao G, Pagliaro L. Natural history and prognostic indicators of survival in cirrhosis: a systematic review of 118 studies. J Hepatol 2006;44: 217–31.

41. Augustin S, Muntaner L, Altamirano JT, et al. Predicting early mortality after acute variceal hemorrhage based on classification and regression tree analysis. Clin Gastroenterol Hepatol 2009;7:1347–54.

42. Lee H, Hawker FH, Selby W, et al. Intensive care treatment of patients with bleeding esophageal varices: results, predictors of mortality, and predictors of the adult respiratory distress syndrome. Crit Care Med 1992;20:1555–63.

43. Sarin SK, Kumar A, Angus PW, et al. Diagnosis and management of acute variceal bleeding: Asian Pacific Association for Study of the Liver recommendations. Hepatol Int 2011;5:607–24.

44. Kim GH, Kim JH, Kim YJ, et al. Value of the APASL severity score in patients with acute variceal bleeding: a single center experience. Hepatol Int 2013;7:1058–64.

45. Reverter E, Tandon P, Augustin S, et al. A MELD-based model to determine risk of mortality among patients with acute variceal bleeding. Gastroenterology 2014; 146:412–9.e3.

46. Mallet M, Rudler M, Thabut D. Variceal bleeding in cirrhotic patients. Gastroenterol Rep (Oxf) 2017;5:185–92.

47. Cárdenas A, Ginès P, Uriz J, et al. Renal failure after upper gastrointestinal bleeding in cirrhosis: incidence, clinical course, predictive factors, and short-term prognosis. Hepatology 2001;34:671–6.

48. Villanueva C, Colomo A, Bosch A, et al. Transfusion strategies for acute upper gastrointestinal bleeding. N Engl J Med 2013;368:11–21.

49. Kulkarni AV, Rabiee A, Mohanty A. Management of Portal Hypertension. J Clin Exp Hepatol 2022;12:1184–99.

50. Chavez-Tapia NC, Barrientos-Gutierrez T, Tellez-Avila FI, et al. Antibiotic prophylaxis for cirrhotic patients with upper gastrointestinal bleeding. Cochrane Database Syst Rev 2010;2010:Cd002907.
51. Augustin S, Altamirano J, González A, et al. Effectiveness of combined pharmacologic and ligation therapy in high-risk patients with acute esophageal variceal bleeding. Am J Gastroenterol 2011;106:1787–95.
52. Seo YS, Park SY, Kim MY, et al. Lack of difference among terlipressin, somatostatin, and octreotide in the control of acute gastroesophageal variceal hemorrhage. Hepatology 2014;60:954–63.
53. de Franchis R, Bosch J, Garcia-Tsao G, et al. Baveno VII - Renewing consensus in portal hypertension. J Hepatol 2021;76(4):959–74.
54. Lin L, Cui B, Deng Y, et al. The Efficacy of Proton Pump Inhibitor in Cirrhotics with Variceal Bleeding: A Systemic Review and Meta-Analysis. Digestion 2021;102: 117–27.
55. Lau JYW, Yu Y, Tang RSY, et al. Timing of endoscopy for acute upper gastrointestinal bleeding. N Engl J Med 2020;382:1299–308.
56. Guo CLT, Wong SH, Lau LHS, et al. Timing of endoscopy for acute upper gastrointestinal bleeding: a territory-wide cohort study. Gut 2022;71:1544–50.
57. Boike JR, Thornburg BG, Asrani SK, et al. North American Practice-Based Recommendations for Transjugular Intrahepatic Portosystemic Shunts in Portal Hypertension. Clin Gastroenterol Hepatol 2022;20:1636–62, e36.
58. Majeed A, Majumdar A, Bailey M, et al. Declining mortality of cirrhotic variceal bleeding requiring admission to intensive care: a binational cohort study. Crit Care Med 2019;47:1317–23.
59. Romcea AA, Tanţău M, Seicean A, et al. The etiology of upper gastrointestinal bleeding in cirrhotic patients. Clujul Med 2013;86:21–3.
60. Kumar M, Ahmad J, Maiwall R, et al. Thromboelastography-Guided Blood Component Use in Patients With Cirrhosis With Nonvariceal Bleeding: A Randomized Controlled Trial. Hepatology 2020;71:235–46.
61. Kalafateli M, Triantos CK, Nikolopoulou V, et al. Non-variceal gastrointestinal bleeding in patients with liver cirrhosis: a review. Dig Dis Sci 2012;57:2743–54.
62. González-González JA, García-Compean D, Vázquez-Elizondo G, et al. Nonvariceal upper gastrointestinal bleeding in patients with liver cirrhosis. Clinical features, outcomes and predictors of in-hospital mortality. A prospective study. Ann Hepatol 2011;10:287–95.
63. Marmo R, Koch M, Cipolletta L, et al. Predictive factors of mortality from nonvariceal upper gastrointestinal hemorrhage: a multicenter study. Am J Gastroenterol 2008;103:1639–47 [quiz: 48].
64. Stewart CA, Malinchoc M, Kim WR, et al. Hepatic encephalopathy as a predictor of survival in patients with end-stage liver disease. Liver Transpl 2007;13: 1366–71.
65. Vilstrup H, Amodio P, Bajaj J, et al. Hepatic encephalopathy in chronic liver disease: 2014 Practice Guideline by the American Association for the Study of Liver Diseases and the European Association for the Study of the Liver. Hepatology 2014;60:715–35.
66. Fichet J, Mercier E, Genée O, et al. Prognosis and 1-year mortality of intensive care unit patients with severe hepatic encephalopathy. J Crit Care 2009;24: 364–70.
67. Bajaj JS, Tandon P, O'Leary JG, et al. Admission Serum Metabolites and Thyroxine Predict Advanced Hepatic Encephalopathy in a Multicenter Inpatient Cirrhosis Cohort. Clin Gastroenterol Hepatol 2022. S1542-3565(22)00388-00393.

68. Katsounas A, Canbay A. Intensive Care Therapy for Patients with Advanced Liver Diseases. Visc Med 2018;34:283–9.
69. Ahmed S, Premkumar M, Dhiman RK, et al. Combined PEG3350 plus lactulose results in early resolution of hepatic encephalopathy and improved 28-day survival in acute-on-chronic liver failure. J Clin Gastroenterol 2022;56:e11–9.
70. Montagnese S, Rautou P-E, Romero-Gómez M, et al. EASL clinical practice guidelines on the management of hepatic encephalopathy. J Hepatol 2022;77: 807–24.
71. Sharma BC, Sharma P, Lunia MK, et al. A randomized, double-blind, controlled trial comparing rifaximin plus lactulose with lactulose alone in treatment of overt hepatic encephalopathy. Am J Gastroenterol 2013;108:1458–63.
72. Jain A, Sharma BC, Mahajan B, et al. L-ornithine L-aspartate in acute treatment of severe hepatic encephalopathy: A double-blind randomized controlled trial. Hepatology 2021;75(5):1194–203.
73. Bajaj JS, Salzman NH, Acharya C, et al. Fecal microbial transplant capsules are safe in hepatic encephalopathy: a phase 1, randomized, placebo-controlled trial. Hepatology 2019;70:1690–703.
74. Kobashi-Margáin R, Gavilanes-Espinar J, Gutiérrez-Grabe Y, et al. Albumin dialysis with molecular adsorbent recirculating system (MARS) for the treatment of hepatic encephalopathy in liver failure. Ann Hepatol 2011;10:S70–6.
75. Bañares R, Nevens F, Larsen FS, et al. Extracorporeal albumin dialysis with the molecular adsorbent recirculating system in acute-on-chronic liver failure: the RELIEF trial. Hepatology 2013;57:1153–62.
76. Maiwall R, Bajpai M, Singh A, et al. Standard-Volume Plasma Exchange Improves Outcomes in Patients With Acute Liver Failure: A Randomized Controlled Trial. Clin Gastroenterol Hepatol 2022;20:e831–54.
77. Larsen FS, Schmidt LE, Bernsmeier C, et al. High-volume plasma exchange in patients with acute liver failure: An open randomised controlled trial. J Hepatol 2016;64:69–78.
78. Vora M, Kulkarni A, Rakam K, et al. Standard volume plasma exchange is safe and effective for patients with acute liver failure. J Clin Exp Hepatol 2022;12: S11–2.
79. Ginès P, Schrier RW. Renal Failure in Cirrhosis. N Engl J Med 2009;361:1279–90.
80. Angeli P, Garcia-Tsao G, Nadim MK, et al. News in pathophysiology, definition and classification of hepatorenal syndrome: a step beyond the International Club of Ascites (ICA) consensus document. J Hepatol 2019;71:811–22.
81. Rajakumar A, Appuswamy E, Kaliamoorthy I, et al. Renal dysfunction in cirrhosis: critical care management. Indian J Crit Care Med 2021;25:207–14.
82. Ginès A, Escorsell A, Ginès P, et al. Incidence, predictive factors, and prognosis of the hepatorenal syndrome in cirrhosis with ascites. Gastroenterology 1993; 105:229–36.
83. Caregaro L, Menon F, Angeli P, et al. Limitations of serum creatinine level and creatinine clearance as filtration markers in cirrhosis. Arch Intern Med 1994; 154:201–5.
84. Kulkarni AV, Premkumar M, Reddy DN, et al. The challenges of ascites management: an Indian perspective. Clin Liver Dis (Hoboken) 2022;19:234–8.
85. Kulkarni AV, Ravikumar ST, Tevethia H, et al. Safety and efficacy of terlipressin in acute-on-chronic liver failure with hepatorenal syndrome-acute kidney injury (HRS-AKI): a prospective cohort study. Sci Rep 2022;12:5503.
86. EASL Clinical Practice Guidelines for the management of patients with decompensated cirrhosis. J Hepatol 2018;69:406–60.

87. Wong F, Pappas SC, Reddy KR, et al. Terlipressin use and respiratory failure in patients with hepatorenal syndrome type 1 and severe acute-on-chronic liver failure. Aliment Pharmacol Ther 2022;56:1284–93.

88. Kulkarni AV, Kumar P, Rao NP, et al. Terlipressin-induced ischaemic skin necrosis. BMJ Case Rep 2020;13(1):e233089.

89. Mackle IJ, Swann DG, Cook B. One year outcome of intensive care patients with decompensated alcoholic liver disease. Br J Anaesth 2006;97:496–8.

90. Williams R, Aspinall R, Bellis M, et al. Addressing liver disease in the UK: a blueprint for attaining excellence in health care and reducing premature mortality from lifestyle issues of excess consumption of alcohol, obesity, and viral hepatitis. Lancet 2014;384:1953–97.

91. Kelly EM, James PD, Murthy S, et al. Health Care Utilization and Costs for Patients With End-Stage Liver Disease Are Significantly Higher at the End of Life Compared to Those of Other Decedents. Clin Gastroenterol Hepatol 2019;17:2339–23346.e1.

92. Gola A, Davis S, Greenslade L, et al. Economic analysis of costs for patients with end stage liver disease over the last year of life. BMJ Support Palliat Care 2015;5:110.

93. Hudson BE, Ameneshoa K, Gopfert A, et al. Integration of palliative and supportive care in the management of advanced liver disease: development and evaluation of a prognostic screening tool and supportive care intervention. Frontline Gastroenterol 2017;8:45–52.

94. Bergenholtz H, Weibull A, Raunkiær M. Supportive and palliative care indicators tool (SPICT™) in a Danish healthcare context: translation, cross-cultural adaptation, and content validation. BMC Palliat Care 2022;21:41.

95. Kim S, Lee K, Kim C, et al. How do we start palliative care for patients with end-stage liver disease? Gastroenterol Nurs 2022;45:101–12.

96. Rogal SS, Hansen L, Patel A, et al. AASLD practice guidance: palliative care and symptom-based management in decompensated cirrhosis. Hepatology 2022;76:819–53.

97. Potosek J, Curry M, Buss M, et al. Integration of palliative care in end-stage liver disease and liver transplantation. J Palliat Med 2014;17:1271–7.

98. Mehtani R, Premkumar M, Kulkarni AV. Nutrition in Critical Care Hepatology. Curr Hepatol Rep 2022.

Sarcopenia and Frailty in Cirrhosis

Assessment and Management

Chalermrat Bunchorntavakul, MD

KEYWORDS

- Liver cirrhosis • Malnutrition • Sarcopenia • Frailty • Nutrition therapy
- Micronutrients • Branched-chain amino acids • Exercise

KEY POINTS

- Sarcopenia and frailty are frequent in cirrhosis, and both lead to an increase in mortality and complications in various aspects.
- The complex pathogenesis of sarcopenia in cirrhosis is mainly determined by hyperammonemia and malnutrition.
- All cirrhotic patients should be periodically assessed for sarcopenia and/or frailty. Frailty tests are useful in the ambulatory settings, whereas a computed tomography scan is the gold standard for defining sarcopenia.
- To manage sarcopenia/frailty, a multidisciplinary team should develop a personalized care plan that includes patient education, protein/calorie intake goals, late evening meals, exercise programs, and micronutrient replenishment. branched-chain amino acid and L-carnitine supplementations, as well as testosterone replacement, may be beneficial for selected patients.

INTRODUCTION

Malnutrition, sarcopenia, and frailty are increasingly common among patients with cirrhosis, particularly in those with decompensated liver disease, and all three contribute to physical deconditioning, increased morbidity, and mortality.[1] Malnutrition is a general term used to describe a nutrition-related disorder (deficiency or excess) that causes measurable adverse effects on tissue/body form (body shape, size, composition) or function and/or clinical outcome.[1,2] Sarcopenia is a progressive and generalized skeletal muscle disorder associated with an increased likelihood of adverse outcomes including falls, fractures, disability, and mortality.[2] Frailty is a multidimensional clinical state of decreased physiologic reserve and increased vulnerability to health stressors.[1,2] Although these three conditions partly overlap, the key phenotypic representations of

Division of Gastroenterology and Hepatology, Department of Medicine, Rajavithi Hospital, College of Medicine, Rangsit University, 2 Phaya Thai Road, Ratchathewi, Bangkok 10400, Thailand
E-mail address: dr.chalermrat@gmail.com

Med Clin N Am 107 (2023) 589–604
https://doi.org/10.1016/j.mcna.2022.12.007
medical.theclinics.com

sarcopenia and frailty in cirrhosis are loss of muscle mass and impaired muscle contractile function, respectively[2] (**Fig. 1**).

The pathogenesis of sarcopenia in cirrhosis is complex and multifactorial, not just a simple reduction of calorie and protein intake. Hyperammonemia appears to be the main driver of sarcopenia in cirrhosis, mainly through myostatin-mediated signaling pathway and muscle autophagy, whereas other potential contributing mediators include endotoxemia, gut dysbiosis, decreased follistatin, branched-chain amino acids (BCAAs), testosterone and growth hormone.[1,3-6] In addition, studies have revealed a substantial correlation between sarcopenia and/or frailty and several micronutrient deficiencies (such as zinc, magnesium, vitamin D, and thiamine), which are increasingly prevalent in cirrhosis, particularly those caused by alcohol[2,7,8] (**Fig. 2**).

Malnutrition, sarcopenia, and frailty are prevalent in patients with cirrhosis, affecting approximately 70% of patients with end-stage liver disease, and are associated with increased morbidity and mortality, as well as the quality of life.[1,2,9,10] It has been proven that prompt diagnosis and care of malnutrition and sarcopenia by a multidisciplinary team can improve bad results to varying degrees.[1,2,9,10]

ASSESSMENT AND DIAGNOSIS OF MALNUTRITION, SARCOPENIA, AND FRAILTY IN CIRRHOSIS

The Royal Free Hospital Nutrition Prioritizing Tool (RFH-NPT) has been the most validated screening and diagnostic tool for malnutrition in patients with cirrhosis.[11-13] Patients are classified into three nutritional risk categories (low, moderate, and high) based on a combination of (1) the presence of acute hepatitis or need for tube feeding; (2) low body mass index (BMI), unplanned weight loss, or maintenance of dietary intake; and (3) whether fluid overload interferes with the ability to eat. Remarkably,

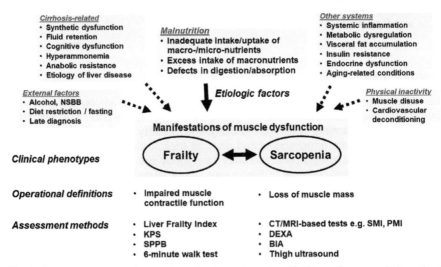

Fig. 1. Assessments and factors contributing to malnutrition, frailty, and sarcopenia in patients with cirrhosis. BIA, bioelectrical impedance analysis; CT, computed tomography; DEXA, dual-energy X-ray absorptiometry; KPS, Karnofsky Performance Scale; MRI, magnetic resonance imaging; NSBB, non-selective beta-blockers; PMI, psoas muscle index; SMI, skeletal muscle index; SPPB, short physical performance battery. (*Adapted from* Lai, J.C., Tandon, P., Bernal, W., Tapper, E.B., Ekong, U., Dasarathy, S. and Carey, E.J. (2021), Malnutrition, Frailty, and Sarcopenia in Patients With Cirrhosis: 2021 Practice Guidance by the American Association for the Study of Liver Diseases. Hepatology, 74: 1611-1644. https://doi.org/10.1002/hep.32049.)

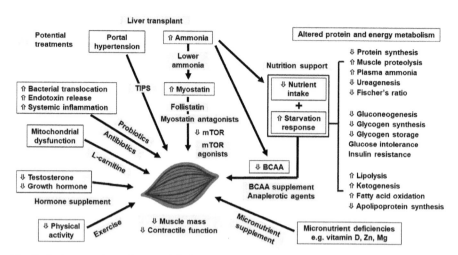

Fig. 2. Pathogenesis and potential therapeutic options of sarcopenia in cirrhosis. BCAA, branched-chain amino acids; mTOR, mammalian target of rapamycin; TIPS, transjugular intrahepatic portosystemic shunt. (Bunchorntavakul, C, Reddy, KR. Review article: malnutrition/sarcopenia and frailty in patients with cirrhosis. Aliment Pharmacol Ther. 2020; 51: 64–77. https://doi.org/10.1111/apt.15571.)

patients with cirrhosis Child-Pugh C and those with BMI <18.5 should be classified routinely as high risk for malnutrition.[9,13]

Most conventional objective methods for identifying sarcopenia, including anthropometric parameters, bioelectrical impedance analysis (BIA), and dual-energy X-ray absorptiometry (DEXA), may have some limitations in their accuracy in patients with decompensated cirrhosis, primarily due to fluid retention in certain body compartments.[1] Methods for assessing muscle mass and functions in patients with cirrhosis are summarized in **Table 1**.[14–17] Notably, except for computed tomography (CT) imaging techniques, the cut-points used to define sarcopenia by the majority of methods were taken from studies of general and older populations with limited validation in patients with cirrhosis.

Skeletal muscle index at L3 (SMI) calculated by special software from CT imaging is currently considered the gold standard for assessment of muscle mass in cirrhosis, as it has been shown to be more accurate and reproducible than anthropometry or DEXA scan in diagnosing sarcopenia in cirrhosis.[1,2,9,13] However, cost and radiation exposure make routine use of CT solely for the purpose of detecting sarcopenia impractical in many clinical settings; but quantification of skeletal muscle mass should be considered when an abdominal CT is obtained as part of clinical care (eg, hepatocellular carcinoma [HCC] surveillance and surgical planning) or in patients in whom assessment of muscle contractile function is not feasible (eg, acutely ill patients, very young children).[2,9] The area of the psoas muscle as determined by CT has also been examined in patients with cirrhosis. However, it has a lesser correlation with total body protein and may misrepresent the risk of death in comparison to SMI.[18,19]

The SMI cut-points of less than 50 cm^2/m^2 in men and 39 cm^2/m^2 in women have been recommended by the US Guidelines for the diagnosis of sarcopenia in patients with cirrhosis.[2,10] These SMI cut-points have been identified to correlate with wait-list mortality in a large multicenter cohort in North America and have also externally validated.[20,21] It should be noted that the mean muscle mass of Asian is approximately 15% lower than that of Western population after height adjustments, and, therefore, ethnicity-specific

Table 1
Screening and diagnostic methods for sarcopenia in cirrhosis

Methods	Advantages	Disadvantages	Comments	Suggested Cut-Points for Sarcopenia
MAMC	Rapid, available, and inexpensive	Low reproducibility; affected by fluid overload and adipose tissue loss	Weak correlation with x-sectional imaging; interpret with cautions	MAMC: men <21.1 cm and women <19.2 cm[13]
BIA	Rapid, available	Less reliable in patients with ascites and/or edema	Proper positioning of inpatients and/or obese patients may be challenging	SMI: men <7 kg/m^2 and women <5.7 kg/m^2 (men <6.6 kg/m^2 and women <5 kg/m^2 for Asians)[14–16]
Ultrasound	Rapid, and available	Operator-dependent, challenging in obese patients	More data are required to standardize the technique	NA
DEXA	Rapid, accurate, and reproducible	Limited availability, low-dose radiation exposure, and limited accuracy in patients with fluid retention	Can perform regional analysis to improve accuracy	ASMI: men <7 kg/m^2 and women <5.5 kg/m^2 (men <6.6 kg/m^2 and women <5 kg/m^2 for Asians)[14–16]
CT/MRI	Rapid (CT), safe, highly accurate, and reproducible	Expensive, limited availability (software), and radiation exposure (CT)	Has the most supporting evidence	SMI at L3: men <50 cm^2/m^2 and women <39 cm^2/m^2 (men <42 cm^2/m^2 and women <38 cm^2/m^2 for Asians)[2,17]

Abbreviations: ASMI, appendicular skeletal muscle index; BIA bioelectrical impedance analysis; CT, computed tomography; DEXA, dual-energy X-ray absorptiometry; MAMC, mid-arm muscle circumference; MRI, magnetic resonance imaging; SMI, skeletal muscle index.

diagnostic criteria for sarcopenia may be required (eg, the Japanese Guideline has suggested using SMI cut-points of 42 cm^2/m^2 for men and 38 cm^2/m^2 for women to define sarcopenia in cirrhosis).[1,17] In addition, sarcopenic obesity (defined as low sex-adjusted SMI and BMI $\geq$ 25 kg/m^2) and myosteatosis (characterized by both a decrease in muscle size and an increase in the proportion of muscular fat) are frequently present in patients with cirrhosis, particularly from metabolic-associated fatty liver disease, and are independently associated with higher long-term mortality.[22,23]

Frailty evaluation methods are frequently arranged in a table from subjective, survey-based instruments assessed by the patient, caregiver, or physician to objective, performance-based tools[2] (**Figs. 1** and **2**). Most of these tools have been studied in the ambulatory setting, mainly in the geriatric population, and there are insufficient data to recommend the use of one frailty tool over another.[2] Notably, some scales have validated thresholds to grade the severity of frailty in patients with cirrhosis specifically the Karnofsky Performance Scale (KPS): KPS 80 to 100 = high performance; KPS 50 to 70 = moderate performance; or KPS 10 to 40 = low performance[24,25]; and the Liver Frailty Index (LFI): LFI <3.2 = robust; LFI 3.2 to 4.3 = prefrail; or LFI $\geq$4.4 = frail.[26,27]

Recommendations for screening and assessment of malnutrition, frailty, and sarcopenia in patients with cirrhosis by the AASLD are summarized in **Fig. 3**.[2] A positive screening for frailty or sarcopenia should prompt an examination of underlying etiologic risk factors and the formulation of an ambulatory, personalized care plan. Reassessment of frailty or sarcopenia (using the same standardized tool as baseline assessment) is crucial and should occur at least annually for patients with well-compensated disease but as frequently as every 8 to 12 weeks for those with decompensated cirrhosis and/or those undergoing active management for these conditions.[2] Of note, frailty testing may be particularly useful in the ambulatory setting and when longitudinal assessments are needed to assess natural progression or response to treatment. Whereas, sarcopenia testing may be particularly useful for patients in whom the administration of tests of frailty is not feasible or is impractical.[2]

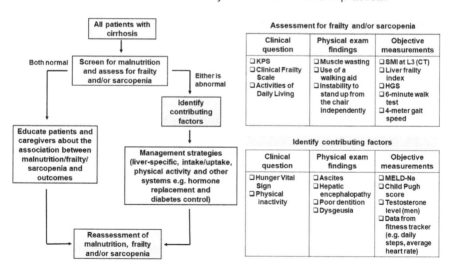

Fig. 3. Algorithm for screening, assessment, and management of malnutrition, frailty, and sarcopenia in patients with cirrhosis. HGS, hand grip strength; KPS, Karnofsky Performance Scale; SMI, skeletal muscle index. (*Adapted from* Lai, J.C., Tandon, P., Bernal, W., Tapper, E.B., Ekong, U., Dasarathy, S. and Carey, E.J. (2021), Malnutrition, Frailty, and Sarcopenia in Patients With Cirrhosis: 2021 Practice Guidance by the American Association for the Study of Liver Diseases. Hepatology, 74: 1611-1644. https://doi.org/10.1002/hep.32049.)

PREVALENCE AND OUTCOMES OF SARCOPENIA AND FRAILTY IN CIRRHOSIS

Sarcopenia is frequent in individuals with cirrhosis and appears to be highly connected with the severity of cirrhosis, with a prevalence of 10% to 20%, 30% to 40%, and 50% to 70% in patients with cirrhosis Child-Pugh A, B, and C, respectively.[20,28–30] Similar to the general population, males with decompensated cirrhosis were approximately two to three times more likely than women to have sarcopenia, and the degree of muscle loss -correlates strongly with the severity of liver disease in men but not in women.[20,28,30] In addition, up to 50% of individuals with alcohol-related liver disease have sarcopenia, which is more prevalent than in patients with other causes of liver disease.[30] Prevalence rates of pre-LT sarcopenia, pre-LT sarcopenic obesity, post-LT sarcopenia, and post-LT sarcopenic obesity were 14% to 78%, 2% to 42%, 30% to 100%, and 88%, respectively, in a systematic review of 35 publications. [31]

Unlike other complications of cirrhosis that are typically improved (or even reversed) after LT, the course of sarcopenia following LT is variable, with either continuing to decline (in most studies), improving, or remaining unchanged.[1,19,23,32–35] Notably, the decrease in skeletal muscle mass after LT is most pronounced during the first year and may reverse thereafter, whereas muscle functions generally improve early after LT and before the improvement in muscle mass.[1] Although the underlying pathophysiology is unclear, Immunosuppressive drugs, particularly corticosteroids and mTOR inhibitors, have a detrimental effect on skeletal muscle and appear to be the primary drivers of post-LT sarcopenia.[1]

Similar to sarcopenia, frailty is common (17% to 43%) among patients with cirrhosis, particularly those with decompensated liver disease, and it tends to worsen over time.[2,3,25,36–38] In addition, the prevalence of frailty appears to be higher in women (than in males; despite comparable MELD scores) and in the presence of hepatic encephalopathy (HE).[37–39] Following LT, LFI scores decreased relative to pre-LT levels in approximately 60%, 40%, and 30% of patients at 3, 6, and 12 months, respectively, and only 20% of patients reached functional "robustness" by 1 year following L.[40,41]

It is well-recognized that the presence of sarcopenia in cirrhosis is associated with worsening clinical outcomes in practically all aspects, such as health-related quality of life, HE, infections, and mortality.[1,2,9,28–31] Further, frailty has recently emerged as a strong predictor of outcomes in patients with cirrhosis, independent of liver functions, both in the ambulatory and post-LT settings.[27,36–38] In the setting of LT, the presence of sarcopenia and/or frailty is(are) predictive of waitlist mortality in addition to MELD score, and both adversely impact LT outcomes in peri-LT and post-LT periods.[1,2,9,10,24–27,29–31,36–38] For instance, in the ambulatory setting, physical frailty (defined as LFI $\geq$4.5) increases the adjusted risk of LT waitlist mortality $\sim$2 folds compared with non-frail patients.[36] Apart from liver-related outcomes, frailty is strongly linked with other general outcomes, including the occurrence of depression, falls, disability, and impaired global quality of life.[42–45] Moreover, frailty appears to be a better predictor of functional capacity and quality of life in LT candidates than sarcopenia.[46] Nevertheless, the presence of frailty and/or sarcopenia at any specific levels should not be considered an absolute contraindication for LT.[2]

MANAGEMENT OF MALNUTRITION, SARCOPENIA, AND FRAILTY IN CIRRHOSIS

To lessen the risk of malnutrition, sarcopenia, and frailty, all cirrhotic patients should ideally receive education, motivation, and behavioral skills support (primary prevention).[2] When possible, a positive frailty or sarcopenia screen should prompt evaluation for underlying etiologic risk factors and the development of an ambulatory personalized management plan by a multidisciplinary team consisting of the patient's primary care provider, gastroenterologist/hepatologist, registered dietician, certified exercise physiologist/physical therapist, and health behavior specialist (if there is a concurrent mental health condition).[2] Comprehensive management of sarcopenia and frailty in cirrhosis are outlined in **Fig. 4** and **Table 1**.

Management of Liver Disease

It is recommended to treat inflammatory disorders that cause cirrhosis, such as HCV, insulin resistance, obesity, and alcohol use disorders, to prevent or lessen malnutrition, frailty, and sarcopenia.[2] Further, the management of cirrhotic complications, especially ascites and HE, should be optimized. Transjugular intrahepatic portosystemic shunt (TIPS) placement for typical indications (eg, variceal hemorrhage, ascites) may have an indirect advantage of improving body compositions with lean body mass gain, decreased visceral fat, and increased total and fat-free muscle mass.[47–50] Because muscle mass changes after LT are highly variable, LT cannot be recommended specifically for the treatment of frailty or sarcopenia.[2,32–35]

Management of Hepatic Encephalopathy

As sarcopenia and HE are pathogenetically connected, the prevention and treatment of HE may also be beneficial for sarcopenia. Long-term ammonia-lowering strategies (eg, L-ornithine-L-aspartate [LOLA], lactulose, rifaximin, and anaplerotic agents) may result in increased muscle mass and strength by down-regulating myostatin-mediated pathway, decreasing muscle autophagy, and improving muscle contractility; however, the data are based on preclinical research and require additional validation in humans.[1,51,52] In hyperammonemic portacaval anastomosis rats, a 4-week LOLA and rifaximin ammonia-lowering therapy improved skeletal muscle mass and function.[51] L-carnitine is an essential nutrient that plays a critical role in mitochondrial fatty acid and energy metabolism. Patients with cirrhosis and sarcopenia/malnutrition are at

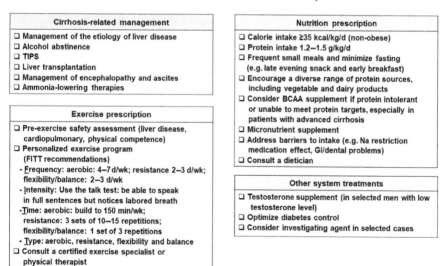

Cirrhosis-related management	Nutrition prescription

❑ Management of the etiology of liver disease
❑ Alcohol abstinence
❑ TIPS
❑ Liver transplantation
❑ Management of encephalopathy and ascites
❑ Ammonia-lowering therapies
	❑ Calorie intake ≥35 kcal/kg/d (non-obese)
	❑ Protein intake 1.2–1.5 g/kg/d
	❑ Frequent small meals and minimize fasting
	    (e.g. late evening snack and early breakfast)
	❑ Encourage a diverse range of protein sources,
	    including vegetable and dairy products
	❑ Consider BCAA supplement if protein intolerant
	    or unable to meet protein targets, especially in
	    patients with advanced cirrhosis

Exercise prescription

❑ Pre-exercise safety assessment (liver disease,
    cardiopulmonary, physical competence)
❑ Personalized exercise program
    (FITT recommendations)
 - Frequency: aerobic: 4–7 d/wk; resistance 2–3 d/wk;
    flexibility/balance: 2–3 d/wk
 - Intensity: Use the talk test: be able to speak
    in full sentences but notices labored breath
 -Time: aerobic: build to 150 min/wk;
    resistance: 3 sets of 10–15 repetitions;
    flexibility/balance: 1 set of 3 repetitions
 - Type: aerobic, resistance, flexibility and balance
❑ Consult a certified exercise specialist or
    physical therapist

Nutrition prescription (cont.)
❑ Micronutrient supplement ❑ Address barriers to intake (e.g. Na restriction   medication effect, GI/dental problems) ❑ Consult a dietician

Other system treatments
❑ Testosterone supplement (in selected men with low   testosterone level) ❑ Optimize diabetes control ❑ Consider investigating agent in selected cases

Fig. 4. Summary of the management of malnutrition, frailty, and sarcopenia in patients with cirrhosis. (*Adapted from* Lai, J.C., Tandon, P., Bernal, W., Tapper, E.B., Ekong, U., Dasarathy, S. and Carey, E.J. (2021), Malnutrition, Frailty, and Sarcopenia in Patients With Cirrhosis: 2021 Practice Guidance by the American Association for the Study of Liver Diseases. Hepatology, 74: 1611-1644. https://doi.org/10.1002/hep.32049.)

high risk for carnitine deficiency (due to decreased intake and biosynthesis), which compromises vital liver metabolic processes such as gluconeogenesis, fatty acid metabolism, albumin biosynthesis, and ammonia detoxification by the urea cycle.[53] According to data from three studies (including one randomized study, $n = 121$), L-carnitine supplementation (1018 to 4000 mg/d) in cirrhotic patients with sarcopenia and/or HE was associated with dose-related reductions in blood ammonia levels, improvement of muscle mass, fatigue, and levels of physical activity.[54–56] Nonetheless, a meta-analysis of four randomized studies ($n = 398$) failed to show the efficacy of L-carnitine in the treatment of HE and its effects on fatigue and quality of life.[57]

Nutrition Intake

A personalized nutrition prescription should be provided to all patients with cirrhosis that is tailored to their current nutritional status.[2] As patients with cirrhosis have increased total energy expenditure and protein requirement,[58,59] It should be emphasized that the optimal daily energy intake should not be lower than 35 kcal/kg/d (in nonobese individuals) and protein intake should not be lower than 1.2 to 1.5 g/kg/d (protein >1.5 g/kg/d can be recommended to replenish malnourished and/or sarcopenic state).[1,2,9] Notably, either dry weight or ideal body weight (whatever is more practical) can be used to determine calorie and protein requirement targets. The daily intake should be divided into frequent small meals and/or snacks (every 3 to 4 h while awake) and, of importance, a late evening meal/snack must be included,[1,2,9] as it is a simple and effective intervention to prevent and to reverse sarcopenia in cirrhosis, resulting in an improvement in quality of life and also liver functions[60–62] (see **Fig. 4**). Sodium restriction has a small-to-moderate benefit in the treatment of ascites but may reduce the palatability of food, representing a barrier to adequate nutrition intake.[1] In a study of 120 outpatients with cirrhosis and ascites, 37 patients adhering to a moderate sodium restriction diet (<2 to 3 g/d) reduced the mean daily calorie intake by 20%.[63] Therefore, sodium restriction should be liberalized if the patient cannot maintain nutritional targets because of diet unpalatability.[2]

Nutritional management of obese cirrhotic patients, particularly with sarcopenia, is more complicated and often requires a specialized multidisciplinary team. In general, a nutritional and lifestyle program to achieve progressive weight loss (>5% to 10%) should be implemented. A tailored, moderately hypocaloric diet (use of caloric targets stratified by BMI: 25 to 35 kcal/kg/d for individuals with BMI 30 to 40 kg/m^2 and 20 to 25 kcal/kg/d for individuals with BMI 40 kg/m^2), including adequate protein intake (1.2 to 1.5 g/kg/d), can be adopted to achieve weight loss in obese cirrhotic patients without compromising protein stores.[2,9]

Branched-Chain Amino Acids Supplementation

The decreased levels of BCAAs (leucine, isoleucine, and valine) in the plasma (also Fischer's ratio) are characteristic of cirrhosis and contribute to the pathogenesis of HE, sarcopenia, and impaired liver regeneration.[1,64] Therefore, BCAAs are likely the preferred source of amino acids in cirrhotic patients, and supplementation with BCAAs seems rational from a theoretical standpoint.[1,64] Several clinical trials have shown the beneficial effects of BCAA supplementation in malnourished cirrhotic patients, including improvements in nutritional status, liver function, HE, quality of life, and event-free survival.[65–68] In these BCAA trials, there were some noteworthy observations, including the following: (1) The BCAA dose ranged from 12 to 30 g/d; (2) The beneficial effects were primarily observed in patients with advanced liver disease and/or prior HE; and (3) Adherence to BCAA supplementation was only moderate (75% to 90%) even in the context of RCT, which may be partially attributed to its unpalatability for some patients.[65–68] In addition, a systematic review (40 articles) and meta-analysis (12 studies) of the effects of BCAA supplementation in patients with cirrhosis found significant benefits on HE, muscle strength, muscle mass, and liver functions, despite the heterogeneity and limited methodological quality of the included studies.[69,70] However, in a meta-analysis of 16 RCTs investigating BCAA supplementation in patients with HE, BCAAs had a favorable effect on HE, but no effect on mortality, quality of life, or nutritional parameters.[71] It should be noted that inconsistencies among guidelines exist. Two European Guidelines on nutrition in liver disease recommend long-term oral BCAA supplementation (0.25 g/kg/d) in patients with advanced cirrhosis, especially when adequate nitrogen intake is not achieved by oral diet,[9,72] whereas the AASLD Guideline does not recommend BCAA supplementation beyond emphasizing the importance of meeting daily protein targets from a variety of protein sources.[2]

Micronutrients Replenishment

Micronutrient deficiencies, particularly folate, thiamine, zinc, magnesium, selenium, vitamin D, and vitamin E, are frequent in patients with alcohol-associated liver disease and decompensated cirrhosis, mainly as a result of inadequate intake, malabsorption, and decreased biosynthesis.[72–75] Hence, deficits in fat-soluble vitamins are well known in patients with cholestatic liver disease.[76,77] Notably, many of these micronutrients are linked to frailty or sarcopenia. Magnesium deficiency is associated with decreased muscle strength in cirrhosis and accelerated bone resorption in children with cholestatic liver disease.[78–81] Zinc deficiency is associated with altered taste and smell, poor appetite, poor wound healing, HE, sarcopenia, and frailty in cirrhosis.[82,83] Vitamin D deficiency is associated with frailty, impaired muscle function, and bone formation in the general population. Taken together, these data suggest that micronutrient replacement (or supplementation) is theoretically justified; nevertheless, there is limited data on the beneficial benefits of micronutrients and vitamin supplementation in cirrhotic individuals, particularly on muscle mass. Of note, research on the elderly suggests that vitamin D supplementation may have beneficial effects on the musculoskeletal system (eg, increased bone density, muscle strength, and physical activity).[8] Uncertainty exists regarding the applicability of these findings to individuals with cirrhosis; however, a pilot randomized clinical trial reported that vitamin D supplementation has a positive effect on muscle mass and strength in patients with decompensated cirrhosis receiving BCAA supplementation.[84] Ideally, Micronutrient deficiencies should be examined at least annually, replenished if deficient, and reevaluated following replenishment.[2] Notably, empiric oral multivitamin supplementation may be a more practical alternative for cirrhotic patients with sarcopenia or sarcopenia.[2] Decisions for prescribing long-term maintenance doses will depend on the assessment of whether the patient is at ongoing risk for malnutrition. For instance, vitamin D levels should be measured in all cirrhotic patients with sarcopenia/frailty, and vitamin D should be administered orally to achieve the goal serum 25(OH) vitamin D level of >30 ng/mL (suggested dose for replacement: 50,000 IU/week vitamin D2 or D3 for 8 weeks, followed by 1500 to 2000 IU/d for maintenance).[1,2,9]

Nutrition Therapy in Hospitalized Patients Setting

In hospitalized patients with cirrhosis who are unable to satisfy their energy needs through volitional intake and oral nutritional supplementation, enteral nutritional supplementation should be considered to reach goals, with caution for aspiration and hyperglycemia.[1,2] The presence of esophageal varices is not a contraindication to the placement of an enteric feeding tube; nonetheless, careful monitoring for signs of rebleeding is necessary if an enteric tube is required following recent banding of esophageal varices as enteral nutrition may increase splanchnic blood flow, which in turn may increase portal pressure and precipitate rebleeding.[1,2,85,86] Parenteral nutrition should be reserved for cirrhotic individuals who are intolerant of enteral nutrition and unable to achieve dietary needs by oral intake alone.[1,2] Notably, a meta-analysis of 13 randomized controlled trials evaluating nutrition therapy by enteral or parenteral route in cirrhosis ($n = 663$) revealed significant beneficial effects on clinical outcomes including mortality, overt HE, and infections, despite the high risk of bias in all included trials.[87] Generally, standard nutrition regimens can be used since specialized regimens (eg, BCAA-enriched or immune-enhancing formulas) have not been shown to improve morbidity or mortality in intervention trials.[1,9,71]

Physical Exercise

Physical inactivity is common and contributes to sarcopenia and frailty in patients with cirrhosis. There is experimental and clinical evidence for the benefits of exercise in cirrhosis, including improvements in muscle health (mass, strength, functional capacity), bone health, quality of life, fatigue, cardiopulmonary fitness, and reductions in hepatic venous pressure gradient and hepatic steatosis, without adverse events; however, caution should be exercised when interpreting these studies in this population as they have been limited by small sample size and inclusion of mostly well-compensated patients (60% to 90% were cirrhosis Child-Pugh A).[88–93] Therefore, physical activity-based interventions are recommended for patients with cirrhosis, including those with decompensated liver disease (whenever possible), and they should consist of three components (1) assessing and reassessing frailty and/or sarcopenia using standardized tools; (2) recommending a combination of aerobic and resistance exercises; and (3) tailoring recommendations based on assessments[2] (see **Fig. 4**). In general, it is reasonable to propose 30- to 60-min sessions of supervised moderate-intensity exercise combining both aerobic and resistance training for a total of $\geq$150 min/week for cirrhotic individuals.[89,91] Aerobic training would be particularly relevant to improve overall fitness, whereas resistance training would help reverse sarcopenia, and improve strength and balance, and bone mineral density.[89,91] Of note, before initiating an exercise program for cirrhosis, the management of portal hypertension-related complications and concomitant cardiopulmonary conditions must be optimized.

Hormone Replacement

Low testosterone levels have been observed in male patients with cirrhosis and sarcopenia compared with patients who are nonsarcopenic, and it is independently associated with adverse outcomes in men with cirrhosis.[94–96] Testosterone therapy has been studied in patients with alcoholic liver disease and cirrhosis to improve nutritional status and muscle mass, but it has not been consistently beneficial.[96–98] In a randomized controlled trial involving 101 male patients with cirrhosis and low testosterone (defined as total testosterone 12 nmol/L or free testosterone 230 pmol/L), testosterone replacement therapy for 1 year was associated with increased muscle mass, bone mass, and hemoglobin, decreased fat mass, and improved glucose metabolism.[99] Despite the controversy, it is advised to exercise caution when taking long-term testosterone replacement therapy because there may be a higher risk of cardiovascular events, venous thromboembolism, polycythemia, cholestasis, prostate cancer, and HCC.[1,100,101] Relative contraindications to the use of testosterone include a history of HCC, other malignancy, or thrombosis.[2]

SUMMARY

Sarcopenia and frailty are frequent in cirrhosis, and both contribute to increased morbidity and death. Sarcopenia and/or frailty screening and reassessment should be undertaken in all cirrhotic patients. Frailty tests are useful in the ambulatory setting, whereas the CT scan is the gold standard to define sarcopenia. A multidisciplinary team should promptly address sarcopenia/frailty by formulating an individualized care plan that includes patient education on protein/calorie intake targets, late evening meals, exercise programs, and micronutrient replenishment. In selected patients, BCAA supplements, and testosterone replacement may also be beneficial.

CLINICS CARE POINTS

- Patients with cirrhosis are at-risk of sarcopenia and frailty.
- Prompt recognition, appropriate assessment, and multidisciplinary interventions of these conditions are essential as they are both strongly associated with poor quality of life, morbidity, and, mortality in patients with cirrhosis.

CONFLICT OF INTEREST

None.

FUNDING SOURCE

This article received no specific grant from any funding agency in the public, commercial, or not-for-profit sectors.

REFERENCES

1. Bunchorntavakul C, Reddy KR. Review article: malnutrition/sarcopenia and frailty in patients with cirrhosis. Aliment Pharmacol Ther 2020;51(1):64–77.
2. Lai JC, Tandon P, Bernal W, et al. Malnutrition, Frailty, and Sarcopenia in Patients With Cirrhosis: 2021 Practice Guidance by the American Association for the Study of Liver Diseases. Hepatology 2021;74(3):1611–44.
3. Tandon P, Montano-Loza AJ, Lai JC, et al. Sarcopenia and frailty in decompensated cirrhosis. J Hepatol 2021;75(Suppl 1):S147–62.
4. Nishikawa H, Enomoto H, Nishiguchi S, et al. Liver Cirrhosis and Sarcopenia from the Viewpoint of Dysbiosis. Int J Mol Sci 2020;21(15):5254.
5. Jindal A, Jagdish RK. Sarcopenia: Ammonia metabolism and hepatic encephalopathy. Clin Mol Hepatol 2019;25(3):270–9.
6. Kawaguchi T, Izumi N, Charlton MR. Sata M Branched-chain amino acids as pharmacological nutrients in chronic liver disease. Hepatology 2011;54(3):1063–70.
7. Nishikawa H, Yoh K, Enomoto H, et al. Serum Zinc Level Is Associated with Frailty in Chronic Liver Diseases. J Clin Med 2020;9(5):1570.
8. Wintermeyer E, Ihle C, Ehnert S, et al. Crucial Role of Vitamin D in the Musculoskeletal System. Nutrients 2016;8(6):319.
9. EASL Clinical Practice Guidelines on nutrition in chronic liver disease. J Hepatol 2019;70(1):172–93.
10. Lai JC, Sonnenday CJ, Tapper EB, et al. Frailty in liver transplantation: An expert opinion statement from the American Society of Transplantation Liver and Intestinal Community of Practice. Am J Transplant 2019;19(7):1896–906.
11. Georgiou A, Papatheodoridis GV, Alexopoulou A, et al. Evaluation of the effectiveness of eight screening tools in detecting risk of malnutrition in cirrhotic patients: the KIRRHOS study. Br J Nutr 2019;122(12):1368–76.

12. Wu Y, Zhu Y, Feng Y, et al. Royal Free Hospital-Nutritional Prioritizing Tool improves the prediction of malnutrition risk outcomes in liver cirrhosis patients compared with Nutritional Risk Screening 2002. Br J Nutr 2020;124(12):1293–302.

13. Tandon P, Raman M, Mourtzakis M, et al. A practical approach to nutritional screening and assessment in cirrhosis. Hepatology 2017;65(3):1044–57.

14. Chen LK, Woo J, Assantachai P, et al. Asian Working Group for Sarcopenia: 2019 Consensus Update on Sarcopenia Diagnosis and Treatment. J Am Med Dir Assoc 2020;21(3):300–7.

15. Cruz-Jentoft AJ, Bahat G, Bauer J, et al. Sarcopenia: revised European consensus on definition and diagnosis. Age Ageing 2019;48(4):601.

16. Yamada Y, Yamada M, Yoshida T, et al. Validating muscle mass cutoffs of four international sarcopenia-working groups in Japanese people using DXA and BIA. J Cachexia Sarcopenia Muscle 2021;12(4):1000–10.

17. Nishikawa H, Shiraki M, Hiramatsu A, et al. Japan Society of Hepatology guidelines for sarcopenia in liver disease (1st edition): Recommendation from the working group for creation of sarcopenia assessment criteria. Hepatol Res 2016;46(10):951–63.

18. Ebadi M, Wang CW, Lai JC, et al. Poor performance of psoas muscle index for identification of patients with higher waitlist mortality risk in cirrhosis. J Cachexia Sarcopenia Muscle 2018;9(6):1053–62.

19. Wells CI, McCall JL, Plank LD. Relationship Between Total Body Protein and Cross-Sectional Skeletal Muscle Area in Liver Cirrhosis Is Influenced by Overhydration. Liver Transpl 2019;25(1):45–55.

20. Carey EJ, Lai JC, Wang CW, et al. A multicenter study to define sarcopenia in patients with end-stage liver disease. Liver Transpl 2017;23(5):625–33.

21. Georgiou A, Papatheodoridis GV, Alexopoulou A. Validation of cutoffs for skeletal muscle mass index based on computed tomography analysis against dual energy X-ray absorptiometry in patients with cirrhosis: the KIRRHOS study. Ann Gastroenterol 2020;33(1):80–6.

22. Montano-Loza AJ, Angulo P, Meza-Junco J, et al. Sarcopenic obesity and myosteatosis are associated with higher mortality in patients with cirrhosis. J Cachexia Sarcopenia Muscle 2016;7(2):126–35.

23. Carias S, Castellanos AL, Vilchez V, et al. Nonalcoholic steatohepatitis is strongly associated with sarcopenic obesity in patients with cirrhosis undergoing liver transplant evaluation. J Gastroenterol Hepatol 2016;31(3):628–33.

24. Tandon P, Reddy KR, O'Leary JG, et al. A Karnofsky performance status-based score predicts death after hospital discharge in patients with cirrhosis. Hepatology 2017;65(1):217–24.

25. Thuluvath PJ, Thuluvath AJ, Savva Y. Karnofsky performance status before and after liver transplantation predicts graft and patient survival. J Hepatol 2018;69(4):818–25.

26. Kardashian A, Ge J, McCulloch CE, et al. Identifying an Optimal Liver Frailty Index Cutoff to Predict Waitlist Mortality in Liver Transplant Candidates. Hepatology 2021;73(3):1132–9.

27. Lai JC, Covinsky KE, Dodge JL, et al. Development of a novel frailty index to predict mortality in patients with end-stage liver disease. Hepatology 2017;66(2):564–74.

28. Tandon P, Ney M, Irwin I, et al. Severe muscle depletion in patients on the liver transplant wait list: its prevalence and independent prognostic value. Liver Transpl 2012;18(10):209–1216.

29. Merli M, Riggio O, Dally L. Does malnutrition affect survival in cirrhosis? PINC (Policentrica Italiana Nutrizione Cirrosi). Hepatology 1996;23(5):1041–6.

30. Tantai X, Liu Y, Yeo YH, et al. Effect of sarcopenia on survival in patients with cirrhosis: A meta-analysis. J Hepatol 2022;76(3):588–99.

31. Ooi PH, Hager A, Mazurak VC, et al. Sarcopenia in chronic liver disease: impact on outcomes. Liver Transpl 2019;25(9):1422–38.

32. Jeon JY, Wang HJ, Ock SY, et al. Newly developed sarcopenia as a prognostic factor for survival in patients who underwent liver transplantation. PLoS One 2015;10(11):e0143966.

33. Kaido T, Tamai Y, Hamaguchi Y, et al. Effects of pretransplant sarcopenia and sequential changes in sarcopenic parameters after living donor liver transplantation. Nutrition 2017;33:195–8.

34. Tsien C, Garber A, Narayanan A, et al. Post-liver transplantation sarcopenia in cirrhosis: a prospective evaluation. J Gastroenterol Hepatol 2014;29(6):1250–7.

35. Bergerson JT, Lee JG, Furlan A, et al. Liver transplantation arrests and reverses muscle wasting. Clin Transplant 2015;29(3):216–21.

36. Lai JC, Rahimi RS, Verna EC, et al. Frailty associated with waitlist mortality independent of ascites and hepatic encephalopathy in a multicenter study. Gastroenterology 2019;156(6):1675–82.

37. Tapper E, Baki J, Parikh ND, et al. Frailty, Psychoactive medications, and cognitive dysfunction are associated with poor patient-reported outcomes in cirrhosis. Hepatology 2019;69(4):1676–85.

38. Tapper EB, Finkelstein D, Mittleman MA, et al. Standard assessments of frailty are validated predictors of mortality in hospitalized patients with cirrhosis. Hepatology 2015;62(2):584–90.

39. Lai JC, Ganger DR, Volk ML, et al. Association of frailty and sex with wait list mortality in liver transplant candidates in the multicenter functional assessment in liver transplantation (FrAILT) study. JAMA Surg 2021;156(3):256–62.

40. Lai JC, Segev DL, McCulloch CE, et al. Physical frailty after liver transplantation. Am J Transplant 2018;18(8):1986–94.

41. Lai JC, Dodge JL, Kappus MR, et al. Changes in frailty are associated with waitlist mortality in patients with cirrhosis. J Hepatol 2020;73(3):575–81.

42. Cron DC, Friedman JF, Winder GS, et al. Depression and frailty in patients with end-stage liver disease referred for transplant evaluation. Am J Transplant 2016;16(6):1805–11.

43. Lai JC, Dodge JL, McCulloch CE, et al. Frailty and the burden of concurrent and incident disability in patients with cirrhosis: a prospective cohort study. Hepatol Commun 2019;4(1):126–33.

44. Tapper EB, Nikirk S, Parikh ND, et al. Falls are common, morbid, and predictable in patients with cirrhosis. J Hepatol 2021;75(3):582–8.

45. Tapper EB, Zhao L, Nikirk S, et al. Incidence and bedside predictors of the first episode of overt hepatic encephalopathy in patients with cirrhosis. Am J Gastroenterol 2020;115(12):2017–25.

46. Yadav A, Chang YH, Carpenter S, et al. Relationship between sarcopenia, six-minute walk distance and health-related quality of life in liver transplant candidates. Clin Transplant 2015;29(2):134–41.

47. Allard JP, Chau J, Sandokji K, et al. Effects of ascites resolution after successful TIPS on nutrition in cirrhotic patients with refractory ascites. Am J Gastroenterol 2001;96(8):2442–7.

48. Artru F, Miquet X, Azahaf M, et al. Consequences of TIPSS placement on the body composition of patients with cirrhosis and severe portal hypertension: a

large retrospective CT-based surveillance. Aliment Pharmacol Ther 2020;52(9): 1516–26.

49. Benmassaoud A, Roccarina D, Arico F, et al. Sarcopenia does not worsen survival in patients with cirrhosis undergoing transjugular intrahepatic portosystemic shunt for refractory ascites. Am J Gastroenterol 2020;115(11):1911–4.

50. Tsien C, Shah SN, McCullough AJ, et al. Reversal of sarcopenia predicts survival after a transjugular intrahepatic portosystemic stent. Eur J Gastroenterol Hepatol 2013;25(1):85–93.

51. Kumar A, Davuluri G, Silva RNE, et al. Ammonia lowering reverses sarcopenia of cirrhosis by restoring skeletal muscle proteostasis. Hepatology 2017;65(6): 2045–58.

52. Sinclair M, Gow PJ, Grossmann M, et al. Review article: sarcopenia in cirrhosis–aetiology, implications and potential therapeutic interventions. Aliment Pharmacol Ther 2016;43(7):765–77.

53. Hanai T, Shiraki M, Imai K, et al. Usefulness of carnitine supplementation for the complications of liver cirrhosis. Nutrients 2020;12(7):1915.

54. Malaguarnera M, Vacante M, Giordano M, et al. Oral acetyl-L-carnitine therapy reduces fatigue in overt hepatic encephalopathy: a randomized, double-blind, placebo-controlled study. Am J Clin Nutr 2011;93(4):799–808.

55. Hiramatsu A, Aikata H, Uchikawa S, et al. Levocarnitine use is associated with improvement in sarcopenia in patients with liver cirrhosis. Hepatol Commun 2019;3(3):348–55.

56. Ohara M, Ogawa K, Suda G, et al. L-Carnitine suppresses loss of skeletal muscle mass in patients with liver cirrhosis. Hepatol Commun 2018;2(8):906–18.

57. Martí-Carvajal AJ, Gluud C, Arevalo-Rodriguez I, et al. Acetyl-L-carnitine for patients with hepatic encephalopathy. Cochrane Database Syst Rev 2019;1(1): CD011451.

58. Córdoba J, López-Hellín J, Planas M. Normal protein diet for episodic hepatic encephalopathy: results of a randomized study. J Hepatol 2004;41(1):38–43.

59. Greco AV, Mingrone G, Benedetti G, et al. Daily energy and substrate metabolism in patients with cirrhosis. Hepatology 1998;27(2):346–50.

60. Chen CJ, Wang LC, Kuo HT, et al. Significant effects of late evening snack on liver functions in patients with liver cirrhosis: a meta-analysis of randomized controlled trials. J Gastroenterol Hepatol 2019;34(7):1143–52.

61. Plank LD, Gane EJ, Peng S, et al. Nocturnal nutritional supplementation improves total body protein status of patients with liver cirrhosis: a randomized 12-month trial. Hepatology 2008;48(2):557–66.

62. Tsien CD, McCullough AJ, Dasarathy S. Late evening snack: exploiting a period of anabolic opportunity in cirrhosis. J Gastroenterol Hepatol 2012;27(3):430–41.

63. Morando F, Rosi S, Gola E, et al. Adherence to a moderate sodium restriction diet in outpatients with cirrhosis and ascites: a real-life cross-sectional study. Liver Int 2015;35(5):1508–15.

64. Holecek M. Three targets of branched-chain amino acid supplementation in the treatment of liver disease. Nutrition 2010;26(5):482–90.

65. Marchesini G, Bianchi G, Merli M, et al. Nutritional supplementation with branched-chain amino acids in advanced cirrhosis: a double-blind, randomized trial. Gastroenterology 2003;124(7):1792–801.

66. Muto Y, Sato S, Watanabe A, et al. Effects of oral branched-chain amino acid granules on event-free survival in patients with liver cirrhosis. Clin Gastroenterol Hepatol 2005;3(7):705–13.

67. Les I, Doval E, García-Martínez R, et al. Effects of branched-chain amino acids supplementation in patients with cirrhosis and a previous episode of hepatic encephalopathy: a randomized study. Am J Gastroenterol 2011;106(6):1081–8.
68. Kawaguchi T, Shiraishi K, Ito T, et al. Branched-chain amino acids prevent hepatocarcinogenesis and prolong survival of patients with cirrhosis. Clin Gastroenterol Hepatol 2014;12(6):1012–8.
69. Ooi PH, Gilmour SM, Yap J, et al. Effects of branched chain amino acid supplementation on patient care outcomes in adults and children with liver cirrhosis: A systematic review. Clin Nutr ESPEN 2018;28(41):41–51.
70. Ismaiel A, Bucsa C, Farcas A, et al. Effects of branched-chain amino acids on parameters evaluating sarcopenia in liver cirrhosis: systematic review and meta-analysis. Front Nutr 2022;9(749969):1–3.
71. Gluud LL, Dam G, Les I, et al. Branched-chain amino acids for people with hepatic encephalopathy. Cochrane Database Syst Rev 2015;9:CD001939.
72. Plauth M, Bernal W, Dasarathy S, et al. ESPEN guideline on clinical nutrition in liver disease. Clin Nutr ESPEN 2019;38(2):485–521.
73. Warner ER 2nd, Aloor FZ, Satapathy SK. A narrative review of nutritional abnormalities, complications, and optimization in the cirrhotic patient. Transl Gastroenterol Hepatol 2022;7:5.
74. Rossi RE, Conte D, Massironi S. Diagnosis and treatment of nutritional deficiencies in alcoholic liver disease: Overview of available evidence and open issues. Dig Liver Dis 2015;47(10):819–25.
75. Wu J, Meng QH. Current understanding of the metabolism of micronutrients in chronic alcoholic liver disease. World J Gastroenterol 2020;26(31):4567–78.
76. Jorgensen RA, Lindor KD, Sartin JS, et al. Serum lipid and fat-soluble vitamin levels in primary sclerosing cholangitis. J Clin Gastroenterol 1995;20(3):215–9.
77. Phillips JR, Angulo P, Petterson T, et al. Fat-soluble vitamin levels in patients with primary biliary cirrhosis. Am J Gastroenterol 2001;96(9):2745–50.
78. Aagaard NK, Andersen H, Vilstrup H, et al. Decreased muscle strength and contents of Mg and Na,K-pumps in chronic alcoholics occur independently of liver cirrhosis. J Intern Med 2003;253(3):359–66.
79. Aagaard NK, Andersen H, Vilstrup H, et al. Muscle strength, Na,K-pumps, magnesium and potassium in patients with alcoholic liver cirrhosis – relation to spironolactone. J Intern Med 2002;252(1):56–63.
80. Rocchi E, Borella P, Borghi A, et al. Zinc and magnesium in liver cirrhosis. Eur J Clin Invest 1994;24(3):149–55.
81. Heubi JE, Higgins JV, Argao EA, et al. The role of magnesium in the pathogenesis of bone disease in childhood cholestatic liver disease: a preliminary report. J Pediatr Gastroenterol Nutr 1997;25(3):301–6.
82. Grüngreiff K, Reinhold D, Wedemeyer H. The role of zinc in liver cirrhosis. Ann Hepatol 2016;15(1):7–16.
83. Mohammad MK, Zhou Z, Cave M, et al. Zinc and liver disease. Nutr Clin Pract 2012;27(1):8–20.
84. Okubo T, Atsukawa M, Tsubota A, et al. Effect of Vitamin D supplementation on skeletal muscle volume and strength in patients with decompensated liver cirrhosis undergoing branched chain amino acids supplementation: a prospective, randomized, controlled pilot trial. Nutrients 2021;13(6):1874.
85. de Lédinghen V, Beau P, Mannant PR, et al. Early feeding or enteral nutrition in patients with cirrhosis after bleeding from esophageal varices? A randomized controlled study. Dig Dis Sci 1996;42(3):536–41.

86. Sidhu SS, Goyal O, Singh S, et al. Early feeding after esophageal variceal band ligation in cirrhotics is safe: Randomized controlled trial. Dig Endosc 2019;31(6): 646–52.

87. Fialla AD, Israelsen M, Hamberg O, et al. Nutritional therapy in cirrhosis or alcoholic hepatitis: a systematic review and meta-analysis. Liver Int 2015;35(9): 2072–8.

88. Berzigotti A, Albillos A, Villanueva C, et al. Effects of an intensive lifestyle intervention program on portal hypertension in patients with cirrhosis and obesity: The SportDiet study. Hepatology 2017;65(4):1293–305.

89. Duarte-Rojo A, Ruiz-Margáin A, Montaño-Loza AJ, et al. Exercise and physical activity for patients with end-stage liver disease: Improving functional status and sarcopenia while on the transplant waiting list. Liver Transpl 2018;24(1):122–39.

90. Kruger C, McNeely ML, Bailey RJ, et al. Home exercise training improves exercise capacity in cirrhosis patients: role of exercise adherence. Sci Rep 2018; 8(1):99.

91. Tandon P, Ismond KP, Riess K, et al. Exercise in cirrhosis: translating evidence and experience to practice. J Hepatol 2018;69(5):1164–77.

92. Williams FR, Berzigotti A, Lord JM, et al. Review article: impact of exercise on physical frailty in patients with chronic liver disease. Aliment Pharmacol Ther 2019;50(9):988–1000.

93. Zenith L, Meena N, Ramadi A, et al. Eight weeks of exercise training increases aerobic capacity and muscle mass and reduces fatigue in patients with cirrhosis. Clin Gastroenterol Hepatol 2014;12(11):1920–6.

94. Moctezuma-Velázquez C, Low G, Mourtzakis M, et al. Association between low testosterone levels and sarcopenia in cirrhosis: a cross-sectional study. Ann Hepatol 2018;17(4):615–23.

95. Sinclair M, Gow PJ, Grossmann M, et al. Low serum testosterone is associated with adverse outcome in men with cirrhosis independent of the model for end-stage liver disease score. Liver Transpl 2016;22(11):1482–90.

96. Sinclair M, Grossmann M, Gow P, et al. Testosterone in men with advanced liver disease: abnormalities and implications. J Gastroenterol Hepatol 2015;30(2): 244–51.

97. Rambaldi A, Gluud C. Anabolic-androgenic steroids for alcoholic liver disease. Cochrane Database Syst Rev 2006;2006(4):CD003045.

98. Yurci A, Yucesoy M, Unluhizarci K, et al. Effects of testosterone gel treatment in hypogonadal men with liver cirrhosis. Clin Res Hepatol Gastroenterol 2011; 35(12):845–54.

99. Sinclair M, Grossmann M, Hoermann R, et al. Testosterone therapy increases muscle mass in men with cirrhosis and low testosterone: A randomised controlled trial. J Hepatol 2016;65(5):906–13.

100. Grech A, Breck J, Heidelbaugh J. Adverse effects of testosterone replacement therapy: an update on the evidence and controversy. Ther Adv Drug Saf 2014; 5(5):190–200.

101. Johnson FL, Lerner KG, Siegel M, et al. Association of androgenic-anabolic steroid therapy with development of hepatocellular carcinoma. Lancet 1972; 2(7790):1273–6.

Liver Transplantation for the Nonhepatologist

Bethany Nahri So, BA[a], K. Rajender Reddy, MD[b],*

KEWORDS

- Liver transplantation • UNOS • MELD-Na

KEY POINTS

- Liver transplantation can be curative or life-prolonging for appropriately selected patients.
- The main indications for liver transplantation are acute liver failure, complications of cirrhosis, and liver-based metabolic diseases.
- Alcoholic liver disease has emerged as a leading indication for liver transplantation.
- A complete evaluation involves multidisciplinary specialists knowledgeable in transplant candidate selection, calculation of a MELD/MELD-Na score, and assessment for major comorbidities.
- Complications after liver transplantation early on are recognized and managed by the transplant team, whereas long-term care may require the involvement of the primary care physician, particularly in the management of comorbidities such as hypertension and diabetes mellitus.

INTRODUCTION

The management of advanced liver diseases has been revolutionized by liver transplantation (LT). The vast majority of LTs are orthotopic, meaning a new liver is placed in the same anatomic location of the native liver. Since the first liver transplantation in 1963, there has been an increase in the number of successful outcomes, including increases in patient survival and graft survival rates.[1] Today, the outcomes of LTs extend beyond amelioration of liver complications by extending life expectancy and improving quality of life.[2,3] LT can be curative or life-prolonging for appropriately selected patients with acute and chronic end-stage liver disease in whom medical therapies have failed.[3] LT is most notably performed in patients with decompensated cirrhosis (DC), a steady deterioration of liver function that may take the form of various complications such as jaundice, ascites, hepatic encephalopathy, hepatorenal

a Division of Gastroenterology and Hepatology, University of Pennsylvania Perelman School of Medicine, Philadelphia, PA, USA; b Division of Gastroenterology and Hepatology, University of Pennsylvania Perelman School of Medicine, University of Pennsylvania, 2 Dulles, 3400 Spruce Street, HUP, Philadelphia, PA 19104, USA
* Corresponding author.
E-mail address: reddyr@pennmedicine.upenn.edu

Med Clin N Am 107 (2023) 605–621
https://doi.org/10.1016/j.mcna.2023.01.004
0025-7125/23/© 2023 Elsevier Inc. All rights reserved.

syndrome, or variceal hemorrhage.[4] Upward of 80% of liver transplantations are for DC.[5] The United Network for Organ Sharing (UNOS) is in charge of revising liver allocation and distribution policies continuously on the principles of justice and utility. Historically, UNOS has allocated livers to the sickest patients while waiting on transplant lists. The number of total organ transplants in 2021 set an all-time record at 41,356 organ transplants, of which 9236 were liver transplants (based on Organ Procurement and Transplantation Network [OPTN] as of December 21, 2022).

Although the delivery and maintenance following liver transplants have seen substantial progress, several areas of uncertainty still remain. Current allocation policy gives highest priority to patients listed as Status 1A by the OPTN. This status indicates the patient has highest urgency due to sudden and severe onset of liver failure and will likely die without transplant in a few days. Although the liver allocation system prioritizes highest short-term mortality risk, inequality in access to liver transplantation continues to be addressed. Although advances in pretransplant and posttransplant critical care, technical skills, and pharmacologic interventions have been made, challenges to long-term management following surgery, immunosuppression, and recurrence of disease remain.[6] In light of the changing landscape for LT intervention, this article provides insight into indications and contraindications for LT, different prognostic and organ allocation models, and guidelines for long-term care after LT.

LIVER TRANSPLANTATION: INDICATIONS/CONTRAINDICATIONS

All LTs begin with determination of indications, followed by an evaluation process. The American Association for the Study of Liver Diseases outlines 4 major categories of indications: (1) acute liver failure, (2) complications of cirrhosis, (3) liver-based metabolic diseases, and (4) systemic complications of chronic liver disease.[3] The presence of hepatic artery thrombosis within 14 days of LT, and leading to graft failure, is also an infrequent indication. These primary indications are listed and further defined in **Box 1**.

Box 1
Indications for liver transplantation

Acute liver failure

One or more complications of cirrhosis
- Ascites; hepatorenal syndrome
- Hepatic encephalopathy
- Hepatocellular carcinoma
- Variceal hemorrhage
- Synthetic dysfunction

Liver-based metabolic diseases
- Alpha-1 antitrypsin deficiency
- Wilson disease
- Familial amyloidosis
- Glycogen storage disease
- Hemochromatosis
- Primary hyperoxaluria
- Hepatic involvement in cystic fibrosis

Extrahepatic complications of chronic liver disease
- Hepatopulmonary syndrome
- Portopulmonary hypertension

Until recently, the most common indication for LT in the United States was cirrhosis due to chronic hepatitis C viral (HCV) infection.[3] Globally, hepatitis B virus (HBV)-related liver disease is also a dominant indication. Although active pre-LT HCV infection had been associated with high rates of graft dysfunction due to recurrent HCV and progression to cirrhosis within 5 to 10 years of LT, the outcomes more lately have been considerably good due to the advent of safe and effective oral therapies for HCV.[7] Now, the leading indication for LT in the United States is alcoholic liver disease (ALD), whereas nonalcoholic fatty liver disease as a cause accounts for a significant proportion of cases[8] (**Fig. 1**; Kwong and colleagues[9]).

The number of those with ALD is further projected to increase.[10] Over the years, the comorbidity profile among patients admitted for ALD has also worsened, with increases in type 2 diabetes and coronary artery disease as noted in a study spanning 2000 to 2011.[10] The same study showed that ALD was associated with a significantly higher mortality compared with all other admission diagnoses. Although hepatocellular carcinoma (HCC) remains a major indication for LT, among the US adult recipient population, liver transplants for HCC have declined from 17.2% in 2010% to 12.6% in 2020.[9]

Contraindications to LT may be absolute or relative, and the latter vary according to centers' experience and policy (**Table 1**).

LIVER TRANSPLANTATION: EVALUATION PROCESS

Once LT is indicated, evaluation should be promptly completed because onset of hepatic decompensation can cause a patient's clinical course to worsen rapidly. An evaluation for LT should be considered once a patient with cirrhosis experiences one or more of index complications as outlined in **Box 1**.[3] Potentially treatable components

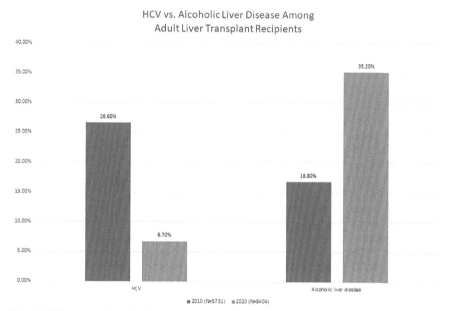

Fig. 1. HCV versus alcoholic liver disease: liver transplants. (*Data from* Kwong AJ, Ebel NH, Kim WR, et al. OPTN/SRTR 2020 Annual Data Report: Liver. Am J Transplant. Mar 2022;22 Suppl 2:204-309. https://doi.org/10.1111/ajt.16978.)

Table 1 Contraindications for liver transplantation	
Absolute Contraindications	**Relative Contraindications**
• Severe cardiopulmonary disease • Active malignancy outside of liver • Persistent noncompliance (ie, ongoing alcohol or illicit substance abuse) • Intrahepatic cholangiocarcinoma (although this is being increased considered in select centers under a defined management protocol) • Active, uncontrolled infection (sepsis) • Lack of adequate social support system	• Advanced age • Cigarette smokers • Severe coronary artery disease • Acute alcoholic hepatitis • HIV infection • BMI at extremes ○ BMI ≥40 (class 3 obesity) • Psychiatric disorders

Abbreviations: BMI, body mass index; HIV, human immunodeficiency virus.

of a patient's hepatic decompensation should be addressed concurrently while moving forward with an evaluation for LT.

Although specific evaluation processes vary across different transplant centers, there are features shared among all. Key features of a complete evaluation include an initial assessment of liver disease severity with the Child-Pugh-Turcotte (CPT) or Model for End-stage Liver Disease (MELD) score. The psychosocial state of a potential LT candidate must also be considered, such as the presence of adequate social support or issues that may complicate the patient's ability to follow a rigorous post-LT regimen after enduring a major surgical procedure. Another important feature is the presence of major comorbid conditions that are likely to preclude a successful LT.[3] **Table 2** outlines several medical comorbidities frequently presented by potential candidates (see **Table 2**; Martin and colleagues,[3] Arguedas and colleagues,[11] Gupta and colleagues[12]).

Other important elements include laboratory testing, hepatology and transplant surgery consultation, cardiopulmonary evaluation, hepatic imaging, general health assessment, infectious disease assessment, anesthesia and dietician evaluation, financial screening, and social work assessment.

A partial liver or whole liver comes from a living or deceased donor, respectively. In a living donor liver transplantation (LDLT), usually the right lobe of the liver from a living adult donor is transplanted into an adult recipient. Deceased donor liver transplantations (DDLT) are more often performed, and the number of DDLTs has been trending upward each year with 8667 performed in 2021; in contrast, LDLT rates have seen a less consistent increase with 569 performed in 2021 (based on OPTN as of November 18, 2022). A comparison of the trends in DDLT (blue) and LDLT (pink) over the years is depicted in **Fig. 2.**

Intended to shorten the long waitlist times and mortality, LDLT was performed as a promising alternative to DDLT for the first time in the United States in 1989. LDLT was initially developed to provide suitable liver grafts for pediatric patients with end-stage liver disease.[13] The procedure was soon expanded to adult-to-adult LDLT. The safety and efficacy of LDLT compared with DDLT have steadily increased over time as experience was gained, and now there is convincing evidence that LDLT is a viable option for expanding the liver donor pool.[14–16]

A complete evaluation of the living donor includes assessment and education of medical risks, psychological risk factors, and suitability of the donor liver graft in regard to quality, size, vascular, and biliary anatomy.[17]

Table 2
Important comorbidities in liver transplantation evaluation

Medical Comorbidity	What to Know
Older age	• Associated with cardiopulmonary risk factors • Older patients require thorough evaluation to rule out absolute contraindications, particularly of cardiovascular disease, and malignancy, to LT
Obesity	• Obesity in LT recipients has been associated with an increased risk of perioperative complications and reduced long-term survival • Obese patients should receive dietary counseling before LT
Coronary artery disease	• Cardiopulmonary disorders preclude a good long-term outcome of LT • Noninvasive testing with stress echocardiography is needed for all adult LT candidates. With associated comorbidities such as DM, even coronary angiography and any needed intervention would need to be pursued • Surgical cardiac revascularization may need to be considered in those with significant stenosis, although there might be a surgical risk due to background of advanced cirrhosis[3]
Portopulmonary hypertension	• Defined as an elevation of mean pulmonary artery pressure ≥ 25 mm Hg in setting of portal hypertension • Moderate to severe portopulmonary hypertension is associated with increased mortality following LT • Routine echocardiography and vasodilator therapy evaluation is recommended
Hepatopulmonary syndrome	• Defined by liver failure, abnormal arterial oxygenation, and intrapulmonary vascular dilatations • Screening by pulse oximetry is recommended and bubble echocardiogram is diagnostic • Association between severity of hepatopulmonary syndrome and increased mortality post-LT has mixed opinions[11,12]
Renal dysfunction	• Thorough evaluation is required to determine cause and prognosis, including estimation of glomerular filtrate rate • Simultaneous liver-kidney transplantation may be indicated for qualified candidates
Osteoporosis (bone disease)	• Characterized by low bone mineral density and susceptibility to fracture • Common complication in patients with cirrhosis • Bone densitometry and treatment of osteoporosis is recommended before LT
HIV	• For HIV-infected candidates to be eligible for LT, immune function must be adequate and virus should be undetectable by time of LT

Abbreviations: DM, diabetes mellitus; HIV, human immunodeficiency virus.

PROGNOSIS MODELS

Allocation models for listing potential LT candidates and predicting waiting list mortality must be based on unbiased criteria. The first system developed was the CPT score, which was originally designed for predicting the outcome of surgery for portal hypertension in patients with cirrhosis.[18] The CPT score was historically used for liver transplant allocations.[19] The CPT score is based on grades or measurements of 5 criteria:

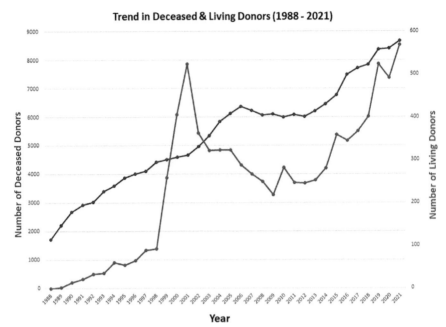

Fig. 2. DDLT and LDLT trends (1988–2021). (*Data from* OPTN as of November 18, 2022.)

encephalopathy, ascites, bilirubin, albumin, and prothrombin time.[19] Often, the international normalized ratio (INR) is used in the place of prothrombin time because it allows for test results to be compared between different laboratories. However, the CPT score does not come without limitations. One of the major limitations is that it does not have precise differentiating capability of the severity of cirrhosis.[18] Another is that it does not account for specific variables that have been shown to have significant impact on cirrhosis prognosis, such as serum creatinine.[20] Finally, it is subjective in assessing certain variables such as ascites and hepatic encephalopathy.

A more comprehensive score that followed was the MELD score, which uses a broader range of more continuous variables.[19] The MELD score could be applied to patients with various causes of cirrhosis and varied degrees of severity.[18] Consisting of serum bilirubin, creatinine, and INR, the MELD score is a continuous variable that ranges from 6 to 40. Even though bilirubin, creatinine, and INR are meant to be objective variables, the MELD score still is subject to variation.[18,21] For instance, one study has shown a downward trend in the c-statistic of the MELD score with 90-day waitlist mortality, beginning at around 0.80 in 2002 and decreasing to 0.73 in 2015.[22] This trend may be due to the declining incidence in the number of listed patients with hepatitis C, a diagnosis associated with high correlation between MELD and mortality.[22]

Since the implementation of MELD, various improved versions have followed. One of the more critical derivatives is the MELD-Na score, which as is suggested includes serum sodium to provide a more accurate survival prediction than MELD alone. The addition of sodium was based off the observation that hyponatremia is a strong independent predictor of mortality in patients with cirrhosis.[23,24] Using OPTN data between 2005 and 2006, Kim and colleagues[25] proposed the MELD-Na model as a way to decrease waitlist mortality. Since its introduction in the United States in 2016, MELD-Na is now the most widely adopted allocation model in the field.[21] The

MELD-Na score provides 1 to 11 additional points to the MELD score. Several studies have shown that liver allocations based on the MELD-Na were associated with a decreased waitlist mortality, including one that saw a 33.5% decrease in the MELD-Na period compared with the MELD period.[26] However, the MELD-Na score does not come without limitations and still includes several of those in the original MELD score. For instance, MELD-Na and MELD use serum creatinine to measure renal function, but this value may not necessarily be a precise marker for renal function in LT candidates. Women, in particular, are observed to have lower creatinine-derived MELD points than men with similar renal dysfunction, which then increases the waitlist time for women.[27] This disadvantage in women is due to their generally lower muscle mass, and thus reduced creatinine levels, compared with that of men.

With these limitations in mind, another model called the MELD 3.0 was developed by Kim and colleagues[28] in 2021. MELD 3.0 adds 2 additional variables to the MELD-Na model: female sex and serum albumin. The MELD 3.0 was determined to have significantly higher discriminative capability than MELD-Na.[28] However, it is important to note that the accuracy of this model, in addition to that of other MELD-Na alternatives, must continue to be tested. Other alterations to the MELD score continue to be explored today, including replacing current MELD-Na measurements or introducing more variables.

MODEL FOR END-STAGE LIVER DISEASE EXCEPTION POINTS

A critical aspect of MELD scoring is delegation of exception points. The purpose of exception points is to reflect a patient's waitlist mortality and thus provide prioritization for LT.[29] For many conditions, the underlying liver disease is not characterized by a high-enough risk of short-term mortality, so the prediction of a short-term LT according to MELD may not be entirely accurate.[30] If a clinician feels a potential candidate has a risk of death not captured by the exception score criteria, an appeal for consideration of nonstandard exception points can be submitted. MELD score exception requests are submitted to the National Liver Review Board, which reviews requests on an anonymous basis to ensure fair and objective consideration of all patients. The medical condition must first be indexed at a level of urgency similar to those without exceptions. This index is based on the median of MELD scores, called the Median MELD at Transplant (MMaT), for people who have recently received LTs in the area surrounding the hospital where there is a liver donor. An exception request consists of the request itself for an adjustment of a certain number of points higher than MMaT or a specific MELD, and the justification behind such request. To qualify for an exception, the potential candidate's medical conditions must meet criteria outlined in OPTN policy. Much consideration of MELD exception scoring has gone toward HCC, an increasingly important indication for LT. A critical study by Mazzaferro and colleagues[31] from Milan showed that LT is an effective treatment of small, unresectable HCC in patients with cirrhosis in a prospective study on 48 subjects. As such, patients with HCC receive MELD exception points, although over the years there have been several adjustments made to the policy.

WAITLIST OUTCOMES

LT candidates are removed from waitlist for several reasons, the most common being for DDLT or LDLT, followed by death on the waiting list, or being too sick for transplant.[9] Morbidity- and mortality-related reasons for waitlist removal over the past decade are depicted in **Fig. 3**. In 2020, the pre-LT mortality rate reached an all-time low of 12.2 per 100 patient-years on waitlist.[9] Pre-LT mortality was found to be highest

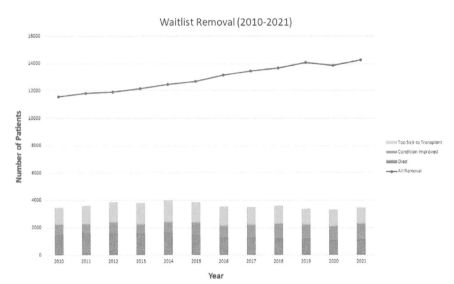

Fig. 3. Waitlist removal reasons. (*Data from* OPTN as of November 18, 2022.)

in candidates with acute liver failure and the lowest in those with HCV or HCC.[9] An active area of research is on determining how waitlist outcomes differ according to liver disease cause. In keeping with ALD as the top indication for LT, it has been suggested that due to alcohol abstinence, LT candidates with ALD may experience lower risk of waitlist removal for death or being too sick compared with patients with other chronic liver diseases such as nonalcoholic steatohepatitis (NASH).[32] In a retrospective study using OPTN/UNOS registry data from 2016 to 2018, 90-day and 1-year waitlist mortality were found to be significantly higher in NASH compared with ALD.[33] In the same study, HCV was found to have similar low risk as ALD, suggesting the efficacy of antiviral therapies in reducing waitlist mortality. Owing to such documented differences in waitlist outcomes, careful monitoring of MELD-Na score and comorbidities is recommended for separate liver disease etiologies.

LONG-TERM CARE AND MANAGEMENT

Complications may arise early or later after LT. Key complications are listed according to the general timeline in **Fig. 4**.

The early complications are primarily addressed by the transplant center. Primary nonfunction of the allograft, the most serious complication, often presents with lack of bile production or clear bile production. A new graft is required for patient survival. Shortly after LT is performed, liver tests are routinely monitored and immunosuppressive medications are administered and adjusted to prevent graft dysfunction. Although the incidence of chronic rejection has decreased over the years, acute cellular rejection is still common.[34] Rejection is reliably diagnosed by liver histology. Biliary complications are managed in a center with expertise in radiology and biliary endoscopy.[35] Bile leaks are more common in immediate postoperative period, whereas biliary strictures are more common weeks to months after surgery[36] (**Fig. 5**).

The purpose of long-term immunosuppression is to balance the risk of graft rejection against the risk of immunosuppression-related complications. The immunosuppressive medications generally fall into 4 groups.

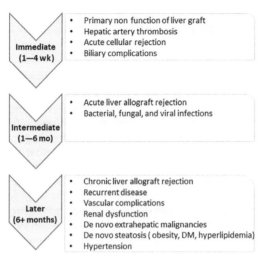

Fig. 4. Post-LT complications. DM, diabetes mellitus.

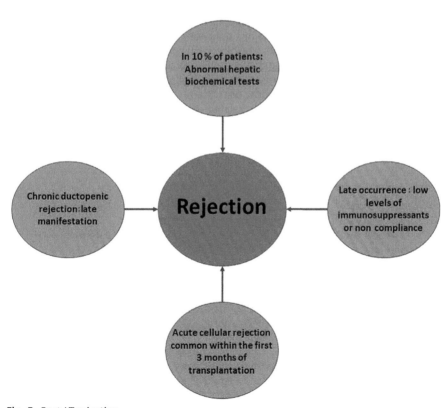

Fig. 5. Post-LT rejection.

- Calcineurin inhibitors
- Mammalian target of rapamycin (mTOR)
- Antimetabolites
- Corticosteroids

The most commonly prescribed immunosuppressive agents are tacrolimus and cyclosporine, both of which are calcineurin inhibitors.[37] Higher levels of calcineurin inhibitors are needed in the initial post-LT period to prevent graft rejection; lower levels are preferred later to reduce the severity of adverse effects. Tacrolimus is used more often than cyclosporine because it has been shown to be superior in the context of survival, graft loss, acute rejection, and steroid-resistant rejection in the first year of administration.[37,38] However, diabetes mellitus and bone marrow suppression are encountered in more patients on tacrolimus compared with those on cyclosporine.[37]

Unlike calcineurin inhibitors, mTORs have lower risks of nephrotoxicity, neurotoxicity, or hypertension. The most commonly used mTORs, which inhibit the proliferation of lymphocytes, are sirolimus and everolimus. Known complications of sirolimus include hepatic artery thrombosis and wound dehiscence.[39] Compared with sirolimus, everolimus has more potent antiproliferative effects and has not been associated with hepatic artery thrombosis.[40–42] Studies on the safety and efficacy of everolimus have mainly supported use of everolimus in combination therapy to minimize post-LT renal dysfunction.[41,43] Everolimus complications include dose-dependent dyslipidemia, hematologic abnormalities, skin rashes, and mouth ulcers.[44]

Mycophenolate mofetil and azathioprine are commonly prescribed antimetabolites, but these are not potent enough to be administered alone.[37] At present, most LT centers have replaced azathioprine with mycophenolic acid.[45] Corticosteroids may also be administered in combination with a calcineurin inhibitor as part of standard therapy. It has been observed in several studies that the use of steroids during postoperative immunosuppression may be associated with a higher risk of developing posttransplant diabetes mellitus in a dose-dependent manner.[46]

The most common complications related to immunosuppression toxicity are chronic kidney disease, diabetes mellitus, hypertension, obesity, and dyslipidemia. The key care points for long-term management of immunosuppression-induced complications are outlined in **Fig. 6.**

Clinics Care Points for Immunosuppression-Related Complications

- Bone disease
  - Osteoporosis and osteopenia are most common
  - Osteoporosis risk increases by long-term use of corticosteroids and poor nutrition[1]
  - For LT recipient with osteopenia: weight-bearing exercise, calcium, and vitamin D supplements recommended[35]
  - For LT recipients with osteoporosis:
    - Reduction of corticosteroid dosage and bisphosphonate therapy recommended[35]
    - Raloxifene, an estrogen agonist in bones that decreases bone resorption and bone turnover, may benefit patients with cirrhosis[47]
    - Denosumab, recently recommended by the American Association of Clinical Endocrinologists/American College of Endocrinology, may be a viable therapeutic option for LT recipients with kidney failure or intolerance to bisphosphonates[48,49]

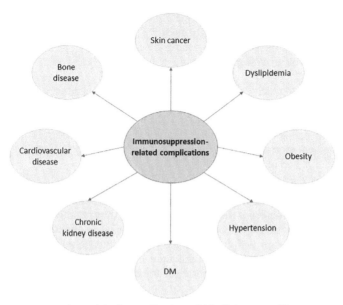

Fig. 6. Immunosuppression-related complications. DM, diabetes mellitus.

- Hormone therapy is not recommended out of concerns for malignancy and availability of other effective nonhormonal agents with fewer adverse effects[50]
- Cardiovascular disease
  - Artherosclerosis-related cardiovascular disease is a major cause of long-term mortality post-LT
  - Risk must be monitored especially in cigarette smokers
- Chronic kidney disease
  - Most common causes include diabetic nephropathy and calcineurin inhibitor toxicity
  - Renal function should be monitored regularly by microalbuminuria screening and glomerular filtration rate measurements[1]
  - Immunosuppression may need to be modified in those who develop renal dysfunction
- Diabetes mellitus
  - Insulin is universally used shortly after LT, but optimal timing of transition to noninsulin therapy is unclear
  - Lifestyle changes recommended first, followed by antidiabetic agents
  - Treatment goal: hemoglobin A_{1c} less than 7.0%[35]
- Hypertension
  - Typically caused by increased system vascular resistance post-LT
  - Treatment goal: 130/80 mm Hg[35]
- Obesity
  - Ongoing dietary counseling recommended
  - Bariatric surgery may be considered for LT recipients who become severely or morbidly obese[35]
- Dyslipidemia
  - Most LT recipients have abnormal lipid metabolism

- o Most common type: Hypertriglyceridemia
  - o First treated with omega-3 fatty acids[35]
  - o Often persists despite dietary changes
  - o Primary choice of medication: statins[1]
- Skin cancer
  - o Nonmelanoma skin cancer is the most common malignancy post-LT[51]
  - o Squamous cell carcinoma is more aggressive in LT recipients compared with the general population[51]
  - o Regular screening by a dermatologist is essential to minimize morbidity and occasional mortality
  - o Additional sun exposure should be avoided[45]
  - o Skin protective agents should be applied

Other long-term complications include recurrent disease and de novo malignancies. In the context of LT, recurrent HBV is a concern, and thus effective prophylactic strategies are pursued while HCV is of little to no concern given effective antivirals. Long-term prophylactic therapy with a combination of antiviral agents and low-dose hepatitis B immune globulin, used for a variable time, can prevent HBV recurrence.[35] Other recurrent diseases include NASH, primary biliary cirrhosis, primary sclerosing cholangitis, and HCC. De novo malignancies, a major cause of death in post-LT recipients in the long-term, may arise from immunosuppression, viral infections, continued alcohol use, cigarette smoking, and older age.[45] Common de novo malignancies are shown in **Fig. 7**. Reducing to the lowest possible level of calcineurin inhibitors in patients with de novo malignancies may improve post-LT outcomes.[45]

Drug-Drug Interactions in the Liver Transplant Recipients

Whenever new medications are begun, it is important to check for possible interactions between the new and concomitant drugs, particularly tacrolimus, cyclosporine,

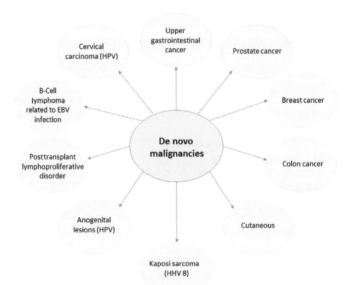

Fig. 7. Common de novo malignancies. EBV, Epstein-Barr virus; HHV 8, human herpesvirus 8; Kaposi sarcoma-associated herpesvirus; HPV, human papillomavirus.

and sirolimus. Tacrolimus, cyclosporine, and sirolimus are metabolized by cytochrome P450 3A4 (CYP3A4), so they may interact with drugs that induce or inhibit this enzyme. The 3 immunosuppressants are all also substrates for P-glycoprotein, a cell membrane-associated transporter protein that influences drug absorption and elimination. It is recommended to avoid medication agents that would affect the metabolism of these immunosuppressants, including those primarily metabolized by the CYP3A4 or P-glycoprotein pathways. **Fig. 8** shows several common CYP3A4 inhibitors and inducers that may impact the plasma concentrations of tacrolimus, cyclosporine, and sirolimus.[52] Some drug interactions are almost universal, whereas others may be seen in rare cases, so a transplant pharmacist should be consulted for specific guidance.

Vaccination in the Liver Transplant Candidates and Recipients

In the posttransplant period, a maximal state of immunosuppression is often observed in the first 6 months, thus increasing risk of infection (see **Fig. 4**). It is recommended that required vaccination schedules be implemented as early as possible before LT due to low immunogenicity after transplantation. When available, vaccine serology after vaccination should be performed. For immunizations after LT, in the absence of any ongoing graft rejection, an interval of 3 to 6 months is usually recommended to improve vaccine immunogenicity.[53] A notable exception is inactivated influenza vaccine, which may be administered as early as 1 month after LT.[53] Common vaccines safe in post-LT patients and household contacts include those for invasive pneumococcal disease, hepatitis A virus, HBV, human papillomavirus, and diphtheria, tetanus, poliomyelitis and acellular pertussis.[54] Except for selected patients with confirmed risk factors, live attenuated vaccines are contraindicated after transplantation, and thus must be administered with at least 4 weeks between vaccination and transplantation.[53] Of note, the live attenuated varicella vaccine has been implemented safely in selected long-term LT recipients on low-dose immunosuppression.[54]

In light of the coronavirus disease 2019 (COVID-19) global pandemic since March 2020, much attention has surrounded the effectiveness and safety of the COVID-19 vaccine in LT recipients, who are particularly vulnerable to severe COVID-19. Based on favorable outcomes in recent studies, LT recipients are strongly recommended

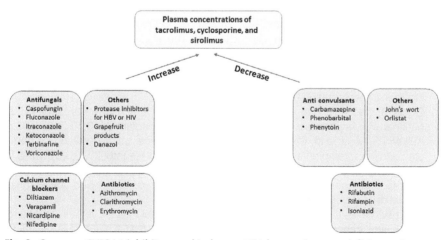

Fig. 8. Common CYP3A4 inhibitors and inducers. HIV, human immunodeficiency virus.

to receive COVID-19 vaccination to reduce morbidity and mortality.[55,56] LT candidates should receive a COVID-19 vaccine before LT whenever possible. If not possible, the optimal time to administer the vaccine is after 3 months post-LT.[57] However, immunization may begin as early as 4 weeks post-LT in high-risk individuals.[57] COVID-19 vaccination should be avoided in LT recipients with active acute cellular rejection.[57]

After 6 months, most patients' immunosuppression levels reach maintenance level, decreasing the risk of opportunistic infections. At this time, patients usually present with infections common among patients without a history of transplantation, such as pneumonias and influenza.

DISCLOSURE

No disclosure relevant to this work.

REFERENCES

1. Oustecky DH, Riera AR, Rothstein KD. Long-term management of the liver transplant recipient: pearls for the practicing gastroenterologist. Gastroenterol Clin North Am 2011;40(3):659–81.
2. Desai R, Jamieson NV, Gimson AE, et al. Quality of life up to 30 years following liver transplantation. Liver Transpl 2008;14(10):1473–9.
3. Martin P, DiMartini A, Feng S, et al. Evaluation for liver transplantation in adults: 2013 practice guideline by the American Association for the Study of Liver Diseases and the American Society of Transplantation. Hepatol 2014;59(3):1144–65.
4. Mansour D, McPherson S. Management of decompensated cirrhosis. Clin Med (Lond) 2018;18(Suppl 2):s60–5.
5. Seaberg EC, Belle SH, Beringer KC, et al. Liver transplantation in the United States from 1987-1998: updated results from the Pitt-UNOS Liver Transplant Registry. Clin Transpl 1998;17–37.
6. Ganschow R, Pollok JM, Jankofsky M, et al. The role of everolimus in liver transplantation. Clin Exp Gastroenterol 2014;7:329–43.
7. Rubin A, Aguilera V, Berenguer M. Liver transplantation and hepatitis C. Clin Res Hepatol Gastroenterol 2011;35(12):805–12.
8. Dababneh Y, Mousa OY. Liver transplantation. Treasure Island (FL): StatPearls Publishing; 2022.
9. Kwong AJ, Ebel NH, Kim WR, et al. OPTN/SRTR 2020 annual data report: liver. Am J Transplant 2022;22(Suppl 2):204–309.
10. Nguyen TA, DeShazo JP, Thacker LR, et al. The worsening profile of alcoholic hepatitis in the United States. Alcohol Clin Exp Res 2016;40(6):1295–303.
11. Arguedas MR, Abrams GA, Krowka MJ, et al. Prospective evaluation of outcomes and predictors of mortality in patients with hepatopulmonary syndrome undergoing liver transplantation. Hepatol 2003;37(1):192–7.
12. Gupta S, Castel H, Rao RV, et al. Improved survival after liver transplantation in patients with hepatopulmonary syndrome. Am J Transplant 2010;10(2):354–63.
13. Kulkarni S, Malago M, Cronin DC 2nd. Living donor liver transplantation for pediatric and adult recipients. Nat Clin Pract Gastroenterol Hepatol 2006;3(3):149–57.
14. Thuluvath PJ, Yoo HY. Graft and patient survival after adult live donor liver transplantation compared to a matched cohort who received a deceased donor transplantation. Liver Transpl 2004;10(10):1263–8.
15. Liang W, Wu L, Ling X, et al. Living donor liver transplantation versus deceased donor liver transplantation for hepatocellular carcinoma: a meta-analysis. Liver Transpl 2012;18(10):1226–36.

16. Hoehn RS, Wilson GC, Wima K, et al. Comparing living donor and deceased donor liver transplantation: a matched national analysis from 2007 to 2012. Liver Transpl 2014;20(11):1347–55.
17. Broering DC, Sterneck M, Rogiers X. Living donor liver transplantation. J Hepatol 2003;38(Suppl 1):S119–35.
18. Durand F, Valla D. Assessment of prognosis of cirrhosis. Semin Liver Dis 2008; 28(1):110–22.
19. Tsoris A, Marlar CA. Use of the child Pugh score in liver disease. Treasure Island (FL): StatPearls Publishing; 2022.
20. Fernandez-Esparrach G, Sanchez-Fueyo A, Gines P, et al. A prognostic model for predicting survival in cirrhosis with ascites. J Hepatol 2001;34(1):46–52.
21. Burra P, Samuel D, Sundaram V, et al. Limitations of current liver donor allocation systems and the impact of newer indications for liver transplantation. J Hepatol 2021;75(Suppl 1):S178–90.
22. Godfrey EL, Malik TH, Lai JC, et al. The decreasing predictive power of MELD in an era of changing etiology of liver disease. Am J Transplant 2019;19(12): 3299–307.
23. Biggins SW, Rodriguez HJ, Bacchetti P, et al. Serum sodium predicts mortality in patients listed for liver transplantation. Hepatol 2005;41(1):32–9.
24. Ruf AE, Kremers WK, Chavez LL, et al. Addition of serum sodium into the MELD score predicts waiting list mortality better than MELD alone. Liver Transpl 2005; 11(3):336–43.
25. Kim WR, Biggins SW, Kremers WK, et al. Hyponatremia and mortality among patients on the liver-transplant waiting list. N Engl J Med 2008;359(10):1018–26.
26. Nagai S, Chau LC, Schilke RE, et al. Effects of allocating livers for transplantation based on model for end-stage liver disease-sodium scores on patient outcomes. Gastroenterol 2018;155(5):1451–62.e3.
27. Allen AM, Heimbach JK, Larson JJ, et al. Reduced access to liver transplantation in women: role of height, MELD exception scores, and renal function underestimation. Transplantation 2018;102(10):1710–6.
28. Kim WR, Mannalithara A, Heimbach JK, et al. MELD 3.0: the model for end-stage liver disease updated for the modern era. Gastroenterology 2021;161(6): 1887–95.e4.
29. Parikh ND, Singal AG. Model for end-stage liver disease exception points for treatment-responsive hepatocellular carcinoma. Clin Liver Dis (Hoboken) 2016; 7(5):97–100.
30. Freeman RB Jr, Gish RG, Harper A, et al. Model for end-stage liver disease (MELD) exception guidelines: results and recommendations from the MELD Exception Study Group and Conference (MESSAGE) for the approval of patients who need liver transplantation with diseases not considered by the standard MELD formula. Liver Transpl 2006;12(12 Suppl 3):S128–36.
31. Mazzaferro V, Regalia E, Doci R, et al. Liver transplantation for the treatment of small hepatocellular carcinomas in patients with cirrhosis. N Engl J Med 1996; 334(11):693–9.
32. Giard JM, Dodge JL, Terrault NA. Superior wait-list outcomes in patients with alcohol-associated liver disease compared with other indications for liver transplantation. Liver Transpl 2019;25(9):1310–20.
33. Nagai S, Safwan M, Kitajima T, et al. Disease-specific waitlist outcomes in liver transplantation - a retrospective study. Transpl Int 2021;34(3):499–513.

34. Choudhary NS, Saigal S, Bansal RK, et al. Acute and chronic rejection after liver transplantation: what a clinician needs to know. J Clin Exp Hepatol 2017;7(4): 358–66.

35. Lucey MR, Terrault N, Ojo L, et al. Long-term management of the successful adult liver transplant: 2012 practice guideline by the American Association for the Study of Liver Diseases and the American Society of Transplantation. Liver Transpl 2013;19(1):3–26.

36. Ayoub WS, Esquivel CO, Martin P. Biliary complications following liver transplantation. Dig Dis Sci 2010;55(6):1540–6.

37. Issa DH, Alkhouri N. Long-term management of liver transplant recipients: a review for the internist. Cleve Clin J Med 2015;82(6):361–72.

38. McAlister VC, Haddad E, Renouf E, et al. Cyclosporin versus tacrolimus as primary immunosuppressant after liver transplantation: a meta-analysis. Am J Transplant 2006;6(7):1578–85.

39. Montalbano M, Neff GW, Yamashiki N, et al. A retrospective review of liver transplant patients treated with sirolimus from a single center: an analysis of sirolimus-related complications. Transplant 2004;78(2):264–8.

40. Jin YP, Valenzuela NM, Ziegler ME, et al. Everolimus inhibits anti-HLA I antibody-mediated endothelial cell signaling, migration and proliferation more potently than sirolimus. Am J Transplant 2014;14(4):806–19.

41. De Simone P, Nevens F, De Carlis L, et al. Everolimus with reduced tacrolimus improves renal function in de novo liver transplant recipients: a randomized controlled trial. Am J Transplant 2012;12(11):3008–20.

42. Rodriguez-Peralvarez M, Perez-Medrano I, Guerrero-Misas M, et al. Everolimus is safe within the first month after liver transplantation. Transpl Immunol 2015;33(2): 146–51.

43. Guan TW, Lin YJ, Ou MY, et al. Efficacy and safety of everolimus treatment on liver transplant recipients: a meta-analysis. Eur J Clin Invest 2019;49(12):e13179.

44. Di Maira T, Little EC, Berenguer M. Immunosuppression in liver transplant. Best Pract Res Clin Gastroenterol 2020;46-47:101681.

45. Colmenero J, Tabrizian P, Bhangui P, et al. De novo malignancy after liver transplantation: risk assessment, prevention, and management-guidelines from the ILTS-SETH consensus conference. Transplant 2022;106(1):e30–45.

46. Pagadala M, Dasarathy S, Eghtesad B, et al. Posttransplant metabolic syndrome: an epidemic waiting to happen. Liver Transpl 2009;15(12):1662–70.

47. Levy C, Harnois DM, Angulo P, et al. Raloxifene improves bone mass in osteopenic women with primary biliary cirrhosis: results of a pilot study. Liver Int 2005;25(1):117–21.

48. Brunova J, Kratochvilova S, Stepankova J. Osteoporosis therapy with denosumab in organ transplant recipients. Front Endocrinol (Lausanne) 2018;9:162.

49. Camacho PM, Petak SM, Binkley N, et al. American association of clinical endocrinologists/american college of endocrinology clinical practice guidelines for the diagnosis and treatment of postmenopausal osteoporosis-2020 update. Endocr Pract 2020;26(Suppl 1):1–46.

50. Rodriguez-Aguilar EF, Perez-Escobar J, Sanchez Herrera D, et al. Bone disease and liver transplantation: a review. Transplant Proc 2021;53(7):2346–53.

51. Herrero JI, Espana A, Quiroga J, et al. Nonmelanoma skin cancer after liver transplantation. Study of risk factors. Liver Transpl 2005;11(9):1100–6.

52. McGuire BM, Rosenthal P, Brown CC, et al. Long-term management of the liver transplant patient: recommendations for the primary care doctor. Am J Transplant 2009;9(9):1988–2003.

53. Valour F, Conrad A, Ader F, et al. Vaccination in adult liver transplantation candidates and recipients. Clin Res Hepatol Gastroenterol 2020;44(2):126–34.
54. Stucchi RSB, Lopes MH, Kumar D, et al. Vaccine recommendations for solid-organ transplant recipients and donors. Transplant 2018;102(2S Suppl 2): S72–80.
55. John BV, Deng Y, Khakoo NS, et al. Coronavirus disease 2019 vaccination is associated with reduced severe acute respiratory syndrome coronavirus 2 infection and death in liver transplant recipients. Gastroenterol 2022;162(2):645–7.e2.
56. Moon AM, Webb GJ, Garcia-Juarez I, et al. SARS-CoV-2 infections among patients with liver disease and liver transplantation who received COVID-19 vaccination. Hepatol Commun 2022;6(4):889–97.
57. Ekpanyapong S, Reddy KR. Liver and biliary tract disease in patients with COVID-19 infection. Gastroenterol Clin North Am 2022.

Drug-Induced Liver Injury due to Biologics and Immune Check Point Inhibitors

Fernando Bessone, MD[a],*, Einar S. Björnsson, MD, PhD[b,c]

KEYWORDS

- Hepatotoxicity • Checkpoint inhibitors • Biologics • Hepatitis
- Drug-induced liver injury

KEY POINTS

- Among biological agents, infliximab is the only drug in Category A with more than 100 cases reported.
- Drug-induced liver injury (DILI) due to infliximab has been reported to occur in 1 out of 120 to 148 users.
- Corticosteroids are frequently needed in patients with infliximab-induced autoimmune-like hepatitis.
- Recurrence of liver injury does not seem to happen in patients with a history of.infliximab DILI who have tried another TNF-alpha antagonist.
- Checkpoint inhibitors-induced hepatotoxicity may occur in up to 17% of treated patients. Its clinical phenotype may present either as hepatocellular, mixed, or cholestatic pattern. Corticosteroid therapy is usually not necessary in approximately 50% of cases.

BIOLOGICS
Risk Factors and Epidemiology

Biological agents have in the last two decades become very important therapeutic agents, particularly for the treatment of various autoimmune disorders. The most widely used biologics are the tumor necrosis factor-α (TNF-α) receptor antagonists: infliximab, adalimumab, and etanercept. Other commonly used biological agents are interleukin (IL)-1 receptor antagonist (Anakinra), interleukin (IL)-6 receptor antagonist (tocilizumab), and CD20 surface antigen antagonist (rituximab). The current review will however focus on TNF-α receptor antagonists. Among these, infliximab is the only drug that belongs to category A in liverTox (https://www.ncbi.nlm.nih.gov/books/)

[a] Facultad de Ciencias Médicas, Hospital Provincial del Centenario, University of Rosario, School of Medicine, Urquiza 3101, Rosario 2000, Argentina; [b] University of Iceland, Hringbraut 101, Reykjavik, Iceland; [c] Division of Gastroenterology and Hepatology, Department of Internal Medicine, Landspitali University Hospital, Reykjavik, Iceland
* Corresponding author.
E-mail address: bessonefernando@gmail.com

Med Clin N Am 107 (2023) 623–640
https://doi.org/10.1016/j.mcna.2022.12.008
0025-7125/23/© 2022 Elsevier Inc. All rights reserved.

which represents an established cause of clinically apparent liver injury and which has been associated with > 100 cases of drug-induced liver injury (DILI).[1] Thus, most of the current review will be about liver injury due to infliximab.

As infliximab is a protein and metabolized within the liver it came as a surprise to many physicians and researchers when postmarketing surveillance by the US Food and Drug Administration (FDA) in 2004 revealed more than 30 reports of suspected liver injury within 5 years of marketing.[2] The type of liver injury induced by infliximab has been mechanistically an indirect liver injury, as it is more related to the action of the drug on the immune system, that is, what it does rather than what it is.[3] The underlying cause of liver injury due to infliximab is not clear which is also the case with most other drugs leading to DILI. It has been proposed that the balance between regulatory and effector T cells might be changed by TNF-α inhibition, which might result in liver injury. Furthermore, TNF-α inhibition leads to an abundance of lymphocytes by impairment of autoreactive B-cell production which might favor antibody production.[4,5] It is unclear why infliximab is more prone to cause liver injury than other TNF-α antagonists. Human leukocyte antigen (HLA) associations have been identified as risk factors for liver injury in users of infliximab.[6,7] In an international study based on 16 patients with a history of DILI due to infliximab and 60 matched controls, a strong association was found with HLA-B*39:01 as a potentially causal risk factor for infliximab-induced DILI.[6] Further but weaker associations have also been reported with other HLA alleles.[6] These results were not reproduced in a recent population-based study from Iceland.[7] The Icelandic study included 36 patients with DILI due to infliximab and compared it with around 50.000 individuals from the general population of Iceland, previously genotyped by deCode genetics (www.decode.com). The study revealed that the genotypes HLA-DQB1*02:01 and HLA-DRB1*03:01 (odds ratio [OR] 2.7, $P = .013$) were associated with increased risk of DILI due to infliximab and HLA-DRB1*04:04 (OR 0.4 [0.14 to 0.96], $P = .041$) was associated with a decreased risk of DILI. In the first study on HLA associations,[6] the association with the strength of the association is probably weaker as corrections for multiple comparisons were not undertaken.[6] In the Icelandic study, none of the patients had the HLA-B*39:01 allele, and it is conceivable that HLA associations might be related to a genetic predisposition to autoimmune disorders in general. Future studies should aim at comparing risk factors in patients treated with infliximab with and without the development of DILI. Previous studies trying to compare patients treated with infliximab who did and did not develop DILI have been limited. A small study of 11 patients with infliximab-induced DILI had patients matched for age, gender, and the indication for infliximab.[8] Neither dose of infliximab given nor ANA positivity before the initiation of infliximab was found to be a risk factor for the development of DILI.[8] However, the use of methotrexate was significantly more frequent in those infliximab users who did not develop DILI. This was suggested to be due to the ability of methotrexate to inhibit antibody formation. Recently, Meunier and colleagues[9] suggested, based on the review of the literature that azathioprine (AZA) might prevent IFX-induced liver injury. Combination of AZA and IFX has been found to decrease the risk for immunization in patients with IBD, as IFX-AZA combination has been found to decrease production of anti-IFX antibodies.[10] The hypothesis of the importance of immunomodulators such as methotrexate and azathioprine for potential prevention of DILI needs to be addressed further in clinical trials.

There are little data on the overall frequency of DILI due to TNF-α inhibitors. In a prospective population-based study from Iceland, four cases of DILI due to infliximab were identified out of 96 DILI patients over a 2-year period.[11] The risk of DILI among infliximab users in 1 out of 148 users.[11] This risk was much higher than for the most common cause of DILI, amoxicillin-clavulanate, occurring in approximately 1 out 2300 users.[11] From the same research group, by expanding the study period to 5 years, an even higher risk was found and one out of 120 patients who were given infliximab developed clinically apparent DILI.[8] Most of the patients with DILI due to infliximab had rheumatological and dermatologic indications for use and few had IBD.[8] Three studies from IBD registries have tried to estimate the risk of liver injury due to biological therapy.[12–14] In a retrospective study from Boston, among approximately 1750 patients initiating anti-TNF-α therapy (2/3 with infliximab), 45 patients had a liver injury (had competing etiologies excluded) and were considered to be associated with infliximab in most, whereas 3 cases were attributed to adalimumab.[12] The only clinical parameter that differed between cases and controls with normal liver enzymes was a lower dose in cases.[12] The median peak ALT elevations were surprisingly low (only 96) and much lower than in other cohorts[7,15,16] and many of the patients continued with infliximab.[12] Thus, it casts some doubt on the likelihood of infliximab being the only cause of liver injury in these patients. More recently, two other studies have tried to identify DILI patients among IBD cohorts and similarly patients who were considered to have DILI often continued therapy and the causality assessment was somewhat unclear.[14,15] Thus, it seems to be difficult to compare the risk factors and frequency of DILI due to infliximab between different cohorts due to lack of consistent definition of liver injury or by excluding non-IBD patients from the studies.[12–14] As mentioned above, other biological agents other than infliximab are less well documented as causes of DILI. Adalimumab has been reported to lead to liver injury.[8,15,16] In a recent systematic analysis on drugs leading to drug-induced autoimmune-like hepatitis (DI-AILH), a total of 11 cases of adalimumab-induced DI-AILH were identified.[17] In all, except in one case, no relapse was observed after cessation of the previous TNF-α of this autoimmune-like hepatitis following adalimumab.[17] Etanercept has also been associated with liver injury and concomitant autoantibodies.[18,19] Discontinuation of etanercept was not enough for the patients to recover as they also required corticosteroids, whereas discontinuation of immunosuppression was not reported.[17] This is important information as in early reports these patients were considered to have autoimmune hepatitis, despite strong drug association and were treated as such with long-term immunosuppression, whereas immunosuppression is very rarely required long-term in patients with DI-AILH.[17]

Clinical Features and Outcomes

The demographics and clinical features of these patients with infliximab DILI are in **Table 1**. One of the studies only included IBD patients.[12] In terms of gender distribution, that study is at odds with the other studies, noting women to be in the minority, whereas the other series, including patients with different indications for TNF-α inhibitors have shown DILI to occur mostly in women (see **Table 1**). From the different series, it is difficult to assess the symptoms of patients diagnosed with DILI. In the largest series, only one-third of patients were symptomatic at presentation (12/36), and who had jaundice (4/36), lethargy, loss of appetite, abdominal discomfort, and joint pain.[7] However, 24 (67%) were asymptomatic. This is line with a study from Portugal where 75% were asymptomatic and 25% were reported to be symptomatic. The proportion of asymptomatic patients ranging from 67% to 75%[7,16] is certainly a higher proportion than in patients with DILI in general. The reason for this is probably due to routine testing for transaminase elevation before anti-TNF initiation and also before each infusion according to clinical guidelines in most countries. In the case series, autoimmune features were in 50% to 88% (see **Table 1**). In the population-based study from Iceland, most of the patients had a hepatocellular injury in 23 cases (64%), mixed in 12

Table 1
Demographics, clinical features, and therapy in four studies in patients with liver injury associated with tumor necrosis factor-α receptor antagonists

	Median Age	Gender (Female %)	Median Latency	Peak ALT	Hepato-Cellular (%)	Liver Biopsy Done	Auto-Antibodies	Cortico-steroid Therapy
Ghabril et al,[15] 2013 (n = 6), infliximab (50%)	35	83%	16 wk	914	83%	67%	50%	83%
Shelton et al,[12] 2015[a] (n = 48), infliximab (94%)	32	44%	18 wk	96	–	12.5%	50%	6.3%
Rodrigues et al,[16] 2015 (n = 8), infliximab (88%)	45	63%	–	433	–	100%	88%	100%
Bjornsson et al,[7] 2022 (n = 36), Infliximab (100%)	46	78%	16 wk	393	64%	17%	67%	47%

[a] Only IBD patients.

cases (33%), and cholestatic in 1 (3%) case.[7] Furthermore, 33% were ANA positive before developing DILI.[7] When the liver injury was detected 67% were ANA positive and 69% had autoimmune features (positive autoantibodies and/or elevated IgG) at diagnosis of liver injury.[7] Although as many as 69% had autoimmune features, many of these patients did not behave like AIH and rather rapidly recovered after the discontinuation of infliximab and did not require corticosteroid therapy. However, in approximately 50% of patients, liver test abnormalities did not resolve by cessation of infliximab therapy. Thus, the decision to treat with corticosteroids was more related to the absence of recovery by discontinuation of infliximab rather than serologic testing with positive autoantibodies. Median time from onset of liver injury to corticosteroid treatment initiation was 44 days (IQR 14 to 69). Corticosteroid treatment was tapered in all patients and no patient had a relapse with elevations of liver enzymes after steroid discontinuation. In the study with only IBD patients, corticosteroid therapy was undertaken in only 6.3%, whereas in other studies DILI patients were considered to require corticosteroids in 88%-100% [15,16] (see **Table 1**). Similarly, the rate of liver biopsies were different between the different studies (see **Table 1**). Liver biopsy was not considered to affect management.[7] Even results of a liver biopsy in patients with AIH have been reported not to influence the decision to treat with corticosteroids.[20] Infliximab-induced liver injury has several phenotypes and at least 5 phenotypes have been reported: (a) Many patients, most with hepatocellular injury, up to 50% recover spontaneously after stopping infliximab although some of them have autoimmune features.[7,15] (b) Another form of hepatocellular injury is in patients with AIH-like phenotype, in whom liver tests do not improve or improve slowly without corticosteroids, most have autoantibodies and/or IgG elevation. (c) Relatively few patients develop cholestatic or mixed liver injury and patients recover spontaneously,[21,22] (d) in line with other types of immunosuppression, infliximab can lead to reactivation of hepatitis B, in patients with HBsAg, and at times resulting in jaundice and mortality.[23–25] It is recommended in clinical guidelines that those who are HBsAg positive receive antiviral prophylaxis while treated with infliximab.[26] Finally, (e) acute liver failure has been reported due to infliximab induces hepatotoxicity.[4,27–35] In many of the cases, patients recovered from the serious liver injury.[29,30,32] However, a total of 9 cases leading to a liver transplantation have been reported (**Table 2**). Interestingly the dose of infliximab administered did not seem to be particularly high; 3 to 5 mg/kg and 400 to 470 mg at each infusion. The median number of weeks from initiation of infliximab was 16 and the median number of infusion was 4 (see **Table 2**), similar to patients who have been reported to have favorable prognosis.[7] However, of particular interest is the lack of an immunomodulator in almost all the cases.[35] It has been reported that concomitant methotrexate use was significantly less often used in patients on infliximab who developed liver injury than those who did not.[8] In at least three cases, infliximab has been reported to cause vanishing bile duct syndrome,[36–38] which in one lead to a need for a liver transplantation.[37]

Checkpoint Inhibitors-Induced Drug-Induced Liver Injury

The emergence of immune checkpoint inhibitors (ICIs) has been one of the milestones in oncology in recent years due to its high therapeutic impact in the management of solid tumors and hematological neoplasias (eg, renal cell carcinoma, Hodgkin lymphoma, melanoma, lung cancer, and also recently hepatocellular carcinoma)[39]

A broad range of immune-related adverse events (irAEs) involve almost every organ but mostly affect the skin, digestive system, lung, endocrine glands, nervous system, kidney, blood cells, and musculoskeletal system. Hepatic adverse reactions usually represent one of the most frequent in clinical practice[40]

Table 2
Patients who have been reported in the literature up to October 15, 2022 and undergone liver transplantation due to infliximab-induced liver injury

Gender and Age F = Female M = Male	Drug	Indication	Dose (mg)	Concomitant Immuno-Modulator Use	Number of Infusions	Latency (weeks)	Outcome	Reference
F39	Infliximab	Rheumatoid arthritis	3 mg/kg	No	6	36	Liver transplant	Tobon et al,[27] 2007
F46	Infliximab	IBD/spondylitis	400	No	2	15	Liver transplant	Kinnunen et al,[28] 2012
F38	Infliximab	IBD	5 mg/kg	No	5	22	Liver transplant	Parra et al,[31] 2015
F51	Infliximab	IBD	—	No	—	28	Liver transplant	Kok et al,[33] 2018
F40	Infliximab	Hidradenitis suppurative	400	No	4	20	Liver transplant	Kok et al,[33] 2018
F34	Infliximab	Psoriatic arthritis	300	No	3	16	Liver transplant	Kok et al,[33] 2018
F69	Infliximab	IBD	5 mg/kg	No	3	12	Liver transplant	Wong et al,[34] 2019
M63	Infliximab	IBD	470	No	3	14	Liver transplant	Shah et al,[4] 2020
M25	Infliximab	IBD	400	Yes/no*	4	12	Liver transplant	Alikhan et al,[35] 2021*

* The designator means that YES-methotrexate and No-no immunomodulator at the time of ALF.[35]

Although most of these agents have been approved by the FDA since 2010, this field continues to grow in research, and in indications and approval of new molecules [5,41,42]. These monoclonal antibodies induce an inhibitory effect on the surface receptors of T cells or tumor cells.[5]

According to the inhibitory effect on the targeted receptor, ICIs can be classified as follows: inhibitors of programmed cell death (PD-1), (eg, nivolumab, pembrolizumab, and cemiplimab), inhibitors of its ligand, programmed cell death ligand-1 (PDL-1), triggered by (eg, atezolizumab, avelumab, and durvalumab), and inhibitors of cytotoxic T-lymphocyte associated protein-4 (CTLA-4) induced by (eg, ipilimumab, tremelimumab). A new ICI, relatlimab, targeting the inhibitory receptor lymphocyte-activation gene 3 (LAG3), has recently been approved, to be used in combination with nivolumab for those with unresectable or metastatic melanoma.[43] Six percent of patients had a hepatocellular pattern of DILI in a pivotal clinical trial.[43]

Of note ICIs used to treat hepatocellular carcinoma (HCC) may be associated with a higher rate of both severe DILI and death because these tumors mostly arise in a cirrhotic liver with varying degrees of the hepatic reserve.[44] However, the rate and the nature of hepatoxicity in cirrhotics with HCC vs. non-cirrhotics is unclear at the current time.

Despite the large number of papers and reviews written on these compounds as triggers of hepatotoxicity in recent years, there are many unclear issues that need to be clarified. They include: (a) the actual incidence of DILI, (b) the risk factors linked to an increased risk of hepatotoxicity, (c) the mechanistic pathways of liver injury (d) the appearance of sclerosing cholangiopathy as a new phenotype associated with ICIs, (e) the role of liver biopsy, (f) the therapeutic management once the liver injury occurs and (g) the heterogeneity in criteria defining DILI.

Risk Factors and Epidemiology

ICI-induced liver injury is not a rare event in clinical practice and they are expected to be more frequent with time, as these agents are now often prescribed in the treatment of a spectrum of tumors. The incidence of hepatotoxicity varies has ranged from 2% to 25% and has depended on whether these compounds were used as monotherapy or as combination therapy[45,46]. If we consider patients receiving monotherapy, the highest rate of liver toxicity is associated with CTLA-4 inhibitors (ipilimumab and tremelimumab).[47]

Studies analyzing monotherapy with CTLA-4 inhibitors have shown a rate of DILI between 3% and 15%, and reaching 20% when high doses of these agents were used. As an example, ipilimumab-induced hepatotoxicity was in only 3% to 5% when prescribed at conventional doses of 3 mg/kg compared with 15% to 16% of those who received high doses[48,49] Similar results have been reported with PD-L1 inhibitors (atezolizumab, durvalumab, and avelumab) where the probability of developing DILI ranged from 1% to 17% (3% to 5% grade 3/4).[50]

In contrast, monotherapy with the PD-1 inhibitors (nivolumab, pembrolizumab), showed rates of DILI no higher than 3% (mostly 1%-2%), whereas DILI of grade3/4 was linked to liver toxicity in < 1% of cases. Hepatotoxicity induced by PD-1 and PD-L1 inhibitors does not appear to be dose-related in nature.[51]

Combined regimens associating CTLA-4 and PD-1 inhibitors have not only shown a synergistic antitumor effect but also reported DILI in 18% to 22% of treated patients (8% to 11% of them developing severe hepatitis)[52].

Although 20% of patients can develop severe forms of DILI (grades 3 and 4), acute liver failure, requiring liver transplantation or death, usually are uncommon complications (0.4%). In a meta-analysis from 2018, five fatal cases were reported.[50]

A recent systematic review and meta-analysis that included 43 randomized control trials and 28,905 treated patients, compared the incidence of DILI induced by antitumoral therapies when ICIs were (or not) added to the therapeutic regimen.[53] ICIs linked to DILI based on their mechanisms showed no significant heterogeneity among the various mechanisms for hepatitis (any grade: OR, 2.13, 95% confidence interval [CI] 1.52 to 2.97, grade 3 to 5: OR, 2.66, 95% CI 1.72 to 4.11. A meta-analysis including 17 phase 2 and 3 studies conducted in patients with advanced cancer showed a higher probability of DILI in patients with melanoma compared with other types of cancer (odds ratio 5.66 vs 2.71, respectively).[54]

Even in those with elevated transaminases and pre-existing chronic liver disease at baseline, an increased risk of hepatotoxicity has not been observed. In those with advanced HCC on liver cirrhosis treated with ICIs AST elevation was frequently described as an adverse event (15% to 23% any grade, 6% to 13% grade 3/4).[55,56] However, these data did not represent a higher incidence of DILI compared with patients without cirrhosis. As these observations were in CHILD A patients, they cannot be extrapolated to those with decompensated cirrhosis.

Interestingly, female sex, combination immunotherapy, and the first line of immunotherapy were associated with a higher incidence of ICI-induced liver toxicity in one study analyzing 1096 patients.[57] The most commonly used agents were PD1/L1 inhibitors ($n = 774$) and CTLA-4 inhibitors ($n = 195$). Sixty-four (6%) patients suffered ICIs-induced hepatic events where severity was < grade 3 in 30 and $\geq$ grade 3 in 24 patients (3.1% overall). Hepatotoxicity was also significantly associated with longer therapy when assessing PD1/L1 vs CTLA-4 inhibitors, where a median of 37 months (95% CI 21.4, NR) was observed with PD1/L1 inhibitors, as compared with 11.3 months (95% CI 10, 13, $P < .001$) with CTLA-4 inhibitors.

Another metaanalysis[58] selected 13 studies from 5030 patients and showed that age, history of ICIs treatment, ICIs combination therapy, and aspartate aminotransferase (AST) level were significantly associated with a higher risk of DILI of any grade. Further, age alone was significantly associated with the risk of DILI grade $\geq$3.

Interestingly, the Prospective European DILI Registry in a recent analysis conducted among 226 DILI patients between 2016 to 2021 found that nivolumab/ipilimumab represented the fourth leading cause of liver toxicity. These data reinforce the observation that ICI-induced liver injury is nowadays being commonly described in clinical practice.[59]

Mechanistic Pathways of Liver Injury

ICIs are a subgroup of the broad family of costimulatory molecules, which are essential to control the immune response. Through phosphorylation cascades, they control T-cell receptor signaling. CTLA4, PD1, and PDL1 are the three most noticeable immunologic checkpoints that aid tumors in avoiding the immune response and thereby enhancing self-tolerance.[5]

These proteins' inhibitory functions are disrupted when ICIs bind to these receptors, thus favoring an immunologic response that promotes T cell activation and proliferation, which in turn kills tumor cells. Immune tolerance to self-antigens is also mediated through the PD1 and CTLA4 pathways, and this explains the immune-induced adverse outcomes that can affect practically all human organs and systems.[60] ICI-related DILI is often regarded as an immune-mediated hepatitis caused by this aberrant activation of the immune response.

Clinical Features at Presentation

Because ICIs are molecules that are expressed on T cells and are responsible for activating the immune system, various systems can be targeted, thus resulting in adverse reactions.[61] Various phenotypes and clinical patterns are associated with ICI-induced hepatotoxicity at clinical presentation (**Table 3**).[62] Clinical patterns tend to be hepatocellular rather than cholestatic/mixed, and range from mild disease to acute liver failure. However, asymptomatic and anicteric elevation of hepatic biochemical tests is a common finding in clinical practice.[63] In most cases, autoantibodies are absent. The time to DILI onset after initiating drug therapy usually ranges between 1 and 3 months.[64] However, hepatic reactions have been described to occur more rapidly when using anti-CTLA-4 agents, beginning between 1 to 7 weeks after the start of treatment, whereas this latency was 2 to 49 weeks for those patients receiving PD-1/PD-L1 therapy.[65]

Of note in a Japanese clinical trial, 29 (5.3%) cases of ICI-induced DILI were identified in 546 patients with advanced malignancies treated with monotherapy or a combination strategy.[66] Only 2 patients had positive ANA titers, serum IgG levels were within normal ranges, and the most prevalent form of hepatotoxicity was cholestatic/mixed injury (79%).Of interest is that the presence of fever within 24 hours of starting medication was a risk factor linked to hepatotoxicity. Mild and moderate forms of DILI are the most frequently observed in clinical practice, whereas severe hepatitis, acute liver failure and the need for liver transplantation are uncommon forms of liver damage.[5]

De Martin and colleagues[64] reported the outcomes of 16 patients who received ICIs, of whom anti-PD-1 drugs were responsible for nine 9 cases and anti-CTLA4 agents for seven. Autoantibodies were typically either negative or at low titers in most patients, and the median DILI latency was 5 weeks. Only 3.5% of patients who underwent immunotherapy for metastatic cancer were found to have acute grade 3 hepatitis, as defined by the CTCAE system (cytolysis and/or cholestasis more than 5 times, total bilirubin more than 3 times ULN). Acute liver failure (ALF) was not described in any patients.[64]

Patients receiving anti-CTLA-4 mAbs or combination therapy were younger than those receiving anti-PD-1/PD-L1 mAbs (median age 52 vs 69 years, (P = .029) respectively; hepatitis developed after 14 weeks (range 2 to 49 weeks) after starting anti-PD-1/PD-L1 treatment, as compared with 3 weeks (range 1 to 7 weeks) with anti-CTLA-4 alone or in combination with an anti-PD1 (P = .019). Interestingly, 6 patients had fever at presentation, whereas 5 of them also had a skin rash. Half of the cases in this series required immunosuppressive treatment, whereas the other 50% had a spontaneous remission. None of the treated patients relapsed after corticosteroid-induced remission.[64] According to Wang and colleagues,[50] most fatalities cases were brought on by an acute illness and were frequently associated with fulminant hepatic failure. Fortunately, ALF had a modest death rate (21 out of 3545 patients, or 0.6%).

Secondary Sclerosing Cholangitis Associated with Immune Checkpoint Inhibitors

More recently a novel type of cholestasis induced by ICIs and resembling primary sclerosing cholangitis have been described.[67] Patients developing other phenotypes of DILI have also been found to have this kind of SSC.[68,69] Diffuse dilatation and thickening of the intrahepatic bile ducts were the main observed characteristics. Nearly 80% of patients with dilated bile ducts had no evidence of biliary blockage.[67]

The majority of these biliary ducts had a diffuse hypertrophy in their wall. In 16 individuals, Cohen and colleagues[70] described a predominant cholangitis pattern linked to portal-based inflammation. On cholangiography, this histologic characteristic was more likely to be linked to bile duct dilatation or narrowing. The long-term clinical effects of the biliary involvement that ICIs cause has not yet been fully studied.

Table 3
Features of immune checkpoint inhibitors and clinical patterns of liver damage

Agent/Mechanism	Type of ICI	DILI Incidence	Clinical Pattern	Histology
PDL-1 PD-1 (programmed cell death-1)	Atezolizumab Avelumab Durvalumab Nivolumab, Pembrolizumab, Cemiplimab	1% to 17%	Hepatocellular, mixed or cholestatic	Acute hepatitis + centrilobular necrosis Chronic hepatitis Slight Lobular Hepatitis Confluent necrosis Endothelitis Lobular hepatitis + microgranulomas Ductal damage
CTLA-4 (cytotoxic T-lymphocyte associated protein-4)	Ipilimumab, Tremelimumab	3% to 15%	Hepatocellular or mixed or cholestatic	Acute hepatitis + centrolobular necrosis Subacute hepatitis Periportal and lobular activity Chronic hepatitis Granulomatous hepatitis with lobular and periportal necrosis
LAG3 (lymphocyte-activation gene 3)	Combined scheme: Relatlimab/Nivolumab	6%*	Hepatocellular*	No histologic descriptions*

* The designator means Pivotal study data.[43]

Data from Opdualag Prescribing Information. Opdualag US Product Information. Last updated: March 2022. Princeton, NJ: Bristol-Myers Squibb Company. https://news.bms.com/news/details/2022/U.S.-Food-and-Drug-Administration-Approves-First-LAG-3-Blocking-Antibody-Combination-Opdualag-nivolumab-and-relatlimab-rmbw-as-Treatment-for-Patients-with-Unresectable-or-Metastatic-Melanoma/default.aspx

In a systematic review of 19 studies, including 5 case series and 14 case reports, A total of 31 cases of SSC caused by PD-1 inhibitors were assessed[71]. The median age of PD-1 inhibitor-related SSC was 67 years at the time of onset (range, 43 to 89). Men appeared to have higher rates of PD-1 inhibitor-related SSC, with a male-to-female ratio of 21:10. Non-small cell lung cancer (20 cases), melanoma (4 cases), gastric cancer (3 cases), bladder cancer (2 cases), small cell lung cancer (1 case), and epithelioid mesothelioma (1 case) were the patients' primary diseases for treatment. Nivolumab (19 cases), pembrolizumab (10 cases), avelumab (1 case), and durvalumab (1 case) were the agents that induced PD-1 inhibitor-related SSC[71]. The median number of cycles before the development of SSC linked to PD-1 inhibitors was 5.5 (range, 1 to 27). The most frequent symptom was abdominal pain (35.5%, 11/31) followed by fever (19.4%, 6/31) and jaundice (12.9%, 4/31). Although 8 patients (25.8%, 8/31) did not have any symptoms, they also had evidence of liver injury. Unfortunately, it has been observed that only 11.5% of patients with SSC induced by ICIs responded to steroids[71]

All patients who develop clinical patterns of cholestasis associated with the use of ICIs should undergo a thorough imaging investigation of the biliary tract to rule out SSC induced by these compounds.

Role of Liver Biopsy

Although there are histologic features that can mimic autoimmune hepatitis (AIH), there are clinicopathologic differences supporting the notion that ICI–induced DILI is a distinct entity from AIH[40] (**Table 4**) Centrilobular necrosis and acute hepatitis with lobular inflammation, and acidophil bodies have been the most frequent findings in DILI-induced by ICIs, whereas ductal injury and hepatocanalicular cholestasis have also been observed.[64](see **Table 4**).

The indication for liver biopsy (LB) in this setting is still controversial, whereas it may be useful as a diagnostic tool to rule out pre-existing liver disease and also describe different patterns of DILI induced by ICIs such as endothelitis and granulomas.[62] De Martin and colleagues[64] examined 16 patients who had liver damage induced by

Table 4
Characteristics differentiating autoimmune hepatitis from immune checkpoint inhibitor-induced drug-induced liver injury

Variable	AIH	ICI-Induced DILI
Gender	Mainly Female	Equal gender incidence
Clinical pattern	Mainly Hepatocellular	Hepatocellular, mixed and cholestatic
Autoantibodies	Usually positive	Usually negative
IgG presence	Usually elevated	Usually negative
Gamma globulin level	Usually elevated	Usually normal
Histologic features	Interface hepatitis, plasma cells, rossettes	Centrolobular necrosis, granulomas, endothelitis
Type of liver infiltration	Plasma cell: CD4+ CD8+	Histiocyte: CD4+ CD8+
Corticosteroid therapy	Required	Spontaneous remission in about 50% of cases
Relapse after corticosteroid withdrawal	Higher than 60%	Uncommon

Abbreviations: AIH, autoimmune hepatitis; ICI-induced DILI, immune checkpoint inhibitors-induced DILI.

ICIs. Patients receiving anti-CTLA-4 monoclonal antibodies showed a typical pattern of granulomatous hepatitis, characterized by the development of fibrin-ring granulomas in addition to central-vein endothelitis. In 50% of the patients, mild portal fibrosis was found, suggesting a potential progression from acute to chronic hepatitis.

In contrast, a recent retrospective study that examined 60 patients who had suspected ICI-related liver injury revealed a pattern of lobular injury and inflammation, endothelitis, and the development of granulomas. These authors claimed that the histology results did not predict the requirement for corticosteroids, the length of therapy, or the requirement for additional immunosuppression. They questioned the usefulness of LB in therapy decision-making for patients who show typical signs of ICI-induced liver damage[70]

Lastly, Li and colleagues[72] carried out a retrospective analysis including a cohort of 213 patients who experienced hepatitis triggered by ICIs that progressed to grade 3 or higher hepatic injury. The panlobular hepatitis pattern of DILI was the most prevalent histologic pattern. Patients who an LB had a significantly longer median time to ALT normalization (42 vs 33 days, respectively; P 0.01), which might represent a selection bias for LB, and further, delay the initiating of empiric corticosteroids for grade 3 or higher DILI.

Thus, although granulomas and endothelitis may indicate a particular type of hepatitis induced by these compounds, the usefulness of LB in this scenario is debatable and not yet established.

Management of Liver Toxicity-Induced by Immune Checkpoint Inhibitors

The use of corticosteroids for the management of liver damage thought to be caused by ICIs is not supported by evidence. In several oncology societies and consensus-based therapy guidelines, it is proposed that all patients should be assessed for other hepatitis causes and steroids should be used as the first line of treatment.[73–76]

The oncological societies based DILI classification on CTCAEv5 criteria recommend that therapy with ICIs not be stopped and hepatic biochemical tests be monitored if the liver injury is mild (ALT $\geq 3 \times$ ULN). If ALT levels drop to baseline within a week, ICI medication can be restarted and/or oral corticosteroids can be administered. If ALT is 3 to 5 ULN, ICIs can be temporarily stopped.[73–76]

These guidelines also propose to classify grade III hepatitis as ALT levels ≥ 5 to 20 ULN and bilirubin above 3 ULN.[73–76] Patients with these conditions should be closely monitored and treated with corticosteroids if their liver tests do not return to baseline. According to these recommendations, ICI medication should be completely discontinued if the levels of ALT are > 10 ULN (grade IV hepatitis) and/or if the ALT > 5 ULN is accompanied by a rise in serum bilirubin.

However, a comprehensive analysis by Peeraphatdit and colleagues[77] showed that nearly half of these patients improved without needing corticosteroids, even those who have developed severe forms of hepatotoxicity. This is in contrast to the statement made by the oncological guidelines that propose a systematic use of steroids in patients with grade 3 to 4 ICI–induced hepatotoxicity.

A significant number of these patients in observational studies spontaneously improved without the administration of corticosteroids.[78,79] In line with these results, 30% of patients with > grade III hepatitis improved without immunosuppression therapy in a French trial,[80] and 33% of patients in a recent Texas study were found to not need corticosteroids.[78]

Several variables, including the degree of hepatotoxicity, the presence of liver metastases, the type of immunotherapy used, and the time since the onset of hepatotoxicity, may have an impact on how long it takes for hepatic biochemical tests to fully recover following the initiation of corticosteroids.[81] However, we have to take into consideration that liver injury can be serious enough to lead to acute liver failure. In a Barcelona study, two of 28 patients with severe hepatitis (> grade III) evolved on to ALF and one of the two died,[82] Mortality due to hepatotoxicity was also found in a study that examined data from the World Health Organization's pharmacovigilance database (Vigilyze)[82]

Recent AASLD guidelines for patients with DILI-induced by ICIs state that in those with Grade 3 or higher hepatotoxicity (ALT 5 to 20 × ULN and/or bilirubin 3 to 10 × ULN or symptomatic liver dysfunction), the ICI should be permanently discontinued, and iv steroids at a dose of 1 to 1.5 mg/kg per day along with hospitalization for patients with jaundice should be considered[83]

As for the EASL guidelines they state that Decisions regarding corticosteroid treatment of immune-mediated hepatitis associated with ICIs are made by a multidisciplinary team involving hepatologists if DILI is sufficiently severe based on clinical and histologic assessment[84]

Secondary immunosuppression mostly with mycophenolate mofetil has been reported to be helpful in non-responsive patients to corticosteroids.[85] However, in the case of corticosteroid-resistant hepatitis, other agents have been studied and appear to be effective: namely azathioprine, cyclosporin, tacrolimus, and anti-thymocyte globulin. In addition, a case series study has shown that patients with severe steroid-resistant cholestatic hepatitis, induced by anti-PD-1, may benefit from ursodeoxycholic acid (UDCA) treatment.[86] Last but not least, rechallenge with the same ICI following a severe immune-related hepatitis has not been associated with the recurrence of liver injury in up to 65% of patients[81]

In conclusion, patients with ICI-induced hepatoxicity without jaundice and/or coagulopathy need to be closely monitored because many of them will recover once ICIs are stopped. Corticosteroids should be given when patients have ongoing jaundice and/or coagulopathy, particularly after discontinuation of ICIs. A dose of methylprednisolone 1 mg/kg/d might be just as effective as higher doses; however, it is not apparent whether doses of 40 to 60 mg of prednisolone are less effective.

Future Directions

- The importance of immunomodulators for the prevention of infliximab-induced liver injury needs to be explored
- Human leukocyte antigen typing in users of infliximab who develop and do not develop hepatotoxicity needs to be investigated
- Data on rechallenge with infliximab in patients who have experienced liver injury are needed
- The importance of serum infliximab concentration and infliximab antibodies needs to be investigated
- A unified definition of hepatotoxicity induced by immune checkpoint inhibitors should be discussed by an expert panel
- The future implementation of biomarkers as a diagnostic tool needs to be explored
- The role of liver biopsy in terms of treatment selection needs to be validated
- Immunosuppressive treatment criteria and how patients should be monitored needs to be agreed upon by consensus.

AUTHOR CONTRIBUTIONS

Fernando Bessone and Einar S. Bjornsson contributed equally to this paper; Einar S. Bjornsson drafted the part on DILI due to biological agents; Fernando Bessone drafted the part on DILI due to immune checkpoint inhibitors. They both contributed to the writing, and in editing the manuscript and review of literature.

DISCLOSURE

The authors have nothing to disclose.

REFERENCES

1. Björnsson ES, Hoofnagle JH. Categorization of drugs implicated in causing liver injury: critical assessment based upon published case reports. Hepatology 2016; 63:590–603. 2.
2. U.S. Food and Drug Administration. Drug induced liver injury rank (DILIRank) dataset. Available at: https://www.fda.gov/science-resea rch/liver-toxicity-knowledge-base-ltkb/drug-induced-liverinjury-rank-dilirank-dataset. Accessed October 2022.
3. Hoofnagle JH, Bjornsson ES. Drug induced liver injury: types and phenotypes. N Engl J Med 2019;381:264–73.
4. Shah P, Sundaram V, Bjornsson ES. Biologic and checkpoint inhibitor-induced liver injury: a systematic literature review. Hepatol Commun 2020;4:172–84.
5. Hernandez N, Bessone F. Hepatotoxicity induced by biological agents: clinical features and current controversies. J Clin Transpational Hepatol 2022;10:486–95.
6. Bruno Christopher, Fremd Brandon, Church Rachel, et al. HLA Associations with Infliximab-Induced Liver Injury. Pharmacogenomics J 2020;5:681–6.
7. Björnsson HK, Gudbjörnsson B, Björnsson ES. Infliximab-induced liver injury: Clinical phenotypes, autoimmunity and the role of corticosteroid treatment. J Hepatol J Hepatol 2022;76(1):86–92.
8. Björnsson ES, Gunnarsson BI, Gröndal G, et al. The risk of drug-induced liver injury from Tumor Necrosis Factor (TNF)-alpha-antagonists. Clin Gastroenterol Hepatol 2015;13:602–8.
9. Meunier L, Malezieux E, Bozon A, et al. Can azathioprine prevent infliximab-induced liver injury? J Hepatol 2022. S0168- 8278(22)00124-00126.
10. Strik AS, van Den Brink GR, Ponsioen C, et al. Suppression of anti-drug antibodies to infliximab or adalimumab with the addition of an immunomodulator in patients with inflammatory bowel disease. Aliment Pharmacol Ther 2017;45: 1128–34.
11. Bjornsson ES, Bergmann OM, Bjornsson HK, et al. Incidence, Presentation and Outcomes in Patients with Drug-Induced Liver Injury in the General Population of Iceland. Gastroenterology 2013;144:1419–25.
12. Shelton E, Chaudrey K, Sauk J, et al. New onset idiosyncratic liver enzyme elevations with biological therapy in inflammatory bowel disease. Aliment Pharmacol Ther 2015;41:972–9.
13. Koller T, Galambosova M, Filakovska S, et al. Drug-induced liver injury in inflammatory bowel disease: 1-year prospective observational study. World J Gastroenterol 2017;23:4102–11.
14. Worland T, Chin KL, van Langenberg D, et al. Retrospective study of idiosyncratic drug-induced liver injury from infliximab in an inflammatory bowel disease cohort: the IDLE study. Ann Gastroenterol 2020;33:162–9.
15. Ghabril M, Bonkovsky HL, Kum C, et al. Liver injury from tumor necrosis factor-alpha antagonists: analysis of thirty-four cases. Clin Gastroenterol Hepatol 2013;11(5):558–64.

16. Rodrigues S, Lopes S, Magro F, et al. Autoimmune hepatitis and anti-tumor necrosis factor alpha therapy: a single center report of 8 cases. World J Gastroenterol 2015;21:7584.

17. Björnsson ES, Medina-Caliz I, Andrade RJ, et al. Setting Up Criteria Hepatol Commun 2022;6:1895–909.

18. Harada K, Akai Y, Koyama S, et al. A case of autoimmune hepatitis exacerbated by the administration of etanercept in the patient with rheumatoid arthritis. Clin Rheumatol 2008;27:1063–6.

19. Fathalla BM, Goldsmith DP, Pascasio, et al. Development of autoimmune hepatitis in a child with systemic-onset juvenile idiopathic arthritis during therapy with etanercept. J Clin Rheumat 2008;14:297–8.

20. Bjornsson E, Talwalkar J, Treeprasertsuk S, et al. Patients with typical laboratory features of Autoimmune Hepatitis rarely need a liver biopsy for diagnosis. Clin Gastroenterol Hepatol 2010;9:57–63.

21. Lerhardi E, Valle ND, Nacchiero MC, et al. Onset of liver damage after a single administration of infliximab in a patient with refractory ulcerative colitis. Clin Drug Investig 2006;26:673–6.

22. Menghini VV, Arora AS. Infliximab-associated reversible cholestatic liver disease. Mayo Clin Proc 2001;76:84–6.

23. Michel M, Duvoux C, Hezode C, et al. Fulminant hepatitis after infliximab in a patient with hepatitis B virus treated for an adult onset still's disease. J Rheumatol 2003;30:1624–5.

24. Ostuni P, Botsios C, Punzi L, et al. Hepatitis B reactivation in a chronic hepatitis B surface antigen carrier with rheumatoid arthritis treated with infliximab and low dose methotrexate. Ann Rheum Dis 2003;62:686–7.

25. Esteve M, Saro C, González-Huix F, et al. Chronic hepatitis B reactivation following infliximab therapy in Crohn's disease patients: need for primary prophylaxis. Gut 2004;53:1363–5.

26. Reddy KR, Beavers KL, Hammond SP, et al. American Gastroenterological Association Institute guideline on the prevention and treatment of hepatitis B virus reactivation during immunsuppressive drug therapy. Gastroenterology 2015;148:215–9.

27. Tobon GJ, Canas C, Jaller JJ, et al. Serious liver disease induced by infliximab. Clin Rheumatol 2007;26:578–81.

28. Kinnunen U, Färkkilä M, Mäkisalo H. A case report: ulcerative colitis, treatment with an antibody against tumor necrosis factor (infliximab), and subsequent liver necrosis. J Crohns Colitis 2012;6:724–7.

29. Haennig A, Bonnet D, Thebault S, et al. Infliximab induced acute hepatitis during Crohn's disease therapy: absence of cross-toxicity with adalimumab. Gastroenterol Clin Biol 2010;34:7–8. 29.

30. Caussé S, Bouquin R, Wylomanski S, et al. Infliximab-induced hepatitis during treatment of vulvar Crohn's disease [in French]. Ann Dermatol Venereol 2013;140:46–51.

31. Parra RS, Feitosa MR, Machado VF, et al. Infliximab-associated fulminant hepatic failure in ulcerative colitis: a case report. J Med Case Rep 2015;9:249.

32. Forker R, Escher M, Stange EF. A 20-year-old woman with ulcerative colitis and acute liver failure. Internist (Berl) 2017;58:982–9.

33. Kok B, Lester ELW, Lee WM, et al. United States Acute Liver Failure Study Group. Acute liver failure from tumor necrosis factor-a antagonists: report of four cases and literature review. Dig Dis Sci 2018;63:1654–66.

34. Wong F, Ibrahim BA, Walsh J, et al. Infliximab-induced autoim- mune hepatitis requiring liver transplanEiswerthtation. Clin Case Rep 2019;7:2135–9.
35. Mustafa Alikhan M, Mansoor E, Satyavada S, et al. Infliximab-induced acute liver failure in a patient with crohn's disease requiring orthotopic liver transplantation. ACG Case Rep J 2021;8:e00586.
36. Bonkovsky HL, Kleiner D, Gu J, et al. Clinical presentation and outcomes of bile duct loss caused by drugs and dietary supplements. Hepatology 2017;65: 1267–77.
37. Shah P, Larson B, Wishingrad M, et al. Now You See It, Now You Don't: a case report of Infliximab-induced vanishing bile duct syndrome. ACG Case Rep 2019;6:e00134.
38. Eiswerth MJ, Heckroth MA, Ismail A, et al. Infliximab-induced vanishing bile duct syndrome. Cureus 2022;14:e21940.
39. Pennock GK, Chow LQ. The evolving role of immune checkpoint inhibitors in cancer treatment. Oncologist 2015;20:812–22.
40. Malnick SDH, Abdullah A, Neuman MG. Checkpoint inhibitors and hepatotoxicity. Biomedicines 2021;9(2):101.
41. Tawbi HA, Schadendorf D, Lipson EJ, et al. Relatlimab and nivolumab versus nivolumab in untreated advanced melanoma. N Engl J Med 2022;386(1):24–34.
42. André T, Shiu KK, Kim TW, et al. Pembrolizumab in microsatellite-instability-high advanced colorectal cancer. N Engl J Med 2020;383(23):2207–12.
43. *Opdualag prescribing information. Opdualag U.S. Product information*, 2022, Bristol-Myers Squibb Company; Princeton, NJ, Available at: https://news.bms.com/news/details/2022/U.S.-Food-and-Drug-Administration-Approves-First-LAG-3-Blocking-Antibody-Combination-Opdualag-nivolumab-and-relatlimab-rmbw-as-Treatment-for-Patients-with-Unresectable-or-Metastatic-Melanoma/default.aspx. Accessed September 16, 2022.
44. Sangro B, Chan SL, Meyer T, et al. Diagnosis and management of toxicities of immune checkpoint inhibitors in hepatocellular carcinoma. J Hepatol 2020;72(2): 320–41.
45. Lanitis T, Proskorovsky I, Ambavane A, et al. Survival Analysis in Patients with Metastatic Merkel Cell Carcinoma Treated with Avelumab. Adv Ther 2019;36: 2327–41.
46. Wang PF, Chen Y, Song SY, et al. Immune-Related Adverse Events Associated with Anti-PD-1/PD-L1 Treatment for Malignancies: A Meta-Analysis. Front Pharmacol 2017;8:730.
47. Topalian SL, Sznol M, McDermott DF, et al. Survival, durable tumor remission, and long-term safety in patients with advanced melanoma receiving nivolumab. J Clin Oncol 2014;32:1020–30.
48. Ascierto PA, Del Vecchio M, Robert C, et al. Ipilimumab 10 mg/kg versus ipilimumab 3 mg/kg in patients with unresectable or metastatic melanoma: a randomised, double-blind, multicentre, phase 3 trial. Lancet Oncol 2017;18:611–22.
49. Croughan WD, Aranibar N, Lee AG, et al. Understanding and Controlling Sialylation in a CHO Fc-Fusion Process. PLoS One 2016;11:e0157111.
50. Wang DY, Salem JE, Cohen JV, et al. Fatal Toxic Effects Associated With Immune Checkpoint Inhibitors: A Systematic Review and Meta-analysis. JAMA Oncol 2018;4:1721–8.
51. Remash D, Prince DS, McKenzie C, et al. Immune checkpoint inhibitor-related hepatotoxicity: A review World. J Gastroenterol 2021;27(32):5376–91.
52. Intlekofer AM, Thompson CB. At the bench: preclinical rationale for CTLA-4 and PD-1 blockade as cancer immunotherapy. J Leukoc Biol 2013;94:25–39.

53. Fujiwara Y, Horita N, Harrington M, et al. Incidence of hepatotoxicity associated with addition of immune checkpoint blockade to systemic solid tumor therapy: a meta-analysis of phase 3 randomized controlled trials Cancer. Immunol Immunother 2022;71(12):2837–48.

54. Wang W, Lie P, Guo M, et al. Risk of hepatotoxicity in cancer patients treated with immune checkpoint inhibitors: A systematic review and meta-analysis of published data. Int J Cancer 2017;141:1018–28.

55. Finn RS, Qin S, Ikeda M, et al. Atezolizumab plus Bevacizumab in Unresectable Hepatocellular Carcinoma. N Engl J Med 2020;382:1894–905.

56. Finn RS, Ryoo BY, Merle P, et al. Pembrolizumab As Second-Line Therapy in Patients With Advanced Hepatocellular Carcinoma in KEYNOTE-240: A Randomized, Double- Blind, Phase III Trial. J Clin Oncol 2020;38:193–202.

57. Miah A, Tinoco G, Zhao Z, et al. Immune checkpoint inhibitor-induced hepatitis injury: risk factors, outcomes, and impact on survival. J Cancer Res Clin Oncol 2022. https://doi.org/10.1007/s00432-022-04340-3.

58. Pana J, Liua L, Guo X, et al. Risk factors for immune-mediated hepatotoxicity in patients with cancer treated with immune checkpoint inhibitors: a systematic review and meta-analysis. Expert Opin Drug Saf 2022;21(10):1275–87.

59. Björnsson E, Stephens C, Atallah E, et al. A new framework for advancing in drug-induced liver injury research. The Prospective European DILI Registry. Liver Int 2022;00:1–12.

60. FDA approves atezolizumab plus bevacizumab for unresectable hepatocellular carcinoma, Available at: www.fda.gov/drugs/drug-approvals-anddatabases/fda-approves-atezolizumab-plus-bevacizumab-unresectablehepatocellular-carcinoma. Accessed June 1, 2020.

61. Naidoo J, Page DB, Li BT, et al. Toxicities of the anti-PD-1 and anti-PD-L1 immune checkpoint antibodies. Ann Oncol 2015;26:2375–91.

62. Bessone F, Bjornsson ES. Checkpoint inhibitor-induced hepatotoxicity: role of liver biopsy and management approach. World J Hepatol 2022;14(7):1269–76.

63. Weber JS, Kähler KC, Hauschild A. Management of immune-related adverse events and kinetics of response with ipilimumab. J Clin Oncol 2012;30:2691–7.

64. De Martin E, Michot JM, Papouin B, et al. Characterization of liver injury induced by cancer immunotherapy using immune checkpoint inhibitors. J Hepatol 2018; 68:1181–90.

65. Huffman BM, Kottschade LA, Kamath PS, et al. Hepatotoxicity after immune checkpoint inhibitor therapy in melanoma: natural progression and management. Am J Clin Oncol 2018;41:760–5.

66. Kazuyuki M, Takanori I, Matsatoshi I, et al. Real world data of liver injury induced by immune checkpoint inhibitors in Japanese patients with advanced malignancies. J Gastroenterol 2020;55(6):653–61.

67. Hamoir C, de Vos M, Clinckart F, et al. Hepatobiliary AND PANCREATIC: NIVOLUMAB-RELATED CHolangiopathy. J Gastroenterol Hepatol 2018;33:1695.

68. Gudnason HO, Björnsson HK, Gardarsdottir M, et al. Secondary sclerosing cholangitis in patients with drug-induced liver injury. Dig Liver Dis 2015;47:502–7.

69. Ahmad J, Rossi S, Rodgers SK, et al. Sclerosing cholangitis-like changes on magnetic resonance cholangiography in patients with drug induced liver injury. Clin Gastroenterol Hepatol 2019;17:789–90.

70. Cohen JV, Dougan M, Zubiri L, et al. Liver biopsy findings in patients on immune checkpoint inhibitors. Mod Pathol 2021;34:426–37.

71. Onoyama T, Takeda Y, Yamashita T, et al. Programmed cell death-1 inhibitor-related sclerosing cholangitis: A systematic review. World J Gastroenterol 2020;26(3):353–65.

72. Li M, Sack JS, Bell P, et al. Utility of Liver Biopsy in Diagnosis and Management of High-grade Immune Checkpoint Inhibitor Hepatitis in Patients With Cancer. JAMA Oncol 2021;7:1711–4.

73. Brahmer JR, Abu-Sbeih H, Ascierto PA, et al. Society for Immunotherapy of Cancer (SITC) clinical practice guideline on immune checkpoint inhibitor-related adverse events. J Immunother Cancer 2021;9(6):e002435.

74. Haanen JBAG, Carbonnel F, Robert C, et al. Management of toxicities from immunotherapy: ESMO Clinical Practice Guidelines for diagnosis, treatment and follow-up. Ann Oncol 2017;28(suppl 4):iv119–42.

75. Management of immune-related adverse events (irAEs) | eviQ, Available at: https://www.eviq.org.au/clinical-resources/side-effect-and-toxicitymanagement/immunological/1993-management-of-immune-relatedadverse-events#collapse 150419. Accessed March 4, 2022.

76. Brahmer JR, Lacchetti C, Schneider BJ, et al. Management of Immune-Related Adverse Events in Patients Treated With Immune Checkpoint Inhibitor Therapy: American Society of Clinical Oncology Clinical Practice Guideline. J Clin Oncol 2018;36(17):1714–68.

77. Peeraphatdit TB, Wang J, Odenwald MA, et al. Hepatotoxicity from immune checkpoint inhibitors: a systematic review and management recommendation. Hepatology 2020;72:315–29.

78. Miller ED, Abu-Sbeih H, Styskel B, et al. Clinical characteristics and adverse impact of hepatotoxicity due to immune checkpoint inhibitors. Am J Gastroenterol 2020;115:251–61.

79. Huffman BM, Kottschade LA, Kamath PS, et al. Hepatotoxicity after immune checkpoint inhibitor therapy in melanoma: natural progression and management. Am J Clin Oncol 2018;41:760–5.

80. Gauci ML, Baroudjian B, Zeboulon C, et al. Immune-related hepatitis with immunotherapy: are corticosteroids always needed? J Hepatol 2018;69:548–50.

81. Riveiro-Barciela M, Barreira-Díaz A, Vidal-González J, et al. Immune-related hepatitis related to checkpoint inhibitors: clinical and prognostic factors. Liver Int 2020;40:1906–16.

82. Bhave P, Buckle A, Sandhu S, et al. Mortality due to immunotherapy related hepatitis. J Hepatol 2018;69:976–8.

83. Fontana RJ, Liou I, Reuben A, et al. AASLD practice guidance on drug, herbal, and dietary supplement–induced liver injury. Hepatology 2022. https://doi.org/10.1002/hep.32689.

84. European Association for the Study of the Liver; Clinical Practice Guideline Panel: Chair; Panel members; EASL Governing Board representative. EASL Clinical Practice Guidelines: Drug-induced liver injury. J Hepatol 2019;70(6):1222–61.

85. Ueno M, Takabatake H, Hata A, et al. Mycophenolate mofetil for immune checkpoint inhibitor-related hepatotoxicity relapsing during dose reduction of corticosteroid: A report of two cases and literature review. Cancer Rep 2022;5(9):e1624.

86. Doherty GJ, Duckworth AM, Davies SE, et al. Severe steroid-resistant anti-PD1 T-cell checkpoint inhibitor-induced hepatotoxicity driven by biliary injury. ESMO Open 2017;2(4):e000268.

Moving?

Make sure your subscription moves with you!

To notify us of your new address, find your **Clinics Account Number** (located on your mailing label above your name), and contact customer service at:

Email: journalscustomerservice-usa@elsevier.com

800-654-2452 (subscribers in the U.S. & Canada)
314-447-8871 (subscribers outside of the U.S. & Canada)

Fax number: 314-447-8029

**Elsevier Health Sciences Division
Subscription Customer Service
3251 Riverport Lane
Maryland Heights, MO 63043**

*To ensure uninterrupted delivery of your subscription, please notify us at least 4 weeks in advance of move.

Printed and bound by CPI Group (UK) Ltd, Croydon, CR0 4YY

03/10/2024

01040467-0008